Adolf Grünbaum

THE PSYCHOANALYTIC PROCESS

THE PSYCHOANALYTIC PROCESS

Theory, Clinical Observations, and Empirical Research

JOSEPH WEISS
HAROLD SAMPSON
and the
MOUNT ZION
PSYCHOTHERAPY RESEARCH GROUP

Foreword by Morris N. Eagle

THE GUILFORD PRESS
New York   London

© 1986 The Guilford Press

A Division of Guilford Publications, Inc.

200 Park Avenue South, New York, N.Y. 10003

Printed in the United States of America

LIBRARY OF CONGRESS CATALOGING-IN-PUBLICATION DATA

Weiss, Joseph, 1924–
   The psychoanalytic process.

   Includes bibliographies and index.
   1. Psychoanalysis.   2. Psychoanalysis—Research.
I. Sampson, Harold.   II. Title.   [DNLM: 1. Psychoanalytic
Therapy.   2. Psychoanalytic Theory.   WM 460 W431p]
RC504.W45   1986b   150.19′5   85-30548
ISBN 0-89862-670-6

CONTRIBUTORS

JOSEPH WEISS, MD, Co-director, Mount Zion Psychotherapy Research Group, San Francisco; Training Analyst, San Francisco Psychoanalytic Institute; Clinical Professor, Department of Psychiatry, School of Medicine, University of California at San Francisco

HAROLD SAMPSON, PhD, Co-director, Mount Zion Psychotherapy Research Group; Director of Research in Psychiatry, Department of Psychiatry, Mount Zion Hospital and Medical Center, San Francisco; Faculty, San Francisco Psychoanalytic Institute; Clinical Professor, Department of Psychiatry, School of Medicine, University of California at San Francisco

And the following members of the
Mount Zion Psychotherapy Research Group:

ABBOT A. BRONSTEIN, PhD, Chief Psychologist, Psychiatric Services, Children's Hospital of San Francisco; Assistant Professor of Medical Psychology, University of California at San Francisco

SUZANNE BRUMER, PhD, Dean of Academic Affairs, Pacific Graduate School of Psychology, Palo Alto; Clinical Faculty, Department of Psychiatry and School of Dentistry, University of California at San Francisco

MARSHALL BUSH, PhD, Member, San Francisco Psychoanalytic Institute; Department of Psychiatry, Mount Zion Hospital and Medical Center, San Francisco

JOSEPH CASTON, MD, Assistant Clinical Professor, Department of Psychiatry, University of California at San Francisco; Faculty Member, San Francisco Psychoanalytic Institute

JOHN T. CURTIS, PhD, Co-director, Clinical Research Center for Adult Development, Mount Zion Hospital and Medical Center, San Francisco; Assistant Clinical Professor, Department of Psychiatry, University of California at San Francisco

CAROL DRUCKER, PhD, Attending Staff, Mount Zion Hospital and Medical Center, San Francisco; Teaching Staff, California School of Professional Psychology, Berkeley

SUZANNE GASSNER, PhD, Advanced Associate, San Francisco Psycho-analytic Institute; Adjunct Lecturer, Department of Psychology, University of California at Berkeley

RUTH K. GOLDMAN, PhD, Professor, Department of Psychology, San Francisco State University

MARLA ISAACS, PhD, Director, Families of Divorce Project, Philadelphia Child Guidance Clinic; Assistant Professor and Adjunct Faculty, Department of Psychiatry, School of Medicine, University of Pennsylvania; formerly Postdoctoral Fellow in Clinical Psychology, Mount Zion Hospital, San Francisco

ELIZABETH MAYER, PhD, Member, San Francisco Psychoanalytic Institute; Assistant Clinical Professor, Department of Psychiatry, University of California at San Francisco; Lecturer in Psychology, University of California at Berkeley; Private practice, Berkeley

MARY MARGARET McCLURE, DMH, Assistant Clinical Professor, Department of Psychiatry, University of California at San Francisco

PAUL RANSOHOFF, DMH, Assistant Clinical Professor, Department of Psychiatry, University of California at San Francisco; Advanced Associate, San Francisco Psychoanalytic Institute

FRANCES SAMPSON, PhD, Psychologist; Psychotherapist in private practice, Berkeley and San Francisco

CYNTHIA SHILKRET, PhD, Private practice, South Hadley, Massachusetts; Part-time faculty, Smith College School for Social Work, Northampton, Massachusetts; formerly Department of Psychiatry, Mount Zion Hospital and Medical Center, San Francisco

GEORGE SILBERSCHATZ, PhD, Co-director, Clinical Research Center for Adult Development, Mount Zion Hospital and Medical Center, San Francisco; Assistant Clinical Professor, Department of Psychiatry, University of California at San Francisco

LIST OF SCALES AND MEASURES

(Instructions to raters for most of the scales and measures are shown in the appendices. Scales reported in the literature are referenced and not included in the appendices.)

1. Gottschalk–Gleser Content Analysis Scale (used in Chapters 12 and 13)
2. Mahl Speech Disturbance Ratio (used in Chapters 12 and 13)
3. Experiencing Scale (used in Chapters 12, 17, 18, and 22)
4. Clinical Judgment of Anxiety Scale (used in Chapter 12)
5. "D" Scale (Appendix 1; used in Chapter 13)
6. "C" Scale (Appendix 2; used in Chapter 13)
7. Freedom versus Beleaguerment Scale (Appendix 3; used in Chapters 13, 17, and 18)
8. Drivenness Scale (Appendix 4; used in Chapters 13 and 22)
9. Level of Awareness into Irrational Feelings of Responsibility and Guilt (Appendix 6; used in Chapter 14)
10. Analyst Scale: Interpretation of Feelings of Responsibility and Guilt (used in Chapter 14)
11. Plan Diagnosis Reliability Measures (Appendix 7; used in Chapter 16)
12. Dahl Affect Measures (Love, Satisfaction, Anxiety, and Fear) (used in Chapters 17 and 18)
13. Patient Scale of Key Unconscious Wishes (Appendix 8; used in Chapter 18)
14. Analyst Scale of Gratifying versus Frustrating Key Unconscious Wishes (Appendix 9; used in Chapter 18)
15. Patient Scale of Key Tests (Appendix 10; used in Chapters 17 and 18)
16. Analyst Scale of Passing versus Failing Tests (Appendix 11; used in Chapters 17 and 18)
17. Plan Compatibility of Interventions Scale (Caston) (Appendix 13; used in Chapter 19)
18. Psychoanalytic Interpretiveness Scale (Appendix 14; used in Chapter 19)

FOREWORD

This is a remarkable book. The authors state that "this book is unique" and, indeed, they are justified in making that claim. As far as I know, it is the only book in which a coherent theory of the psychoanalytic process is presented and is then followed by systematic testing of the implications of that theory. This book is remarkable, in another way also. Most research dealing with psychoanalysis, however interesting (or uninteresting) it might otherwise be, generally has few, if any, implications for psychotherapeutic practice. (See compilations of such research in the Fisher & Greenberg, 1977, and Kline, 1981, volumes.) What distinguishes this work is that it has relatively clear-cut implications for doing psychotherapy as well as for conceptualizing the therapeutic process.

Weiss, in Part I, contrasts two broad psychoanalytic theories of therapy, one based on early Freud's "automatic functioning" hypothesis and the other based on the hypothesis of unconscious higher mental functioning. According to the former hypothesis, psychic life and behavior are determined by the automatic interaction of instinctual impulses seeking gratification and controlling ego defenses, relatively uncoordinated by thought or plan. According to the latter hypothesis, a person may exert unconscious control over a wide range of his or her behavior and is capable of making unconscious plans, unconscious assessments of safety and danger, and unconscious decisions regarding which mental contents are to be warded off (repressed) and which are to be brought forth. Weiss derives this approach from Freud's later writings, but elaborates and extends it to a degree and in a manner unanticipated by Freud or his followers.

In the traditional psychoanalytic conception of the psychotherapeutic process, patients come to treatment seeking gratification of unconscious instinctual impulses. These are mobilized and frustrated by the analyst's neutrality and are mainly experienced through the transference. This traditional view is contrasted with a conception of treatment in which patients enter treatment not as passive victims of the psychic forces of instinctual impulse and defense, but as active agents capable of evaluating conditions of safety and danger, of developing unconscious plans, and of exerting some degree of control over unconscious material. According to this conceptualization, patients harbor unconscious pathogenic beliefs, based on early traumas. These beliefs are grim and distressing and interfere with patients' abilities to lead satisfying lives. These beliefs are usually rooted in unconscious guilt that makes pursuing gratifications and leading an independent and satisfying life unconsciously equivalent to such taboo acts as abandoning or destroying one or both parents. Patients in treatment seek conditions in which it is safe for them to bring forth warded-off material relating to pathogenic beliefs, and they have unconscious plans regarding how they can accomplish this and disconfirm the unconscious pathogenic beliefs. In successful treatment, these beliefs are disconfirmed and a patient is then able to modify them and/or give them up—a process Weiss sees as the essential one of psychotherapy.

This very brief description cannot begin to do justice to the richness of the clinical and research material and the ideas contained in this book. I can give just a few brief examples: Evidence is reported that warded-off contents can emerge without interpretation as long as the therapist does not do anything to confirm the patient's pathogenic beliefs. Different clinical judges can reliably diagnose a patient's unconscious plans. Therapist interventions compatible with the patient's unconscious plan lead to more positive immediate effects than do plan-incompatible interventions. When a patient experiences that the therapist does nothing to confirm his pathogenic beliefs or even helps to disconfirm these beliefs, this facilitates the bringing forth of warded-off material and also constitutes an implicit interpretation that these beliefs need no longer be maintained. Hence, one need not draw a dichotomy between insight and the experience of the therapeutic relationship.

Much research on psychoanalytic hypotheses is essentially of an illustrative kind. Experiments and studies are carried out that are intended to illustrate or demonstrate this or that psychoanalytic hypothesis or concept (e.g., that repression exists or that a cluster of traits exists that fits the "oral character"). Very rarely, if at all, do the results of these studies do anything more than illustrate or demonstrate (or fail to illustrate or to demonstrate). They do not help one select between opposing hypotheses nor do they serve the truly heuristic function of modifying the original psychoanalytic formulations that generated the study. In contrast to these sorts of studies, research reported in this book is always framed in terms of two alternative conceptions of the psychoanalytic process and the results reported are always discussed in the context of the relative support given to each of these conceptions. I know of no other program of psychoanalytic research that has even attempted such a project. Because this research is directly relevant to the psychoanalytic process, the clinically oriented reader will find that he or she will be as interested in the research findings as in the clinical and theoretical material. The reader will also find that almost the entire content of the book will be of importance in influencing clinical understanding and therapeutic approach.

One final comment should be noted regarding one of the main themes of the book. It has always struck me, since I first became familiar with the work of Weiss, Sampson, and their colleagues, that the search for conditions in which it is safe enough to bring forth warded-off material, in order to test and disconfirm one's deepest fears, guilts, and pathogenic beliefs, is a basic motive and yearning in all interpersonal relations, not just the therapeutic one. This is only one reason that the appearance of this book is an important event.

Morris N. Eagle

PREFACE AND
ACKNOWLEDGMENTS

The theory and clinical approach presented in this book were developed by Weiss. The research, in its overall organization, was carried out by both authors, who share equally the responsibility for it.

Weiss began the work that eventuated in this book in 1958 and continued it on and off for many years. He studied the process notes of a number of analyses to develop and test certain hypotheses about the psychoanalytic process. His studies were not completely rigorous or systematic. Nonetheless, in their general approach and in a number of their conclusions, these studies prepared the way for the formal, quantitative research that Weiss and Sampson were later to organize and direct.

In the early informal studies (as in the later rigorous ones organized in collaboration with Sampson), Weiss, using the single-case method, investigated the psychoanalytic theory of therapy by testing one psychoanalytic hypothesis against another, competing, hypothesis. Moreover, in the early studies, Weiss tested some of the same hypotheses that he and Sampson were to test in the later studies. For example, Weiss tested the hypothesis that the coming to consciousness of a previously repressed mental content (impulse, affect, idea, memory, etc.) is typically controlled by the patient, against the alternative hypothesis that its coming to consciousness typically takes place beyond the patient's control. In these studies, Weiss found evidence for the hypothesis of unconscious control (Weiss, 1971). Weiss also tested the hypothesis that when a patient makes an unconscious demand on the therapist, he is primarily testing the therapist rather than attempting to gratify an unconscious impulse. Weiss (1971) here found evidence for the hypothesis of unconscious testing. In still other studies, Weiss found evidence that the patient's psychopathology is rooted in unconscious pathogenic beliefs and that in treatment the patient works in accordance with certain unconscious plans to change these beliefs. The hypotheses that Weiss developed and tested in the study of process notes were carefully tied to observation, and so, readily testable by the formal, empirical research methods that Weiss and Sampson were later to employ.

In 1964, we (Weiss and Sampson) began a collaboration on formal, rigorous research into the psychoanalytic process. We were in agreement from the start about the need for such research. Our philosophy of science and our approach to psychoanalytic research were much the same. Throughout our collaboration we have met regularly to discuss hypotheses about the therapeutic process and to develop research methods by which these hypotheses may be tested. Our collaboration has been rich and rewarding.

After the completion of our first empirical work (published in 1972), we recognized the need for a group of capable co-workers familiar with the hypotheses we wished to test and with the methods we envisioned for testing them. We invited interested colleagues to join us in forming the Mount Zion Psychotherapy Research Group, which was established in 1972 with 10 members. This research group has grown steadily. Over the years, some 50 people have participated in the group, and nearly 40 of them are active members at this time. Among these are psychoanalysts, psychiatrists, psychologists, social workers, statisticians, and other mental health professionals. All of the research presented here has been organized and carried out by members of the Mount Zion Psychotherapy Research Group.

We present here a list of our current and past members: Edward Ballis, Sandra Bemesderfer, Kay Blacker, Abbot Bronstein, Suzanne Brumer, Martel Bryant, Marshall Bush, Lynn Campbell, Joseph Caston, Lowell Cooper, John Curtis, Jack Dolhinow, Carol Drucker, Lewis Engel, Steven Foreman, Polly Fretter, Michael Friedman, Suzanne Gassner, Jess Ghannam, John Gibbins, Ruth Goldman, Irwin Gootnick, Seppe Graupe, Harriette Grooh, Forrest Hamer, Arthur Hoffman, Leonard Horowitz, Marla Isaacs, Cynthia Kale, Thomas Kelly, Anya Lane, Georgine Marrott, Elizabeth Mayer, Terry McCall, Mary Margaret McClure, Harvey Peskin, Paul Ransohoff, Owen Renik, Saul Rosenberg, Eleanor Sampson, Frances Sampson, Cynthia Shilkret, Robert Shilkret, Ellen Siegelman, George Silberschatz, Alan Skolnikoff, Ronald Spinka, Thomas Stein, Stanley Steinberg, Estelle Weiss, Michael Windholz, Abby Wolfson, and Neil Young.

The members of the research group differ in their training, experience, and outlook. They differ, too, in their ideas about psychoanalytic theory and research methods. These differences are evident in the research chapters, each of which reflects the point of view of the principal author. Our weekly research discussions have benefited from our differences. Through participation in our weekly meetings, each member of the group has contributed to the clarification of hypotheses, the design of studies, and the interpretation of research findings.

Several members of the research group deserve special mention for their particular contributions:

Abby Wolfson and Stanley Steinberg carried out a valuable study of how psychoanalysts conceptualize the therapeutic process. They worked with Milton Bronstein (of the Los Angeles Psychoanalytic Institute), who devoted much time and effort to this project.

Leonard Horowitz helped in the development of some of our research designs and in the application of certain research methods.

Neil Young contributed to our philosophical understanding of certain issues in single-case research.

Saul Rosenberg and Lynn Campbell classified all the analyst's interventions in the first 100 sessions of the case we studied into such categories as "clarifications," "suggestions," "questions," and "interpretations," thus providing us with a broad overview of the analyst's activities during this time.

John Curtis and Suzanne Gassner helped in the editing of this entire book.

Estelle Weiss critiqued thoroughly all of our writings, and in particular helped us to conceptualize our studies on the acquisition of insight.

Thomas Kelly contributed invaluably to our statistical analyses.

We have received help from many persons outside the research group, whose contributions we gratefully acknowledge:

Emanuel Windholz inspired us by his example. He introduced us to psychotherapy research and taught us to follow the therapeutic process by close study of process notes. He alerted us to the importance in therapy of the unconscious motives of the ego. It was a privilege to work closely with him.

Robert Wallerstein encouraged us directly, and by the example of his own pioneering work, to undertake the arduous but rewarding task of formal research on the psychoanalytic process. As a consultant to our work from 1966 to the present, he has generously shared with us his experience and wisdom in psychoanalytic research. In addition, as Chief of the Department of Psychiatry, Mount Zion Hospital and Medical Center, he gave full administrative support to our work.

James Faircloth and Robert Wallerstein each studied from process notes the first 100 sessions of the analysis of Mrs. C, the patient whose treatment we studied by formal research methods. Their conclusions about the therapeutic process during these sessions complemented ours and provided us with an important corroboration of certain of our research findings.

We benefited also from the frequent opportunity to exchange ideas about psychotherapy research with Mardi Horowitz. His presence in this city and his readiness for open scientific dialogue provided constant stimulation and valuable assistance to us. We were proud to participate in the Center for the Study of Neuroses, which he directs.

We have also benefited from the thoughtful critiques and suggestions of many other colleagues, both locally and nationally. We can only mention here a few persons whose detailed response to aspects of our work has helped us to clarify and advance our thinking: Hartvig Dahl, Morris Eagle, Merton Gill, Robert Holt, Lester Luborsky, Herbert Schlesinger, Calvin Settlage, Lloyd Silverman, and Philip Spielman. We are grateful to each of them.

James Blight was the first editor of this book. We were stimulated by his enthusiasm, and we benefited from his insightful suggestions.

Our present editor, Bertram Cohler, has contributed in many important ways to the final organization of the book. We owe him special thanks for many improvements that he suggested.

Lisa Buchberg and Jess Ghannam did library research for us. Lisa Buchberg helped us to trace the development in Freud's writings of the higher mental functioning hypothesis. Jess Ghannam helped us to trace, in the work of recent psychoanalytic writers, the development of concepts about unconscious guilt.

Our research also required the efforts of numerous raters and judges. We appreciate their indispensable contributions. We have made use of so many raters and judges that the following list is necessarily incomplete:

Joseph Afterman, Adrienne Applegarth, Michael Bader, Edward Ballis, Peter Banys, Renee Binder, David Black, Spencer Bloch, Morris Brock, Jessica Broitman, Abbot Bronstein, Suzanne Brumer, Lisa Buchberg, Marshall Bush, Lynn Campbell, Roy Carry, Joseph Caston, Marilyn Caston, Phyllis Cath, Samuel Chase, Karen Cliffe, Donald Cliggett, Peter Cohen, Lauren Cunningham, John Curtis, William Dickman, Marcia Dillon, James Dimon, Jane Dixon, Alan Dreifus, Carol Drucker, Jacqueline Ferraro, Leslie Fink, Charles Fisher, Robert Friend, Erik Gann, Maxine Gann, Suzanne Gassner, Jess Ghannam, Jane Ginsberg, Steven Goldberg, Ruth Goldman, Thea Goldstine, Irwin Gootnick, Kenneth Gottlieb, Norman Gottreich, Daniel Greenson, Harriette Grooh, Roy Gryler, Forrest Hamer, Toni Heinemann, Arthur Hoffman, Jill Horowitz, Laura Howard, Roberta Huberman, Marla Isaacs, Lester Isenstadt, Elsa Johnson, Jane Jordan, Raoul Kaufman, Thomas Kelly, Susan Kolodny, Ronald Krasner, David Lake, Larry Lanes, Albert Levy, Frank Lossy, Ramana Mabutas, Elinor Martin, Elizabeth Mayer, Mary Margaret McClure, Arnold Milstein, Ilana Myers, Susan Opsvig, Rebecca Palley, Morris Peltz, Jon Peterson, Kristine Pfleiderer, Andrew Propper, Sheryl Rand, Paul Ransohoff, Owen Renik, David Ritvo, Diane Rockloff, Pat Roddy, Saul Rosenberg, Janet Roth, Susan Roviaro, Joel Saldinger, Frances Sampson, Melvin Schupack, Carol Shapiro, Cynthia Shilkret, Robert Shilkret, George Silberschatz, Judith Sills, Earl Simburg, Robert Smither, Carl Sommers, Mary Sparks, Patricia Stamm, Donald Stanford, Thomas Stein, Stanley Steinberg, Jeffrey Weiner, Anita Weinshel, Estelle Weiss, Judith Wilson, Michael Windholz, Myra Wise, Neil Young, and Carl Zlatchin.

We are also grateful for the financial help we received from various sources. Our initial empirical work was supported in part, from 1967 to 1976, by Research Grant MH-13915 from the National Institute of Mental Health, NIMH, some of the current work mentioned briefly in Chapter 22 was supported in part by NIMH Grants MH-34052 and MH-35230. As already noted, Mount Zion Hospital and Medical Center provided administrative support for the project from its inception to the present. Mount Zion has also generously contributed research funds, which have provided partial support for our project from 1973 to the present. The Chapman Research Fund has provided partial financial support for some of the studies reported in this book (Chapters 17, 18, 20, and 22) as well as for related work reported elsewhere. In addition, we have recieved partial support for particular studies (Chapter 22) from the Fund for Psychoanalytic Research. We are grateful to each of these institutions for their indispensable help.

Finally, we are especially grateful to Janet Bergman, the executive secretary of our research group for many years. She has taken a great deal of initiative in helping us to carry out the research and to put this book together. Her reliability, efficiency, dedication, and good humor have been invaluable. We know that if Janet takes on a task it will be done properly and well.

This book is unique in that it presents in one volume a particular psychoanalytic theory of the mind along with clinical observations and research to support it. The book will be more useful to the reader if he or she reads the part on theory and clinical observation before the part on research. However, enough theory has been included in the part on research to enable the reader interested primarily in research to read this part separately.

Joseph Weiss
Harold Sampson

CONTENTS

II. RESEARCH FINDINGS
A. Introduction

B. The Patient Studied

THEORY AND
CLINICAL OBSERVATIONS

1

INTRODUCTION

JOSEPH WEISS

The main purpose of this book is to propose a particular psychoanalytic theory and to support it by a variety of observations, including observations obtained by rigorous empirical research. The theory is broad and general. Indeed, it is a psychoanalytic theory of the mind. However, it will be applied here mainly (but not exclusively) to the understanding of the behavior of the patient during psychoanalysis or psychoanalytic psychotherapy.

The book contains three parts. In Part I, I shall propose the theory. Part II presents a series of formal quantitative research studies on the psychoanalytic process, which both support the theory and have influenced it. In Part III, we will discuss the theory and research in a broad context and point to certain implications of both.

The theory presented in Part I is broader than the research presented in Part II. Part I contains certain theoretical ideas that are not tested directly in Part II, as well as certain observations that support the theory but that are not presented in Part II. This is the case because proposing and developing a theory is a different kind of enterprise than is testing a theory by formal empirical research. In developing a broad theory, the investigator should cast a wide net. He[1] should, in his theorizing, take account of a wide variety of observations. A theory of the psychoanalytic process would be unconvincing unless it were able to explain the behaviors of various kinds of patients, and unless, in addition, it were able to account adequately for significant behaviors other than those of the analytic patient.

In contrast, the investigator who tests a psychoanalytic theory must focus on a narrow range of observations. This is because it is possible to test a broad theory in only a few areas. The investigator must do considerable work to discover just those areas in which the theory may predict

1. For the sake of brevity and readability the masculine pronoun is used in the generic sense throughout this book. The reader should always keep in mind the missing feminine pronoun.

testable consequences. Then he must make many careful observations in these areas. Thus, the research reported in Part II does not (and need not) test directly all the major tenets of the theory proposed in Part I. Testing certain consequences of the theory tests the theory as a whole and hence lends support to all of its basic ideas.

Part I thus contains a relatively full account of the theory and a variety of observations to support it. It supports the theory with certain clinical observations made by Freud and a number of other analysts, including myself. It supports it with observations I have made in the careful though informal study, by means of process notes, of the analyses of a number of analytic patients. It provides evidence for the theory from certain significant observations not connected directly with analysis, including Niederland's study of Holocaust survivors (1981), Beres's study of children placed in foster homes (1958), and Balson's study (1975) of the dreams of soldiers before, during, and after internment as prisoners of war.

Although the theory is based on a wide variety of observations, the research studies are all concerned with one patient, Mrs. C. They are all concerned with investigations (from process notes and transcripts) of her behavior as a patient. Indeed, they are all concerned with a few significant aspects of her behavior.

We have limited our research studies to the analysis of this patient for practical reasons. We have not had the time and resources to replicate the research with another patient, although we have done less complete and less rigorous studies on several other analytic patients. Our research on the analysis of Mrs. C took a number of years. Despite its limitations, we consider it a significant step. It is one of all-too-few attempts to test and support a particular psychoanalytic theory by formal empirical methods, and it has been relatively successful. Ours is a kind of work that must be replicated and developed in various directions if psychoanalysis is to mature as a science.

INTRODUCTION TO THE THEORY

Let us now turn to the theory itself. The theory is both Freudian and new. It is Freudian in that its basic ideas were developed by Freud or strongly implied by him. It is new in that it relies heavily on, and indeed expands and develops, certain fundamental ideas that Freud developed mainly in his late writings. It expands and applies certain ideas that Freud presented in brief outline form, and it makes explicit certain ideas that Freud strongly implied but did not spell out. Thus it expands the ideas, which Freud presented briefly in the *Outline* (1940a, p. 199), that a person is able unconsciously to exert some control over his behavior, that he regulates it unconsciously in accordance with thoughts, beliefs, and assessments of current reality, and that he attempts, by his regulation of behavior, to avoid putting himself in dangerous situations. It spells out the idea, which Freud strongly implied in *Inhibitions, Symptoms and Anxiety* (1926a), that a person maintains his psychopathology primarily in obedience to certain compelling grim beliefs, which he acquires in early childhood by inference from experience.

In the language of Freud's structural model, the theory proposed here emphasizes the great part played by the unconscious ego and the unconscious superego in the maintenance of psychopathology, in the therapeutic process, and in a wide range of psychological processes.

The theory proposed here contrasts with Freud's early views about the nature of unconscious mental life as Freud presented them in *The Interpretation of Dreams* (1900). There Freud minimized a person's capacity to exert control over his unconscious mental life and to unconsciously either think or make use of any of his higher mental functions. Freud assumed there that the unconscious mind consists of psychic forces, which are instinctual impulses (wishes) and defenses. The impulses seek immediate gratification; the defenses oppose their coming forth. The impulses and defenses interact automatically, uncoordinated by thought or plan, and by their interactions they determine behavior. Two equal and opposite forces may nullify each other, a strong force may overwhelm a weaker one, or two tangential forces may give rise to compromise behavior, that is, behavior that gratifies both.

Thus, in *The Interpretation of Dreams*, Freud more or less based his theory of the unconscious mind on what I shall refer to as the "hypothesis of automatic functioning." According to this hypothesis, all or almost all unconscious mental life is derived from the dynamic interplay of psychic forces, beyond the patient's control and without regard for his thoughts, beliefs, or assessments of his current reality. In those parts of his ego psychology from which the theory proposed here is derived, Freud relied on what I shall refer to as the "hypothesis of higher mental functioning." This hypothesis does not rule out unconscious automatic functioning. However, it assumes that a person may exert a certain degree of control over his unconscious mental life, and that he may regulate it in accordance with his *unconscious* thoughts and beliefs and his assessments of his current reality.

Very few analysts today assume implicitly or explicitly that unconscious mental life is regulated entirely either automatically or by higher mental functions. *Most analysts assume both kinds of regulation.* However, as will be seen, the automatic functioning hypothesis still exerts a powerful, perhaps predominant, influence on psychoanalytic thinking.

In the following few pages I shall introduce several basic tenets of the theory that is the subject of this book. These tenets, each of which assumes the unconscious use of certain higher mental functions, are concerned with a person's unconscious control of his repressions (and of certain other behaviors as well), with his unconscious pathogenic beliefs, and with the work he unconsciously performs in an effort to overcome his problems.

A PERSON'S UNCONSCIOUS CONTROL OF HIS REPRESSIONS

According to a basic tenet of the theory proposed here, a person (in everyday life or in analysis) may exert some control over his repressions, the degree of which varies from one person to another. He may, as Freud stated in the *Outline* (1940a, p. 199) repress a particular impulse if, in his unconscious judgment, he is endangered by it. He may maintain the repression of the impulse as long as he considers it dangerous, and he may lift the repression of this impulse and bring it forth when, in his unconscious judgment, he can safely do so.

A patient may exert control unconsciously not only over his repressions but over other unconscious behaviors as well. Indeed, he may unconsciously plan and carry out a variety of behaviors. Moreover, he regulates these behaviors by the criteria of safety and danger. Thus, he ordinarily lifts his repressions and carries out his unconscious plans only if in his unconscious judgment he may safely do so. As Freud wrote, "The ego is governed by considerations of safety" (1940a, p. 199).

PATHOGENIC BELIEFS

A person, in unconsciously deciding whether he may safely carry out a course of action, is governed by certain unconscious beliefs. It is in obedience to such beliefs that he maintains his repressions and, indeed, his psychopathology. Since such beliefs play a crucial part in the development and maintenance of psychopathology, they are here termed "pathogenic." The familiar example of a pathogenic belief is the male's belief that if he maintains a sexual interest in his mother he will be punished by castration by his father. A person acquires pathogenic beliefs in early childhood by normal inference from experience, albeit subjective experience.

Though Freud did not develop a theory of pathogenic beliefs, he laid the foundation for such a theory in his discussions of the boy's belief in castration. This belief, which, according to Freud, underlies much of the male's psychopathology, should be distinguished from fantasy as Freud defined it in, for instance, *Formulations on the Two Principles of Mental Functioning* (1911). There Freud wrote that a person's fantasies are wishful. They are regulated by the pleasure principle and are not subject to reality testing:

With the introduction of the reality principle, one species of thought-activity was split off; it was kept free from reality-testing and remained subordinated to the pleasure principle alone. This activity is *phantasying*, which begins already in children's play, and later, continued as *day-dreaming*, abandons dependence on real objects. (p. 222, italics Freud's)

Pathogenic beliefs, in contrast to fantasies, are not wishful but instead grim and constricting. They are not opposed to reality; they represent reality. They are, in the language of Freud's structural model, part of the unconscious ego. The id or primary process as described by Freud cannot create beliefs. The id simply turns away effortlessly (automatically) from painful realities (Freud, 1900, p. 600).

Freud stated explicitly in *Inhibitions, Symptoms and Anxiety* (1926a) that from the point of view of the boy, castration is a real danger. There he wrote about castration fear as follows: "It was therefore a realistic fear, a fear of danger that was impending or was judged to be a real one" (1926a, p. 108). Freud also stressed that the belief in castration, rather than causing pleasure, is shocking. Indeed, he assumed that the experiences from which a boy infers the belief in castration provide him with "the severest trauma of his young life" (1940a, p. 190).

Freud repeatedly referred to the belief in castration as a belief or conviction, and only on a few occasions as a fantasy. For example, he wrote that after a boy who has been threatened with castration perceives the female genitals, "he cannot help *believing* in the *reality* of the danger of castration" (1940b, p. 277, italics mine).

A young boy may acquire a variety of pathogenic beliefs (not just the belief in castration) by inferring them from certain traumatic experiences with his parents. He may, by such inference, come to believe that almost any impulse, attitude, or goal is dangerous in that he would, by expressing the impulse or attitude or by pursuing the goal, risk the disruption of his ties to a parent and thus leave himself insufficiently protected or cared for. For example, the boy may come to believe that, by expressing the impulse or pursuing the goal, he would either provoke punishment or rejection from the parent, or worry, injure, or even kill the parent.

THE PATIENT'S UNCONSCIOUS WORK

The analytic patient suffers a great deal unconsciously from his problems and, indeed, from the pathogenic beliefs in which they are rooted. He is made miserable by his pathogenic beliefs; he is frightened, weakened, constricted, weighed down, or made to feel guilt, shame, or remorse by them. Therefore he unconsciously wishes to disconfirm them. Moreover, he works unconsciously to disconfirm them by testing them in relation to the analyst (Weiss, 1971). He tests them by the use of certain trial actions, hoping by such actions to demonstrate to himself that he does not affect the analyst in ways predicted by his pathogenic beliefs. For example, a patient whose pathogenic beliefs warn him that if he is rivalrous with the analyst he will provoke punishment from him may test this belief unconsciously by a trial expression of rivalry. He hopes unconsciously to demonstrate to himself that he will not provoke the analyst and, thus, that the belief is false.

As a patient, by repeatedly testing a particular pathogenic belief, succeeds in loosening its hold on him, he may lift the repressions he had been maintaining in obedience to the belief and begin both to experience and to express the motives he had repressed in obedience to the belief. Thus he may become bolder and more insightful.

EVIDENCE FOR THE THEORY

CRYING AT THE HAPPY ENDING

The explanatory power of the idea that a person may regulate certain repressions in accordance with unconscious assessments of danger and safety was suggested to me years ago by a familiar and paradoxical observation—that a person may weep at a moment of great joy (Weiss, 1952, 1971). As he weeps, he may feel little or no sadness, he may experience a brief but not unpleasant sense of sadness not connected to any particular idea, or he may experience profound sadness connected with painful memories which, until the joyful moment, had been deeply repressed. A good example of a person's weeping at a happy ending is as follows:

A person watching a movie about a love story experienced little or no emotion when the lovers quarreled and left each other. However, he was moved to tears when they resolved their difficulties and were reunited. He became happy, experienced a brief but not unpleasant sense of sadness, and wept.

To explain the moviegoer's paradoxical behavior, I assumed that he identified unconsciously with one of the lovers, so that when the lovers separated, he was in danger of feeling sad, not only for the lovers, but also for himself. He felt endangered, however slightly, by the sadness, and so intensified his defenses against it. (He certainly did not repress his sadness deeply. He merely suppressed or isolated it.) Later, when the lovers were reunited at the happy ending, the moviegoer became happy, both for the lover with whom he identified and for himself. He no longer had reason to feel sad, and so was no longer threatened by the sadness which he had previously warded off. He decided unconsciously that he could safely experience the sadness and so lifted the defenses opposing it and brought it forth. He made it fully conscious, not for gratification, as the experience of sadness is not gratifying, but to gain relief from the effort he had been making to keep it warded off.

My explanation of the moviegoer's weeping at the happy ending was inspired by Freud's theory of wit, as he presented it in *Jokes and Their Relation to the Unconscious* (1905b). From this work I got the idea of examining an everyday phenomenon in which a warded-off mental content comes forth. However, my explanation was based more directly on the concept, developed by Freud in his late theorizing, that a person may lift his defenses and bring forth a warded-off mental content when he unconsciously or preconsciously perceives that he may safely experience it (1940a, p. 199).

The assumption of unconscious automatic functioning as developed in *The Interpretation of Dreams* cannot account for crying at the happy ending. According to this assumption, the moviegoer could exert no control over his defenses. He could not lift them. His unconscious sadness could come forth only if it became intensified relative to the defenses opposing its emergence, that is, if the defenses became weaker or if the sadness became stronger. Yet the assumption of automatic functioning can account neither for a weakening of the moviegoer's defenses, nor for an intensification of his sadness. Nor can it explain why either of these things would occur precisely when the moviegoer became happy.

Moreover, according to the automatic functioning hypothesis, the only impetus to consciousness of a warded-off content is the blind, uncontrolled pursuit of gratification, and the sadness could have no such impetus to consciousness. The experience of sadness is not gratifying, as gratification is defined in the automatic functioning hypothesis. The coming forth of the moviegoer's sadness is an example of the kind of process that Freud (*Beyond the Pleasure Principle*) described as contradicting his earlier assumption that unconscious mental life is regulated exclusively by the search for pleasure (1920, p. 32).

Though the example of the moviegoer's crying at the happy ending is intriguing, it is not completely satisfying as evidence that a person may bring forth *deeply repressed* sadness at a happy ending. In the case of the moviegoer, the sadness was not deeply repressed. Moreover, since in this case a mere feeling came forth unconnected to a particular idea or memory, its coming forth may not have reflected an important unconscious process.

THE SPONTANEOUS RETRIEVAL OF NEW MEMORIES: THE CASE OF DR. N

As the next example makes clear, a person in everyday life may, at a happy ending, bring forth intensely sad memories which previously had been deeply repressed.

Dr. N, a physician and colleague, was intensely moved by the birth in her second marriage of a son. When he was brought to her room after the delivery, she not only wept profusely but also retrieved memories of another son from her first marriage who had died 9 years before at the age of 2. Earlier, Dr. N had scarcely been able to remember the dead boy. Indeed, on one occasion she had startled her mother by not recognizing him in the mother's family album. However, after the birth of this second boy, she not only remembered the dead child vividly but also remembered how happy she had been with him and how devastated she had been by his death. Moreover, she brought these memories forth without being overwhelmed by them.

My explanation of her weeping, with which Dr. N agreed, was similar to my explanation of the moviegoer's weeping: Dr. N had been unable to face her sadness at the loss of her son and so, at the time of his death, had repressed it. Moreover, in order to avoid facing her sense of loss, she repressed not only her sadness but almost all memory of her son.

Dr. N was overjoyed by the birth of her second son, partly because she had experienced his birth as making up for her earlier agonizing loss.

His birth therefore not only made her intensely happy, it also enabled her to tolerate her sadness at the earlier loss without being overwhelmed by it.

Dr. N's joy and weeping at the birth of her second son may have depended on another factor, which I did not discuss with Dr. N (who was not a patient) but which, on the basis of my experience with certain patients, I consider likely: She may have unconsciously experienced the death of her son as a kind of punishment. She may have inferred from the fact that her son was taken from her that she did not deserve to have a son. Perhaps she concluded that she was a bad or at least an unlucky person or that God had turned his back on her. If Dr. N did feel that way, she may have repressed her sadness partly because she may have felt that in her son's death she was simply receiving her just desserts. Thus, Dr. N may have been overjoyed by the birth of her second son partly because his birth disconfirmed her earlier idea that she had been undeserving. If the birth of her second son convinced her that she was not in fact unworthy, she could perhaps allow herself to experience the death of her first son not as a punishment but as a sad and undeserved loss.

INFORMAL EVIDENCE FROM PROCESS NOTES: STUDIES OF ANALYTIC PATIENTS

I studied, from process notes, long segments of the analyses of a number of analytic patients to investigate how and in what circumstances the analytic patient becomes conscious of previously repressed mental contents, particularly if these contents have not been interpreted. My findings, as illustrated by the two examples presented below, are compatible with my explanation of Dr. N's retrieval of previously repressed memories. I found that a patient may keep a variety of mental contents (impulses, affects, ideas, memories, and transferences) repressed until he unconsciously decides that he may safely experience them. Then he may lift his repressions and bring them forth.

THE CASE OF MISS P

Miss P, an analytic patient, behaved more or less as did Dr. N. Both wept at a happy ending, and both brought forth previously repressed memories of sad experiences. Dr. N's happy ending came about as a consequence of a particular change in her circumstances: the birth of a son. Miss P's happy ending came about as a consequence of a successful piece of analytic work:

Miss P was an unmarried lawyer in her early 30s. She was inhibited, depressed, plodding, and unimaginative. She had low self-esteem. She thought of herself as boring, but attempted, by a dogged kind of cheerfulness, to make herself interesting. She expected to be left out and rejected.

Miss P appeared detached and isolated. She pictured her childhood home life as bleak. Her mother, as she remembered it, made no effort to cook dinner, merely opening cans of food and serving the food in the cans. At dinner everyone was silent.

The patient pictured both of her parents as withdrawn, burdened by her demands for care and attention, and rejecting. She received little from her parents and gave little to them. She was afraid that if she offered her parents something they would reject it. She spoke of her parents' neglect of her without showing sadness or anger.

Miss P made slow progress in her analysis. With the analyst she was restrained, correct, and undemanding. She was careful with him not to voice her feeling that he was rejecting her. Indeed, she retained a forced cheerfulness. She did complain, mildly at first, about her parents' rejection of her. (Later she complained more bitterly about it.) Moreover, she did become aware that she was afraid the analyst would reject her. As she faced these feelings, she became somewhat less depressed and withdrawn, acquired a few friends, and began to date occasionally.

Then one day during the fourth year of her analysis, Miss P surprised the analyst by announcing in a matter-of-fact way that she planned to stop treatment in about 3 months. She had, she stated, accomplished a lot and was now able to progress on her own. The analyst neither agreed nor disagreed with Miss P about her plan to stop treatment, but instead attempted to investigate it analytically. In attempting to help Miss P understand her wish to stop, the analyst offered her a number of interpretations about it, all concerned with a few themes. Thus on several occasions he attempted to show Miss P that she wished to stop treatment because she feared that she was draining the analyst by her demands on him. On other occasions the analyst told Miss P that she wished to stop treatment to make certain that she rejected him before he rejected her. Miss P reacted only slightly to these interpretations. Though she considered them plausible, she did not change her mind about stopping. However, she revealed by a slight lightening of her mood that she was pleased by the analyst's interpretations. Particularly, she appeared somewhat moved by the interpretation, which the analyst made several times, that her wish to stop may have stemmed from a belief that she did not deserve help. According to the analyst, Miss P had developed this belief in relation to her parents. She had perceived them as assuming that she was unworthy and undeserving, and she had come to feel that way about herself.

Miss P eventually acknowledged that she had become uncertain about her motives for stopping. As the patient's deadline approached, the analyst suggested that she continue treatment until her motives for stopping, which she acknowledged were obscure, became clearer. The patient protested that there was no need to continue. However, she looked somewhat less tense than usual. Then, at the end of the hour, she said grudgingly that, although she was going against her better judgment, she would continue for a while longer.

During the next few sessions, the patient seemed less depressed and friendlier to the analyst. About a week after she agreed to continue, the patient, in associating to a dream, brought forth a new memory. She brought it forth without its having been interpreted. Moreover, she did not become anxious about it, either while telling it or afterward. The memory was of an occasion in her seventh year when gang warfare with shooting erupted in her neighborhood. Everyone was frightened, and the other mothers in the neighborhood made their children stay inside. However, the patient's mother reacted differently. Instead of making the patient stay home, her mother gave her some money and sent her out to buy groceries. The patient assumed that her mother wanted her to be killed because she (the patient) was too much trouble for the mother. The patient was so overcome by sadness at this memory, which she had not thought of for years, that she wept for 20 minutes.

Miss P's agreeing to stay in analysis and her recovery of the sad memory of her mother's neglect marked a definite, although not sharp, turning point in her treatment. After this point, the treatment became more productive. Miss P never again threatened to leave treatment prematurely. Moreover, she subsequently recovered other memories of feeling deeply rejected by both parents. She kept these memories of parental rejection in mind and used them to understand herself better. She also began to face more directly her feelings that she was a burden to the analyst and her boyfriends and that she deserved to be rejected by them.

Miss P, according to my formulation, had felt traumatized in childhood by her impressions (however subjective) that her mother and, to a lesser extent, her father were either indifferent to her demands or burdened by them. She had assumed that the way she was treated by her parents was the way she deserved to be treated by them, and had complied with this assumption. She had developed the pathogenic belief that she did not deserve her parents' care and attention, and that if she sought more than minimal care from them she would endanger herself either by burdening them or by provoking further rejection from them.

Miss P had reacted to her early experiences of rejection and to the pathogenic beliefs she had inferred from these experiences much as, according to Freud, a young boy in the throes of his Oedipal conflict reacts to the belief in castration as a punishment. The boy, in obedience to this belief, may decide to repress not only his Oedipal impulses but also the belief itself and the experiences (such as castration threats, parental punishments, or the sight of the female genitalia) from which he inferred the belief. Similarly, Miss P repressed her wish for her parents' love, she repressed the belief that she did not deserve their care and would endanger herself by seeking it, and she repressed certain of the experiences of parental rejection from which she had inferred this belief.

As I have emphasized, Miss P also repressed her sadness at her parents' rejection of her. She repressed it not only because she had experienced the parental rejection as traumatic but also because she had unconsciously believed that she deserved their rejection and thus had no right to be sad about it. She had accepted her parents' rejection of her as her due.

In her analysis Miss P quickly developed a mother transference. From the start she unconsciously governed her relations to the analyst in accordance with the pathogenic beliefs she had acquired in childhood: She unconsciously expected to receive little or no help from the analyst, and she unconsciously believed that she did not deserve help from him. She unconsciously assumed that if she were to demand attention or care from him, or that if she were to complain about him, she would burden him and thereby provoke him to reject her.

Miss P did not guide her unconscious behavior entirely in accordance with her pathogenic beliefs. She had significant doubts about them. If she had not intended to struggle against her pathogenic beliefs by testing them, she would not have sought psychoanalytic treatment. Miss P began her testing of her pathogenic beliefs (or of the analyst) cautiously: She complained about the way her parents had treated her. She feared that the analyst would disapprove of her complaining about her parents, for she would have experienced such disapproval as confirming her belief that she had deserved parental rejection. When the analyst did not disapprove, Miss P experienced relief. Also she became more indignant at her parents, and she remembered more about having suffered from their rejection of her.

Miss P did not permit herself to test the analyst directly. She did not criticize him or complain about him. However, over a period of time, she took reassurance from his willingness to listen to her, to take her seriously, to remember what she had told him, and on several occasions to accommodate her requests for changes in her appointment times.

It was not until the fourth year of her analysis, after she had acquired more confidence in the analyst and had begun to change her pathogenic beliefs, that Miss P carried out the large-scale test already described, of announcing without warning that she was much improved, and so planned to stop treatment in three months. Miss P's unconscious purpose in presenting this test was to disconfirm her belief that she deserved to be rejected by the analyst; she hoped to demonstrate to herself that the analyst would refuse to accept her plan to terminate. She unconsciously would have experienced the analyst's accepting this plan as a rejection of her and thus as confirming her belief that she deserved to be rejected.

Miss P, in her own mind, took a big risk. By assuming responsibility for stopping treatment on the grounds that it had helped her, she made it easy for the analyst to reject her in good conscience. The analyst's reaction to Miss P's plan to stop—he simply treated it as something to be investigated analytically—did not affect her much consciously, but it did affect her unconsciously. She revealed this by becoming calmer and friendlier to him. She reacted in much the same way to the analyst's interpretations, all of which were intended to make her aware that her plan to stop stemmed from irrational pathogenic beliefs.

Miss P was especially pleased unconsciously by the analyst's suggestion that she continue her treatment until she understood better her motives for planning to terminate. She unconsciously took this suggestion as evidence against her pathogenic belief that she deserved to be rejected. She revealed her relief at the analyst's suggestion by deciding to continue treatment.

Miss P both weakened her pathogenic belief that she deserved to be rejected and partially resolved a mother transference. She became more aware that she had been unconsciously perceiving the analyst as in childhood she had perceived her mother. She became better able to perceive him as someone who would not find her demands burdensome and who would not reject her. She was better able to trust him and indeed was able to experience with him the happiness which corresponded to Dr. N's happiness at the birth of her second son.

In a sense, the testing Miss P carried out was a kind of reality testing. It enabled her to discriminate between her mother as she remembered her and the analyst as she was then perceiving him. Thus, Miss P's testing here exemplified Freud's idea (1940a, p. 199) that reality testing enables a person to discriminate between memories (in Miss P's case, transferences) and current perceptions.

As Miss P became more secure with the analyst and therefore happier, she decided unconsciously that she could safely bring forth the traumatic memory that I have described. She brought it forth without feeling much anxiety about it. She kept it in consciousness and she used it in her efforts to understand herself better.

The above account assumes that Miss P unconsciously exerted some control over her behavior, indeed that she controlled it unconsciously in accordance with a particular ego purpose or goal, namely, to test a certain pathogenic belief in the hope of disconfirming it. This account explains Miss P's behavior more convincingly than would an account of it based on the assumption that her behavior was regulated automatically by the dynamic interplay of impulse and defense. It ties together and makes sense of a number of events of her treatment, which, in the alternative account, are unconnected and not readily explained. These include Miss P's plan to stop treatment, her unconscious relief at the analyst's attempts to show her that her wish to stop expressed resistance, and her ready acceptance of the analyst's suggestion that she continue until she understood better her wish to stop. It explains, too, the observation that Miss P, shortly after agreeing to continue, brought forth on her own (without its being interpreted) and without feeling anxious, the sad memory of parental rejection. Finally, it explains how Miss P, during this period, made definite gains, which she retained from that time on.

The idea that Miss P lifted her defenses and brought forth the memory of rejection when she unconsciously decided that she could safely experience this memory (as opposed to the idea that it came forth propelled by its own thrust) is supported by the following observations:

- Miss P previously had not been conscious of the memory.
- Miss P recalled the extremely upsetting memory on her own, unhelped by interpretation.
- Miss P appeared relieved rather than anxious before she recalled it. Nor was she anxious about it while she was remembering it or afterward.
- Miss P did not try to re-repress the memory. Instead, she retained it in consciousness and used it in an attempt to understand herself better.
- Miss P did not use her retrieval of the memory to defend herself against, for example, her dependency on her parents or her hostility to them. In fact, after the events reported above, Miss P, rather than becoming more defensive, became more aware of her dependency and her hostility, and expressed them more directly.

According to the automatic functioning hypothesis, the memory of maternal rejection could have come forth either by pushing through the patient's defenses or by emerging opposed by defenses as part of a compromise formation. If it had pushed through the patient's defenses, Miss P would not have behaved as she did. Rather, she would have come into conflict with the memory before, during, and after its emergence into consciousness. Moreover, after its emergence she would have attempted to re-repress it. She would not have calmly retained it in consciousness and used it to understand herself better. If it had emerged as part of a compromise formation, Miss P could have retained it in consciousness. However, she could not have used it to help in understanding herself.

THE CASE OF MRS. G

In another study from process notes, a patient brought forth not an important previously repressed memory but an important previously repressed sexual fantasy.

Mrs. G became aware of a fantasy toward the end of her second year of treatment. She became aware of it in a seemingly casual way and without its having been interpreted by the analyst. She remembered a short dream in which the analyst "does something to her." In associating to the dream, she thought, without conviction, of several things that the analyst might do to her. She then paused and the analyst asked, "Do you have any other ideas about what I might do to you?" She answered with a laugh, "Well, you might turn me over your knee and spank me." (See Chapter 4 for a discussion of beating fantasies.)

Mrs. G had given no evidence earlier of having been aware of this beating fantasy and later, when discussing it with the analyst, she confirmed that she had not been conscious of such a fantasy since adolescence. Yet Mrs. G did not become anxious about it, and, though slightly ashamed of it, made no effort to repress or isolate it. Indeed, she referred to it from time to time and used her knowledge of it constructively in an attempt to understand herself better. For example, in one session she connected the beating fantasy to her behavior at work where, by a provocative display of carelessness, she had induced her employer to reprimand her.

The unobtrusive and apparently nonconflictual emergence of this fantasy suggested to me an informal research study. This was to use the process notes of Mrs. G's analysis to study the process preceding her becoming aware of the fantasy in order to identify those factors that made it possible for her to experience it. I shall summarize my findings below.

In the 150 sessions preceding Mrs. G's becoming conscious of the beating fantasy, she had gradually but steadily brought about a certain significant change in her relationship to the analyst. She had, before this series of sessions, been timid, compliant, and detached with him. However, during this series of sessions, she had gradually become able to assert herself comfortably in relation to him. She had thereby taken a first step toward resolving a particular father transference.

Mrs. G's father (and to a lesser extent her mother) had been perceived by her in early childhood as possessive and vulnerable. According to the patient, her father had been intensely involved with her. He had been pathetically eager for her to admire him and to accept his opinions even in trivial matters.

When Mrs. G disobeyed her father or disagreed with him even in small things, he would become upset. If sufficiently provoked, he would hit her. If not provoked to the point of violence, he would pout and become depressed. By the same token he would become overjoyed if Mrs. G went out of her way to express her admiration for him.

A vivid example of the kind of experience with her father that Mrs. G found so disturbing occurred when she was 6 years old. Her father had asserted that a horse never takes all of its hoofs off the ground even while galloping. Mrs. G responded by showing her father a photograph from an encyclopedia of a horse galloping with all of its hoofs off the ground. He became very upset, whereupon Mrs. G felt guilty about showing him up and went to her room depressed.

As a result of childhood egocentricity, Mrs. G had no doubt greatly exaggerated her power to affect her father. Nonetheless, her impression that she could greatly affect him either by asserting herself with him or by submitting to him was part of her psychic reality. It was from such impressions that Mrs. G had inferred two closely related pathogenic beliefs by which she governed her childhood relationship to her father: She believed that if she were assertive with her father she would hurt him, and that if she were submissive to him she would restore him.

At the beginning of the 150 sessions with which I am concerned, Mrs. G was in the throes of a father transference. She unconsciously regulated her relationship to the analyst in accordance with the pathogenic beliefs she had developed in her relation to her father. As a consequence of her unconscious image that the analyst was vulnerable, she was afraid to be either assertive or submissive to him. She feared that if she were assertive with the analyst she would hurt him, and that if she were submissive to him, or even too cooperative, she would fall into a masochistic relationship with him from which she would be unable to free herself.

Mrs. G's fear of submitting to the analyst was causally connected to her fear of asserting herself with him: Her knowledge that she could not comfortably disagree with the analyst contributed greatly to her fear that if she were to develop a close relationship with him she would be unable to extricate herself from it. She unconsciously feared that she would feel compelled to admire him, accept bad advice from him, and stay in treatment with him even if the treatment was of no value.

Mrs. G, during the 150 sessions that are the subject of this report, worked unconsciously by testing the analyst (and, by the same tests, her pathogenic beliefs) in order to disconfirm the pathogenic belief that if she were assertive with the analyst she would hurt him. She tested the analyst, not as Miss P had done with one grand test, but with numerous small tests. She began her testing by criticizing the analyst in a self-demeaning way, that is, by being petty, mocking, or petulant in her criticisms. She apparently assumed that the analyst would be less challenged by such criticisms than by larger ones that were well thought out and delivered with dignity. For example, early on in these sessions, Mrs. G spent part of an hour making fun of the analyst for having his name on the office door. She complained that its presence there exemplified his bad taste. A few weeks later she complained that the noise made by men working down the hall was disturbing her. She thought the analyst should ask them to stop working, and when he did not she accused him of being a "Caspar Milquetoast."

Mrs. G was anxious or tense while criticizing the analyst, and her voice became shrill. If, however, the analyst did not appear defensive, Mrs. G would assume that she had not hurt him and would relax. Moreover, she would remain relaxed for several sessions. While relaxed, she would be more cooperative. She would also bring forth new material, as, for example, new memories of having hurt her father.

On four or five occasions, the analyst told the patient that she was reluctant to criticize him for fear of hurting him. Each time he made this interpretation, Mrs. G made good use of it. She confirmed it and became more relaxed and more insightful.

Overall, during the 150 sessions prior to the emergence of the beating fantasy, Mrs. G became more assertive, calmer, and less constricted. She came to experience various affects more intensely. She was at times more friendly and at other times more critical. Toward the end of this series of sessions Mrs. G spent an analytic hour reviewing an article (on applied psychoanalysis) written by the analyst. It was in a field that Mrs. G knew quite a bit about. Her discussion of the article was relaxed, humorous, well rounded, and mildly critical. She summarized her opinion by saying, "Well, I'll give you a C+ or a B− on it."

It was only after Mrs. G had established her capacity to be confidently assertive with the analyst that, during an hour in which she was relaxed, she brought forth her sexual fantasy of being beaten by him.

The idea that Mrs. G brought the fantasy forth only after she *decided* unconsciously that she could safely experience it (as opposed to the idea that it pushed forth propelled by its own thrust) is supported by the following observations:

- Mrs. G experienced the fantasy only after she had acquired a means of experiencing it safely.
- She experienced it without conflict and tension, and did not try to re-repress it.
- She applied her knowledge of the fantasy to the understanding of other behavior. She connected it, for example, to her provocative behavior with her employer.

Unless the beating fantasy had emerged as part of a compromise formation, its coming forth beyond Mrs. G's control would have been marked by tension and anxiety, and she would have attempted to repress it. If, on the other hand, it had emerged as part of a compromise formation, its coming forth would not necessarily have aroused anxiety, but neither would she have been able to connect it with other behavior.

The idea that Mrs. G's criticisms of the analyst were not simply the expression of, say, unconscious hostility but, in addition, were intended to test the analyst is supported by the following observation: She became nervous when criticizing the analyst, but if she perceived that he did not react defensively she would relax, and while relaxed might bring forth a previously repressed memory. This sequence is easily accounted for by the hypothesis that Mrs. G, by criticizing the analyst, was testing him, hoping thereby to assure herself that she could not hurt him by criticizing him. According to this hypothesis, Mrs. G became anxious while criticizing the analyst because she feared she would hurt him, but relaxed when she observed that he was not defensive. She inferred then that she had not hurt him, and then temporarily relaxed and stopped worrying about him. Since she was assured temporarily that she could not hurt the analyst by her hostility, she became less guilty for those occasions in her childhood when, as she saw it, she had hurt her father. As she felt less guilty about these episodes, she became able safely to remember them.

An alternative assumption, that Mrs. G's criticisms of the analyst were primarily the uncontrolled expression of aggression, cannot explain the observation that she would relax after she had convinced herself that she had not, by a particular criticism of the analyst, hurt him. According to this hypothesis, Mrs. G should have become more tense rather than more relaxed. Her aggression should have been frustrated and hence intensified. Indeed, her frustrated aggression should have pushed to the surface and come into conflict with the defenses opposing its emergence, causing anxiety and tension.

The idea that Mrs. G was working unconsciously during this period of her treatment explains her behavior better than an alternative idea that she was simply ruminating, using defiance to undo submissiveness and using submissiveness to undo defiance. Mrs. G was no doubt ruminating. However, if she were simply obsessing during those sessions, she would have made no progress, whereas in fact she made a great deal of progress. She became progressively more able to defy the analyst, and progressively more relaxed and comfortable. Also, she became more insightful and made a good start in analyzing a particular father transference. Moreover, she did all of these things more or less on her own, helped only occasionally by the analyst's interpretations about her fear of hurting him.

In this chapter I have introduced a particular psychoanalytic theory of the mind and presented certain observations in support of it. In the next chapter I shall show in some detail how this theory derives from ego psychology as developed by Freud and certain other analysts.

2

TWO PSYCHOANALYTIC HYPOTHESES

JOSEPH WEISS

In the last chapter I pointed out that psychoanalytic theory contains two hypotheses about unconscious mental functioning. According to the first, a person is not able to exert control over his unconscious mental life. According to the second hypothesis, a person may exert some degree of control over at least part of his unconscious mind. All basic psychoanalytic concepts and many basic psychoanalytic clinical observations assume, either explicitly or implicitly, one or the other of these hypotheses.

The first hypothesis—the automatic functioning hypothesis—is much more influential, even today, than may be apparent at first glance. For example, the assumption that changes in behavior reflect changes in the unconscious dynamic equilibria of certain psychic forces (namely, impulses and defenses) is an assumption of the automatic functioning hypothesis. According to that hypothesis, a person's unconscious mental life is regulated automatically by the pleasure principle, without regard for thought, belief, or current reality.

According to the other hypothesis, which I have referred to as the higher mental functioning hypothesis, a person may exert some control over his unconscious mental life, the degree of which varies from person to person. He exerts this control in accordance with thoughts, beliefs, and assessments of current reality. The theory that is the subject of this book is one variant of the higher mental functioning hypothesis.

THE HISTORY OF THE TWO HYPOTHESES

INTRODUCTION

In the last chapter I discussed the two hypotheses by comparing their capacities to explain certain familiar observations, both in everyday life and in analysis. In the present chapter I shall discuss them in another context, that is, in the context of their development by Freud and other writers.

The two hypotheses are contained both in Freud's writings and in current psychoanalytic literature, though, with rare exceptions, neither is set forth, or used clinically, in a pure form. Of the two hypotheses, the automatic functioning hypothesis is considerably more prominent in Freud's writings. It is also more prominent in current psychoanalytic literature. It exerts the greater influence on present-day clinical thinking. As a rapid perusal of a group of current psychoanalytic journals makes clear, the basic concepts of the higher mental functioning hypothesis are used only occasionally, and seldom explicitly. Only a small minority of psychoanalytic writers make regular and explicit use, in their clinical discussions, of such concepts as unconscious control, belief, thought, plan, or goal.

Freud, in his early writings, did explicitly develop the idea that unconscious mental life is regulated automatically. It was not until many years later that he explicitly developed the idea that unconscious mental life (or a part of it, namely, that part arising in the unconscious ego and superego) may be regulated by higher mental functions. When he did explicitly develop the idea of unconscious regulation in accordance with higher mental functions, he found the concept bewildering. However, Freud did not make a point of having developed two different hypotheses about unconscious mental functioning. He tended to stress the continuity in his thinking, and to give the impression of a gradual, purposeful unfolding of theory.

Freud retained throughout his theorizing the idea of unconscious automatic regulation, but he assigned it a progressively less important part in unconscious mental life. Originally he assumed that all or almost all mental life is regulated automatically by the pleasure principle, and later that the system Unconscious is subject to such regulation. After he developed the structural model, he restricted automatic regulation to the id. Then he further limited its sway by progressively assigning to the ego and superego a greater part in unconscious mental life, and to the id a lesser part. In the *Outline* (1940a), which is Freud's last major theoretical work, he assigned the ego and superego quite powerful parts and wrote about the id as almost unknowable.

It is perhaps because Freud stressed the continuity in his thinking and because he did not fully develop the higher mental functioning hypothesis that many analysts have not recognized its importance. Nonetheless, its development, in my opinion, reflects a major and persistent trend if not the predominant trend in Freud's theorizing. However, I shall not attempt to demonstrate that here. To do so would require an extensive presentation. In addition, the demonstration of that trend is not essential to my thesis, which is that the higher mental functioning hypothesis has greater explanatory power than the automatic functioning hypothesis. The value of an hypothesis depends not on the judgment of authority, but on empirical considerations.

My division of Freud's conceptual pie into an automatic functioning hypothesis and a higher mental functioning hypothesis overlaps certain distinctions made by other psychoanalytic writers. George S. Klein, for example, has described two different kinds of psychoanalytic explanation, one based on mechanisms and impersonal regulatory principles, the other based on a clinical theory that assumes intentions and purposes (1976). Gill (1976) has distinguished between Freud's metapsychology, which uses natural science concepts of force, energy, or structure, and Freud's "pure psychology," which is contained in some aspects of Freud's clinical theory. However, neither Klein's clinical theory nor Gill's pure psychology is very much like the higher mental functioning hypothesis, which Freud developed in his late writings, for neither makes much explicit use of such concepts as unconscious thought, belief, and decision, which are central to the higher mental functioning hypothesis, and which, in my opinion, are required by observation.

My comparison of the two hypotheses about unconscious mental functioning also overlaps with comparisons made by Arlow and Brenner between the topographic and the structural theory (1964). However, Arlow and Brenner, in their discussion of the structural theory, hardly refer to Freud's concepts about unconscious belief, thought, anticipation, and decision making, which I consider so important.

In the history of Freud's ideas which I shall unfold below, I am indebted to Hartmann's "The Development of the Ego Concept in Freud's Work" (1956b). In his essay, Hartmann refers to the radical departures and reformulations in Freud's late works. According to Hartmann, the ego psychology of Freud's late works greatly strengthens the psychoanalytic view of unconscious adaptation, control, and integration. It points to "centralized functional control" (p. 291). It points to the importance of unconscious anticipation and thought and to the ego's "command of the pleasure–unpleasure principle" (p. 292). It points to the importance of the development of object relations. It assumes that neuroses may be adaptive.

I am indebted, too, to Rapaport's histories (1956, 1958). Rapaport, like Hartmann, assumed that in Freud's late writings behavior no longer results simply from the dynamic interplay of impulse and defense. Moreover, Rapaport pointed to certain clinical applications of Freud's late theory. He assumed that the late theory alerts the clinician to the part played in unconscious mental life by unconscious identification and by unconscious guilt.

THE AUTOMATIC FUNCTIONING HYPOTHESIS

When Freud developed the automatic functioning hypothesis in *Project for a Scientific Psychology* (1895) and in *The Interpretation of Dreams* (1900), he had been treating patients for almost 10 years. His views, therefore, were informed by a large number of observations of patients. Nonetheless, Freud's approach to the development of the automatic functioning hypothesis was strongly influenced by certain *a priori* considerations, in particular by his wish to develop a scientific psychology along the lines of a natural science. Freud, in his introduction to the *Project*, stated explicitly that he wished to develop such a psychology. He wrote: "The intention is to furnish a psychology that will be a natural science: that is, to represent psychical processes as quantitatively determinate states of specifiable material particles, thus making those processes perspicuous and free from contradiction" (1895, p. 295).

The scientific ideals that animated the *Project* were retained by Freud in Chapter 7 of *The Interpretation of Dreams*. G. S. Klein described Freud's intentions in *The Interpretation of Dreams* as follows: "[Freud sought] to tell, in impersonal terms, how the mind functioned, and tell it without employing the language of purpose, as the purposes were the phenomena that were to be explained . . . its intent was the same [as in the *Project*]—to provide a non-teleological, causal account of the phenomenon of purposefulness as these revealed themselves in the psychoanalytic situation" (1976, p. 45).

The basic elements of the automatic functioning hypothesis are psychic forces, that is, impulses and defenses. The basic law regulating them and indeed all unconscious mental life is the pleasure (or unpleasure) principle. The pleasure principle functions automatically, that is, without regard for thought, belief, or reality. In Freud's words, this principle exerts "an automatic regulation by unpleasure" (1905a, p. 266). Under its regulation the mind automatically and hence effortlessly seeks pleasure and avoids pain. In Freud's words, "as a result of the unpleasure principle, the first system is totally incapable of bringing anything disagreeable into the context of its thought. It is unable to do anything but wish" (1900, p. 600).

Impulses, according to the automatic functioning hypothesis, are closely connected to instinct. They are shaped from instinct automatically by certain experiences of frustration and gratification. Impulses are regulated by the pleasure principle; they seek immediate gratification. They interact with each other and with the defenses dynamically, that is, according to the law of vector addition (Rapaport & Gill, 1959, p. 155).[1] And by their interactions they determine the various phenomena of psychic life. In Freud's words: "Psychoanalysis derives all mental processes (apart from the reception of external stimuli) from the interplay of forces, which assist or inhibit one another, combine with one another, enter into compromises with one another, etc." (1926b, p. 265).

The defenses, too, are regulated automatically by the pleasure principle. Thus, a person cannot lift his defenses. In general, a person does not become aware of a repressed impulse until the impulse or the defense warding it off has been interpreted.

THE HIGHER MENTAL FUNCTIONING HYPOTHESIS

The automatic functioning hypothesis exerted considerable influence on Freud's clinical thinking. Yet, he was never able to adhere to it completely, even in theory. For example, in the *Project*, Freud complained that he could not account for the initiation of primary defense without assuming a homuncular ego that focuses attention and carries out action. In *The Interpretation of Dreams* (1900), Freud theorized a homuncular ego, which makes use of higher mental functions and which is able to inhibit the free discharge of the primary system. Then, "when the second system has concluded its exploratory thought activity, it releases the inhibitions and damming up of excitations and allows them to discharge themselves in movement" (1900, p. 600).

Nor could Freud retain the concept that the mind, in its unconscious functioning, is governed exclusively by the pleasure principle. The hard facts of clinical observation, as Freud later stated, led him eventually to change this view. In *Beyond the Pleasure Principle*, Freud wrote that a particular observation induced him to limit the scope of the pleasure principle; this observation was that a patient may repeat both with the analyst and in dreams experiences that are not pleasurable and never could have been pleasurable (1920, p. 32).

Later still, in *Analysis Terminable and Interminable* (1937), Freud wrote that his observations about the great part played by guilt and masochism in human life were not compatible with his earlier view about the scope of the pleasure principle:

---

1. Gill, in his recent writings (e.g., 1976), has been sharply critical of the automatic functioning hypothesis.

Nothing impresses us more strongly in connection with the resistances encountered in analysis than the feeling there is a force at work which is defending itself by all possible means against recovery and is clinging tenaciously to illness and suffering. We recognize that part of this force is a sense of guilt and a need for punishment. . . . If we consider the whole picture made up of the phenomenon of masochism inherent in so many people, the negative therapeutic reaction, and the neurotic sense of guilt, we will have to abandon the belief that mental processes are governed exclusively by a striving for pleasure. (p. 242)

Long before Freud evolved his structural model, he was by implication endowing the unconscious mind with regulations and contents that do not fit the conceptualizations of the automatic functioning hypothesis. For example, in *The Interpretation of Dreams* (1900), in which Freud was most consistent in his effort to adhere to the automatic functioning hypothesis, he introduced an idea that was later to be a keystone of the higher mental functioning hypothesis—namely, the idea of unconscious regulation by higher mental functions in accordance with the criteria of danger and safety. He introduced this idea to account for the observation that certain unconscious impulses that are repressed in waking life may find expression in dreams. He assumed that the censor permits repressed impulses to find expression in dreams because the sleeper's power of motility has been shut down. Since the sleeper cannot act on his impulses, the censor can safely permit them to be expressed in dreams.

Also in *The Interpretation of Dreams*, Freud implied the existence in unconscious mental life of certain elements such as guilt or grim belief, which cannot readily be conceptualized as impulses or defenses and so cannot be accommodated readily by the mind as it is described in the automatic functioning hypothesis. For example, Freud implied the existence of unconscious guilt in his interpretation of his dream of Irma's injection. His purpose in producing this dream was, he wrote, to assure himself that he was not to blame for Irma's illness. By his reference to castration anxiety, Freud implied that the unconscious mind may contain beliefs or theories, for castration anxiety, as he later made clear, arises in the belief that castration is used as a punishment for sexuality (1900).

The automatic functioning hypothesis cannot accommodate unconscious guilt and unconscious belief because these, as Freud later wrote, are acquired from experience, not automatically but by the use of higher mental functions. They are acquired by a process that might well be described as learning from experience. Additionally, unconscious guilt and unconscious castration anxiety do not fit the automatic functioning hypothesis in that they are not pleasure-seeking motives. They may be directed to self-torture, not to gratification.

During the period between *The Interpretation of Dreams* (1900) and *Beyond the Pleasure Principle* (1920), Freud changed his ideas about unconscious mental functioning gradually and more by implication than explicitly. For example, in his discussions of the boy's Oedipus complex, Freud described certain unconscious motives that are acquired, not by automatic processes, but by inference from experience and that seek, not immediate gratification, but long-term goals. Such a motive is the boy's Oedipal rivalry with his father. The boy learns from experience that his father stands between him and his mother, and thus he learns from experience to be a rival of his father. Also, he may learn from experience that he cannot defeat his father immediately and so may develop the goal of defeating him in the distant future.

Especially important in inducing Freud to alter his views about unconscious mental functioning was his growing conviction about the importance of the castration complex in the mental life of the male. Castration anxiety is a very powerful motive, yet it is neither a defense nor an impulse. It arises in a belief that is acquired not automatically but by inference from experience and represents a "realistic fear, a fear of danger which was actually impending or was judged to be a real one" (1926a, p. 108). As early as 1909, Freud wrote that Little Hans acquired his castration anxiety directly from his mother's threats to have him castrated as a punishment for masturbation (1909, pp. 7-9).

The belief in castration is not like an unconscious fantasy as described by Freud in *Formulations on the Two Principles of Mental Functioning* (1911). Unconscious fantasies are exempt from reality testing, and they are wishful. However, the belief in castration represents reality to the boy who adheres to it, and this belief is horrifying rather than wishful. Finally, the belief in castration does not affect behavior automatically, as, according to the automatic functioning hypothesis, an unconscious impulse is supposed to affect it. A person who is guided unconsciously by a belief in castration is applying a theory to the planning of his behavior. He anticipates a particular course of action, considers whether it might provoke castration, and decides, on the basis of his expectations, whether to carry it out. A man suffering from unconscious castration anxiety who becomes anxious and leaves when a seductive woman approaches him is behaving not automatically but in accordance with a theory which warns him of danger.

The idea that a person may be guided unconsciously by the belief in castration as a punishment played a considerable part in Freud's development of ego psychology, which suggested that a person may be motivated unconsciously by powerful and deeply repressed ideas about reality. The belief in castration must be almost as deeply repressed as the Oedipal strivings, the emergence of which it opposes. Yet this belief cannot be produced by the unconscious mind as conceived of in the automatic functioning hypothesis. According to the automatic functioning hypothesis, the unconscious mind does not produce beliefs; rather, it reacts to a horrible reality, such as the possibility of castration, by automatically turning away from it.

The idea that a person may be guided unconsciously by beliefs makes it necessary to postulate that a part of the executive agency that guides behavior on the basis of beliefs may itself be unconscious and indeed deeply repressed. In *The Ego and the Id* (1923), Freud introduced the concept of such an executive agency, the ego, which guides behavior and may be to a considerable extent unconscious. He also introduced another agency, the superego, which may be largely unconscious and which contains the faculties of guilt and self-criticism. Freud described his new concept of the superego (which, as we shall see, contradicts a number of assumptions of the automatic functioning hypothesis) as bewildering. After writing that certain subtle and difficult intellectual operations can be carried out without coming into consciousness, Freud (1923) added:

There is another phenomenon which is far stranger. In our analyses we discover that there are people in whom the faculties of self-criticism and conscience, *mental activities, that is, which rank as extremely high ones,* are unconscious and unconsciously produce effects of the greatest importance." Freud added, "But this *new* discovery, which compels us, in spite of our better judgment, to speak of an unconscious sense of guilt, *bewilders* us far more than the other. (pp. 26–27, italics mine)

The concepts of unconscious guilt and unconscious self-criticism, as Freud introduced them in *The Ego and the Id,* deviate from the automatic functioning hypothesis in that they imply regulation by higher mental functions. A person who directs his behavior in accordance with the faculties of self-criticism and conscience must assess the behavior he intends to carry out and anticipate its probable effect on others. Furthermore, the unconscious motives that stem from the faculties of self-criticism and conscience, unlike those postulated by the automatic functioning hypothesis, are generally not gratifying.

In *Inhibitions, Symptoms and Anxiety* (1926a), Freud took several new giant steps toward developing the higher mental functioning hypothesis. He stressed even more the centrality of the boy's belief that if he pursues his mother sexually he will be punished by his father by castration. (He also wrote there of the female's belief that if she pursues her father sexually she will be punished by the loss of her mother's love.) In *Inhibitions, Symptoms and Anxiety*, Freud made the male's belief in castration a central building block of his theory by connecting it both with one of his oldest and most basic concepts, repression, and with one of his newest but increasingly important concepts, the superego. Freud assumed that in obedience to the boy's belief in castration he decides unconsciously to repress his sexuality, and Freud assumed that the superego is formed around the belief in castration (1926a, p. 114).

Also in *Inhibitions, Symptoms and Anxiety*, Freud took a big step away from the old idea of unconscious automatic regulation by suggesting that a person may unconsciously regulate repression not automatically but by thought. Several years after he wrote *Inhibitions, Symptoms and Anxiety*, Freud (1933) summarized his new idea about unconscious thought and conveyed his sense of its being a new and surprising idea:

How do we now picture the process of a repression under the influence of anxiety? The answer will, I think, be as follows. The ego notices that the satisfaction of an emerging instinctual demand would conjure up one of the well remembered situations of danger. This instinctual cathexis must therefore be somehow suppressed, stopped, made powerless. We know that the ego succeeds in this task if it is strong and has drawn the instinctual impulse concerned into its organization. But what happens in the case of repression is that the instinctual impulse still belongs to the id and that the ego feels weak. The ego thereupon helps itself by a technique *which is at bottom identical with normal thinking*. Thinking is experimental action carried out with small amounts of energy, in the same way as a general shifts small figures about on a map before setting his large bodies of troops in motion. Thus the ego anticipates the satisfaction of the questionable instinctual impulse and permits it to bring about the reproduction of the unpleasurable feelings at the beginning of the feared situation of danger. With this the automatism of the pleasure–unpleasure principle is brought into operation and now carries out the repression of the dangerous instinctual impulse. . . .

"Stop a moment!" you will exclaim; "we cannot follow you any further there!" You are quite right, I must add a little more before it can seem acceptable to you. First, I must admit that I have tried to translate into the language of our normal thinking what must in fact be a process that is neither conscious nor preconscious, taking place between quotas of energy in some unimaginable substratum. (pp. 89–90, italics mine)

Freud made clear in the above that he was writing about unconscious thinking, not about preconscious or conscious thinking. Also, by his assumption that the reader would be taken aback by his discovery of unconscious thinking, Freud implied that this discovery was new and a surprise to Freud himself.

In the *Outline* (1940a), Freud's last major work, he wrote more directly than before about the ego's unconscious regulation of behavior by the criteria of danger and safety. He stated:

Its [the ego's] constructive function consists of interpolating, between the demand made by an instinct and the action that satisfies it, the activity of thought which, after taking its bearings in the present and assessing earlier experiences, endeavors by means of experimental actions to calculate the consequences of the courses of action proposed. In this way the ego comes to a decision on whether the attempt to obtain satisfaction is to be carried out or postponed or whether it may be necessary for the demand by the instinct to be suppressed altogether as being dangerous. (Here we have the *reality principle*.) Just as the id is directed exclusively to obtaining pleasure, so the ego is governed by considerations of safety. The ego has set itself the task of self-preservation which the id appears to neglect. (p. 199)

Freud, in this passage, indicated that in unconsciously planning behavior the ego makes use of trial actions. Here, thought and decision are clearly not epiphenomena determined by the dynamic interplay of instinct and defense, but instead true determinants of behavior.

Freud elaborated on almost all the ideas of the higher mental functioning hypothesis in the *Outline*. He assigned a much greater part to those agencies of the mind that are acquired by learning from experience, that think and anticipate, make decisions and plans, and direct criticism against the self. He endowed the ego with much greater strength and much greater independence from the id by assigning it a powerful motive of its own: self-preservation, which, he wrote, "the id appears to neglect" (p. 199). Moreover, he assigned the ego a number of important subtasks, which it carries out as part of its task of self-preservation. These include the acquisition of control over the demands of the instincts (p. 146) and the regulation of behavior in terms of safety and danger (p. 199). He assumed that the ego is the great reservoir of the libido "from which libidinal cathexes are sent out onto objects and into which they are withdrawn like the pseudopodia of a body of protoplasm" (p. 151). He thereby implied that object relations are not formed automatically, but that the ego controls their development. The *Outline* assigns a diminished place to the id and thus to the importance in unconscious mental life of the search for pleasure. The id is described as almost unknowable. "It is hard to say anything of the behavior of the libido in the id" (p. 150).

Also in the *Outline*, Freud described more vigorously than earlier how the ego develops the belief in castration by inference from experience. The young boy, he wrote, may not be too impressed at first by his mother's threats to have him castrated as a punishment for masturbation. Later, when he perceives or remembers the perception of the female genitals, he puts two and two together and becomes convinced of the reality of his mother's threats. Freud also wrote explicitly about how the superego develops in relation to parents, and he stated that after its development a person's superego treats him much as his parents had treated him. Finally, Freud assumed that a person's superego contains certain pathogenic beliefs, such as the belief that he must remain ill for he deserves no better.

Before ending my discussion of Freud's development of the higher mental functioning hypothesis, I shall touch on two of its concepts that do not fit readily into the narrative I have presented above. The first is the concept of an unconscious wish for mastery. This was introduced tentatively in *Beyond the Pleasure Principle* (1920) and, as I shall discuss further in Chapter 5, was developed in *Inhibitions, Symptoms and Anxiety* (1926a, p. 167) and in other works, including the *Outline* (1940a, p. 146). According to Freud (1920), a person may repeat unpleasurable traumatic experiences not to attain gratification from them but to master them. The wish for mastery may be observed in the play of children. Children repeat their traumatic experiences in play in order to master them. The wish for mastery takes precedence over the pleasure principle. According to Freud, the mastery of excitation must be accomplished before the pleasure principle may function. In introducing an unconscious wish for mastery, Freud went beyond the automatic functioning hypothesis in several ways: He theorized the existence of a wish that is not directed to gratification but to a certain achievement and that seeks not an immediate but a long-term goal.

The other concept that does not fit readily into my narrative concerns the importance of identification in the development both of the ego and the superego. The ego, Freud suggested, develops by identifying unconsciously with lost love objects (1923, pp. 29–30). A person, through such identification, may develop new motives, such as the wish to acquire certain abilities similar to those of a person he once loved or admired, or to obtain a position such as a loved person once held. The concept that the ego develops by identifying with love objects points to the great part played by experience in the development of motivation. It points, too, to the development of powerful unconscious motives that, unlike the impulses of the automatic functioning hypothesis, may seek not immediate gratification, but the long-term development of certain abilities and capacities.

In each of the ideas of the higher mental functioning hypothesis, Freud postulated an unconscious mental process that is similar to a familiar conscious mental process. Taken together, these ideas constitute the rudiments of a new view of the unconscious mind, according to which a person may do many of the same kinds of things unconsciously as he does consciously. He may unconsciously learn from experience. He may, for example, by inference from experience, acquire beliefs about his relations to the main persons in his life, including beliefs about how he has affected or has been affected by them and how he is likely to affect or be affected by them. He may, on the basis of such beliefs, become inhibited, anxious, or guilty. He may institute repressions, and he may develop certain long-term goals. Furthermore, as a consequence of certain unconscious beliefs, he may torture himself with guilt, shame, or remorse.

INFLUENCE OF THE AUTOMATIC FUNCTIONING HYPOTHESIS ON CLINICAL THINKING

The automatic functioning hypothesis, as I have already pointed out, was developed more fully and explicitly than the higher mental functioning hypothesis. Even in *An Outline of Psychoanalysis* (1940a), the concepts of the higher mental functioning hypothesis are simply outlined in a few pages. In addition, their clinical implications are not spelled out.

The views of most analysts about the therapeutic process and technique are still to a surprising degree dominated by the automatic functioning hypothesis. (There are, of course, exceptions, as I shall later show. A few analysts, most of whom are well known and highly respected, have made considerable use in their clinical writings of the higher mental functioning hypothesis.)

The predominance of the automatic functioning hypothesis in clinical thinking, even today, may be explained by the fact that Freud evolved his theory of therapy and technique long before he explicitly developed the major concepts of the higher mental functioning hypothesis. Freud developed his theory of therapy and technique as early as 1911–1915 in his *Papers on Technique,* and the ideas he put down in these papers remain the basis of much psychoanalytic practice. Lipton, in surveying developments in Freud's ideas about technique between 1920 and 1939, concluded, "Freud considered that by 1920 the fundamental premises of psychoanalytic technique were established and that he directed his efforts to theoretical expansion, to technical refinement, and to the stabilization and preservation of the basic premises against numerous forces that jeopardized them" (1967, p. 91). Coltrera and Ross also concluded that "the general principles of psychoanalytic technique as now practiced are usually dated to around 1913" (1967, p. 38). In a review of psychoanalysis after 1939, Kanzer and Blum delineated a series of important contributions of ego psychology to psychoanalytic therapy, but concluded with the overall judgment: "Nevertheless, classical analysis, as the *innermost core* of analytic theorizing and therapy, *has undergone relatively little change—one that is to be measured more in the analyst's outlook and use of his techniques than in their formal aspects*" (1967, pp. 138–139, italics mine). Weinshel drew a similar conclusion in his review of contemporary contributions to the theory of technique (1970).

THE DEVELOPMENT SINCE FREUD OF
THE HIGHER MENTAL FUNCTIONING HYPOTHESIS

Since Freud, a number of psychoanalytic writers have contributed to the development of the higher mental functioning hypothesis. So have numerous writers in other fields, such as psychology and child development. The recognition and clarification of the importance, in unconscious mental life, of cognition, thought, and decision making, constitute a major trend in present-day psychology. It is a trend which deserves scholarly treatment and documentation. However, I shall not attempt such scholarship in this book. My purpose is to present a particular psychoanalytic theory of the mind and of the psychoanalytic process. Therefore, in discussing the development after Freud of the higher mental functioning hypothesis, I shall merely refer to a few psychoanalytic writers, all of whom are well known to my generation of psychoanalysts.

• Hartmann, in a series of major theoretical contributions (1939, 1956a, 1956b), developed further the concept of the ego's relative independence from the drives. He showed that the ego does not develop entirely from the interactions of the instincts with one another or with the environment. Indeed, adaptation to reality is not imposed upon the individual entirely by the demands of life, but, to some extent, as a consequence of an independent capacity for anticipation and postponement, and a motivation, independent of the drives, toward adaptation ("something in the person speaks out for reality" [1956a, p. 243]).

• Kris, in numerous papers (1947, 1950, 1951, 1956a, 1956b), stressed the capacity of the ego to control unconscious mental life in accordance with higher mental functions. For example, Kris assumed that in artistic production regression may take place in the service of the ego. This concept indicates that the ego may control the coming to consciousness of previously unconscious fantasies, and that it may bring these fantasies forth for a purpose of its own, namely, to produce a work of art. The ego could do these things only if it unconsciously could think, decide, and plan, and, in addition, exert control in accordance with its unconscious thoughts, decisions, and plans. Kris also observed that the coming forth of warded-off memories during analysis is regulated by the ego, which may bring them forth in pursuit of its goal of attaining mastery over the unconscious.

• Rapaport's contributions (1951, 1957) include the further development of the concept of the autonomy of the ego, as well as further exploration of the idea that the ego may unconsciously control both the unconscious expression of certain impulses and their coming to consciousness.

• Erikson's formulations about stages in the development of the ego, as well as his concept of identity, indicate that the ego has powerful motives of its own, unconscious as well as conscious (1950, 1956, 1968). For example, his concept of identity implies that behavior is not completely determined by the dynamic interaction of psychic forces, but rather is guided by organized, coherent motivational systems that may or may not be accessible to consciousness. These motivational systems integrate a person's impulses, defenses, values, identifications, and judgments about reality into coherent, long-term, adaptive purposes and goals.

• Loewenstein (1954) elaborated on the idea (which Freud indicated in *Analysis Terminable and Interminable* [1937, p. 235]) that a patient may, in relation to the analyst, unconsciously do analytic work. Loewenstein proposed that a patient, to help in overcoming the distortions brought about by his impulses and defenses, may rely on the analyst as an autonomous auxiliary ego. A patient could use the analyst in this way only if he were aware unconsciously that his own perceptions were distorted by certain impulses and defenses and if, in addition, he were motivated unconsciously to free himself from these distortions.

• Sandler and Joffe (1969) endowed the ego with a capacity to regulate unconscious impulses not only in accordance with anticipation of danger, but also in accordance with anticipation of safety. Thus, Sandler and Joffe assumed that a person may not only repress an emerging impulse that he decides would endanger him if expressed, but he may also lift the defenses opposed to the emergence of an impulse that he decides he could safely experience.

• Rangell (1968) elaborated and applied clinically concepts that Freud developed in the *Outline* about the ego's use of trial actions to determine in advance whether it may safely carry out a proposed course of action. According to Rangell, the ego of the patient routinely tests both its internal and its external environment before carrying out any significant new behavior or before bringing any new affects or impulses to consciousness. Rangell has stressed the ego's control of the therapeutic process. He has written that regression in the service of the ego is a central dynamic of therapy, and has discussed, in some detail, the decision-making function of the ego. Also, Rangell has pointed to certain clinical applications of Freud's concepts about unconscious cognition and unconscious ideas (1969a, 1969b, 1971).

THE CURRENT STATUS OF THE TWO HYPOTHESES

The concepts of the higher mental functioning hypothesis about unconscious thinking, decision making, and anticipation have, since Freud introduced them, been subject to much discussion. Certain analysts (e.g., Waelder, 1967) who continue to adhere to the scientific ideals that inspired *Project for a Scientific Psychology* (1895) and *The Interpretation of Dreams* (1900) have criticized concepts about unconscious thought, decision making, and anticipation as violating these ideals, and hence as being unscientific. Some of these analysts have criticized the higher mental functioning hypothesis as violating the strict determinism of the automatic functioning hypothesis and as providing pseudoexplanations, that is, explanations that are teleological or tautological or that use the ego as a homunculus. In the opinion of such analysts, explanations in terms of, say, thoughts, decisions, and plans, are not fundamental, for thoughts, decisions, and plans are themselves determined by the dynamic play of forces.

To illustrate the persistence of the views embodied in the automatic functioning hypothesis, I shall quote Robert Waelder (1967), who not long ago vigorously articulated such views. He argued against the concept of anticipation on the grounds that it is teleological, and hence may not be reducible to a mechanical model. "The question is open, of course, whether the process is thereby effectively reduced to mechanical terms because the implicit ability of the ego to anticipate still contains the whole secret: how does the ego do the anticipating?" (p. 17). Waelder (1967) also asserted that "the 'ego' is a concept of a different kind from, say, 'instinct,' 'drive,' or 'id' " (p. 13), and that the ego is in its "higher operations" a teleological concept similar to Aristotle's *entelechy*:

A drive is a force like, say, gravity; it pushes things in a particular direction with a certain intensity. It is what the medieval philosophers called a *vis a tergo*, a force pushing from behind. But the ego can be so-described only on the lowest level of its activities, viz., that of reflex action; in its higher operations it is a *problem-solving agent* and thus a *teleological* concept. It explains psychic activities in terms of the purposes they serve. It is a close relative of Artistotle's *entelechy*, the pre-existing force which guides the development of plant or animal according to nature; or a relative of the medieval physician's *vis mediatrix naturae*, the healing power of nature. (pp. 13–14, italics Waelder's)

Waelder was especially critical of Freud's last work, *An Outline of Psychoanalysis* (1940a), in which, according to Waelder (1967), causal explanations in terms of tensions and pressures are virtually subordinated to explanations in terms of higher mental functions:

The goal-directed expressions abound in this text: "The ego has . . . *at its command* . . . it has the *task* of . . . it *performs* that task . . . by gaining *control* . . . by *deciding* . . . by *postponing* . . . it is guided by *consideration.* . . ." Causal explanations in terms of tensions and pressures still turn up but they appear to be subordinated to the ego rather than determining it. (p. 15, italics Waelder's)

Just as some analysts, such as Waelder, have criticized the higher mental functioning hypothesis for its concepts about thinking, anticipation, and decision making, other analysts have criticized the automatic functioning hypothesis for its concepts about forces, energies, and structures. Such writers, including Klein (1969), Gill (1976), and Holt (1975), have argued that such natural science concepts of the automatic functioning hypothesis are not derived from psychoanalytic data, do not apply to that data, and fail to explain it.

Some analysts have assumed that the automatic functioning hypothesis and the higher mental functioning hypothesis are compatible, and thus that they can be combined into a single, coherent theory. However, other analysts, in particular those who disagree with either the automatic functioning hypothesis or the higher mental functioning hypothesis, have considered the two hypotheses incompatible. For example, Zilboorg, who disagrees with the concepts of the higher mental functioning hypothesis, argued that the development of ego psychology has led to the "fragmentation of psychoanalysis" and the "breaking up of its scientific unity" (1952, p. 21). Similarly, Glover (1968) attributes "confusion" and "schisms" within present-day psychoanalysis to attempts to reconcile Freud's earlier formulations as presented in the *Interpretation of Dreams* (1900) and in his later theorizing.

George S. Klein, who is critical of the metapsychology inherent in the automatic functioning hypothesis, also considers it useless to try to integrate ego psychology and its higher mental functioning concepts into a theory that is saddled "with a foggy language of cathexis, neutralization, and discharge" (1969, p. 523). Holt, who also is critical of the automatic functioning hypothesis, argued that attempts to integrate ego psychology with the basic assumptions of Freud's metapsychology have been "the fatal flaw of psychoanalytic ego psychology" (1975, pp. 572–573).

Arlow (1975) has taken a similar position:

Freud brought over into the new paradigm [i.e., the structural theory] a whole set of metapsychological propositions he had developed in connection with his earlier theory. Energic concepts of bound and free cathexes were foisted upon the newer structural concepts. . . . This blending of metapsychological propositions with clinical theory has, in my opinion, resulted in further confusion as far as psychoanalytic research and treatment are concerned. (pp. 514–515)

Among those analysts who considered the automatic functioning hypothesis and the higher mental functioning hypothesis compatible, and hence capable of being integrated into a single theory, are such major contributors to psychoanalytic ego psychology as Hartmann, Kris, Loewenstein, and Rapaport. However, there is disagreement about how well such integration could be carried out. Hartmann, Kris, and Loewenstein—who, individually and as collaborators, were dedicated to the task of integration—fully recognized its difficulties and the incompleteness with which they themselves had carried out this task. They wrote, "Since a structural viewpoint was introduced into psychoanalytic thinking, *hypotheses previously established must be reintegrated.* The task of synchronization *is larger than it might seem at first*" (1946, p. 12, italics mine). Similarly, Kris (1950) noted:

Freud's thoughts were constantly developing, his writings represent a sequence of reformulations, and one might therefore well take the view that the systematic cohesion of psychoanalytic propositions is only, or at least best, accessible through their history. The clearest instance of such a reformulation was the gradual introduction of structural concepts. *The introduction of these new concepts has never been fully integrated with the broad set of propositions developed earlier.* (p. 219, italics mine)

Kris (1947) also emphasized the extent of the changes Freud introduced in *Inhibitions, Symptoms and Anxiety,* and implied that the task of integration was difficult and not yet accomplished: "In 1926, in *Inhibitions, Symptoms and Anxiety,* Freud reformulated a considerable set of his previous hypotheses. I am convinced that this reformulation reaches further than was realized at the time of publication, possibly by Freud himself" (pp. 25–26).

Rapaport, in attempting to integrate the two hypotheses, devised a particular model of the mind in which behavior is regulated both automatically and by the ego through use of its higher mental functions. His model posits an hierarchical arrangement of impulse–defense layers, in which the deeper layers are governed more or less automatically and the more superficial layers are governed by higher mental functions. However, Rapaport's model has not figured prominently in current theorizing. As Holt (1975) has observed, Rapaport's students have become disenchanted with efforts to combine Freud's early theory with concepts about intention, purpose, and meaning. For example, G. S. Klein, who was once a student of Rapaport, wrote, "Contemporary ego psychology is a reminder to psychoanalysis of theoretical tasks hardly begun" (1969, p. 523).

Those analysts who agree that present-day psychoanalytic theory is not well integrated differ in their attitudes about its lack of integration. Some analysts, such as Peterfreund (1975, pp. 536–537), have emphasized their concern for its lack of integration. Others, such as Abrams (1971), assume that the integration of various psychoanalytic perspectives is not at present possible, and thus that we should be satisfied at present with a loose organization of psychoanalytic ideas. Abrams assumes that it is of heuristic value to the clinician to apply a variety of psychoanalytic models to the understanding of patients.

According to the viewpoint that animates this book, the automatic functioning hypothesis and the higher mental functioning hypothesis, while containing certain ideas in common, are different theories. According to the automatic functioning hypothesis, a patient's unconscious mental life is determined by psychic forces that interact dynamically beyond the patient's control with little or no regard for thought, anticipation, decision making, and so forth. The higher mental functioning hypothesis does not rule out all automatic functioning, but expects that a significant part of the patient's unconscious mental life is not determined automatically. For example, unconscious thoughts and decisions are not determined automatically by the dynamic interplay of psychic forces, and they make a powerful and independent contribution to behavior. The two hypotheses, as will be seen, provide different ideas about how the mind works and indicate different explanations for almost all clinical phenomena. While it is conceivable that the two hypotheses can be integrated at some future time into a coherent, unified theory, this possibility seems unlikely. A number of analysts have attempted such integration, but as I have shown in the preceding pages, those who have carefully studied these attempts believe that this integration has not been successfully carried out. There are some situations in which the two hypotheses, as presently formulated, cannot both be right. It does not make much sense, for example, to state that a patient brought forth a particular transference *both* because he was overpowered by it and hence could not keep it repressed *and* because he became strong enough to bring it forth safely. The principle of overdetermination (or multiple function) does not violate logic when, in the framework of the automatic functioning hypothesis, it is applied to contradictory impulses; however, it does violate logic when it is applied to contradictory explanations. It makes sense (in the framework of the automatic functioning hypothesis) to state that two contradictory impulses both find expression in the same compromise formation. But it does not make much sense to state that the same impulse came forth both because it was strengthened relative to the defenses opposed to its emergence, and because it was weakened relative to these defenses.

EMPIRICAL CONSIDERATIONS

The question of how the unconscious mind functions is empirical. It cannot be settled by arguments or philosophical discussion, only by observation and research. Thus, I disagree with those who object to the automatic functioning hypothesis on philosophical grounds about, say, its use of the energy concept. As we hope to show in Part II of this book, the automatic functioning hypothesis and its energy concept are testable.

If the automatic functioning hypothesis is not as good as the higher mental functioning hypothesis, this is simply because it does not fit observation as well as the higher mental functioning hypothesis.

What I have said about the importance of empirical considerations also applies to the higher mental functioning hypothesis. It should not be dismissed because it is presumed to sacrifice a rigorous determinism or because it is thought to be teleological or tautological. Again, it should be judged by how it fits with observation. A theory need not be strictly deterministic; it need merely make lawful and testable predictions. The higher mental functioning hypothesis, as we shall show in Part II of this book, does make such predictions.

Nor is a theory in which decisions and plans are assumed to be basic determinants of behavior any less scientific than one in which impersonal forces are assumed to be basic. Waelder and others, who assume that impersonal forces should be considered basic and decisions derivative, are arbitrarily upholding certain premises of the automatic functioning hypothesis that are far from commonsense. As Miller, Galanter, and Pribram (1960) have argued, decisions and plans are so basic in mental life that it is impossible to conceive of any human psychological behavior, whether it be a simple motor or perceptual act or a complex piece of behavior such as that studied by psychoanalysts, that is not done in accordance with a plan and hence a decision.

Nor is the decision concept of the higher mental functioning hypothesis any more tautological than the impulse concept of the automatic functioning hypothesis. A critic (in an attempt to discredit the decision concept) might argue that it adds nothing to our understanding of a person's carrying out a certain piece of behavior to state that he is carrying it out because he has decided to do so. However, a critic could attack the impulse concept in precisely the same terms: It adds nothing to our understanding of a person's carrying out a certain piece of behavior to say that he is carrying it out because he has an impulse to do so. Indeed, in the early days of psychoanalysis, the impulse concept was criticized in such terms. This criticism gave way only after the relationship of the impulse concept to a new and powerful theory became clear.

The criticism of the impulse concept in Freud's early theory as tautological was, of course, incorrect. The early theory with its automatic functioning hypothesis, does not use the impulse concept in the simplistic way ascribed to it by its critics. Nor does the higher mental functioning hypothesis use the decision concept in such a way. The automatic functioning hypothesis uses the impulse concept, and the higher mental functioning hypothesis uses the decision concept, not to explain isolated pieces of the patient's behavior, but to explain sequences, changes, and continuities, and thus to link different pieces of behavior to one another.

As I have suggested above, the future development of psychoanalytic theory will depend more on empirical research than on philosophical discussion. Logical completeness and clarity of terms, if these are to be pertinent to observation, must be achieved by the careful coordination, through research, of theory and observation.

3

UNCONSCIOUS GUILT

JOSEPH WEISS

This chapter is concerned with unconscious guilt, shame, fear, anxiety, and other such affects. These are rooted in unconscious beliefs, and hence are not readily accommodated by the unconscious mind as conceptualized by Freud in much of his early theorizing. They are, however, readily accommodated by the unconscious mind as Freud conceptualized it in parts of his ego psychology. Thus, unconscious guilt is scarcely mentioned in *Papers on Technique* (1911–1915), but its importance in mental life is emphasized in the *Outline* (1940a).

According to the theory proposed here, unconscious guilt, as well as the other affects referred to above, play a prominent part in unconscious mental life and in the development and maintenance of psychopathology. The development of such affects in childhood depends on the child's inner and outer worlds, that is, on certain of his motives, and on certain of his experiences. A child may develop guilt, and so forth, not only about motives such as murder and incest, which are generally considered reprehensible, but also about reasonable and generally accepted goals, such as becoming stronger or deriving greater enjoyment from life. Indeed, a person may suffer from guilt or anxiety about relaxing or about feeling healthy and happy.

A COMPARISON OF THE EARLY AND
LATE THEORIES AS REGARDS GUILT

FEAR OF PUNISHMENT IN THE EARLY THEORY
AND IN THE LATE THEORY

In his early writings, in which he relied heavily on the automatic functioning hypothesis, Freud explained by automatic processes observations that he was later to explain by unconscious guilt. Consider, for example, his early attempts to explain an irrational fear of punishment. In these attempts Freud assumed that an irrational fear of punishment develops almost entirely from the automatic functioning, in accordance with the pleasure principle, of certain defenses, namely, denial and projection. For example, a boy, by denying his unconscious wish to punish his father and projecting this wish onto his father, may come to expect punishment from his father.

In his late theorizing, after he developed the idea of Oedipal guilt, Freud assumed that a boy's fear of punishment from his father is mediated by the belief that if he pursues his mother sexually, his father will castrate him. Freud assumed that the boy acquires this belief not by the functioning of automatic processes, but by inference from experience. The experiences from which the boy infers this belief may, according to Freud, be distorted by denial and projection. By denying his rivalry with his father and projecting it onto him, the boy may perceive his father as more threatening than he really is. However, the experiences from which the boy infers the belief in castration may be relatively undistorted by denial and projection. For example, in the typical case which Freud presented in the *Outline* (1940a, pp. 183–194), denial and projection do not play an important part in the boy's development of the belief in castration. In this case, the boy develops the belief in castration from his mother's castration threats and from the sight of the female genitalia. According to Freud a boy may be unimpressed by his mother's castration threats until he remembers or perceives for the first time the female genitalia. Then he puts two and two together and concludes that his mother's threats to have him castrated are to be taken seriously.

The boy's belief in castration is, of course, not objectively warranted. However, it may be a reasonable intellectual achievement, given the boy's limited experience. The belief in castration as a punishment may be false or distorted not primarily because of the boy's use of denial and projection but because of the boy's egocentricity, his dependence on his parents, and his limited knowledge of human relations. The boy has no prior knowledge of human relations by which he may judge his relations to his parents. He may, for example, assume that he is a greater threat to his father than he really is. Moreover, he may, for a variety of reasons, take his parents' actual threats to castrate him far too seriously; he may have developed confidence in his parents' reliability, or he may be reluctant to believe that the persons on whom he must rely for protection are willing to make malicious threats. Even if skeptical, he may be unwilling to ignore such serious threats.

Whether or not the experiences from which the boy inferred his pathogenic belief in castration were distorted by denial and projection, it is the belief, rather than the denial and projection, which fixes the boy's fear of punishment and makes it a persistent part of his unconscious mental life.

WORRY IN THE EARLY THEORY AND IN THE LATE THEORY

Another example of Freud's reliance on the automatic functioning hypothesis in his early theorizing is his explanation of worry. He explained worry by this formula: the unconscious wish is the conscious fear. According to this idea, a hostile impulse, as a consequence of infantile omnipotence, is automatically (as in the formation of dreams) experienced as fulfilled. The hostile child who unconsciously wishes his mother dead consciously worries that she will die.

This formula, which Freud developed prior to his ideas about unconscious guilt, does not explain why a child whose mother gives him good reason to worry about her is more likely to do so than a child whose mother is robust and happy. A child's tormenting worry about his mother, as I shall discuss later, is mediated not automatically, but by an unconscious belief that he has acquired by inference from experience. This belief is that if he attempts to gratify a particular impulse or to reach a particular goal, he will be punished by something harmful happening to his mother.

The experiences from which a child infers and so comes to believe that he will hurt his mother may be distorted by his infantile omnipotence (egocentricity) or by his projections. However, it is the belief which fixes the relationship between the motive and the worry. It is the belief, too, which makes this connection a persistent part of the child's internal mental life.

THE PART PLAYED BY GUILT IN PSYCHOPATHOLOGY ACCORDING TO THE EARLY THEORY AND THE LATE THEORY

In his early theorizing, Freud attempted to explain all psychopathology as resulting from automatic processes that unfold without reference to experience, belief, or guilt. However, in certain brief but explicit theoretical discussions in his late works, Freud assumed that unconscious guilt or the unconscious need for punishment plays a part in all neurotic illness.

He wrote, "It seems that this factor, an unconscious need for punishment, has a place in every neurotic illness" (1933, p. 108).

In the *Outline* (1940a), Freud's last major work, he strongly emphasized the importance of unconscious guilt in psychopathology. He stressed, too, its importance as a resistance:

The further our work proceeds and the more deeply our insight penetrates into the mental life of neurotics, the more clearly two new factors force themselves on our notice, which demand the closest attention as sources of resistance. Both of them are completely unknown to the patient. . . . They may both be embraced under the single name of "need to be ill or to suffer." . . . The first of these two factors is the sense of guilt or consciousness of guilt, as it is called, though the patient does not feel it and is not aware of it. It is evidently the portion of the resistance contributed by a super-ego that has become particularly severe and cruel. The patient must not become well but must remain ill, for he deserves no better. . . .

It is less easy to demonstrate the existence of another resistance, our means of combating which are specially inadequate. There are some neurotics in whom, to judge by all their reactions, the instinct of self-preservation has actually been reversed. They seem to aim at nothing other than self-injury and self-destruction. . . . Patients of this kind are not able to tolerate recovery. (pp. 179–180)

THE CHILD'S DEVELOPMENT OF GUILT IN RELATION TO HIS PARENTS

In two of his late writings (1930, 1940a), Freud, in just a few pages, discussed the development of guilt in such a way as to suggest that the child may develop guilt not simply over Oedipal strivings but over a wide variety of impulses, purposes, attitudes, and goals. In addition, in his description of the child's development of guilt in relation to his parents, he laid the basis of an object relations theory of the kind advocated both by Loewald (1972) and by Settlage (1980).

The child's motive for developing a sense of guilt, as Freud discussed it, stems from his dependency on his parents. The child needs his parents to protect him from a variety of dangers, including the danger of their punishing him. He therefore dares not risk the loss of their love. In order to retain it, he develops a powerful wish to obey his parents, be loyal to them, and be like them. Moreover, he condemns in himself whatever, in his opinion, threatens his ties to his parents. For example, he condemns in himself those motives, traits, and behaviors that seem greatly to upset his parents or that they seem to condemn in him. Thus, Freud (1930) wrote:

As to the origin of the sense of guilt, the analyst has different views from other psychologists; but even he does not find it easy to give an account of it. To begin with, if we ask how a person comes to have a sense of guilt, we arrive at an answer which cannot be disputed: a person feels guilty . . . when he has done something which he knows to be "bad." . . . Perhaps, after some hesitation, we shall add that even when a person has not actually *done* the bad thing but has only recognized in himself an *intention* to do it, he may regard himself as guilty . . . . Both cases, however, presuppose that one had already recognized that what is bad is reprehensible. . . . How is this judgment arrived at? . . . What is bad is often not at all what is injurious or dangerous to the ego; on the contrary, it may be something which is desirable and enjoyable to the ego. Here, therefore, there is an extraneous influence at work, and it is this that decides what is to be called good or bad. Since a person's own feelings would not have led him along this path, he must have had a motive for submitting to this extraneous influence. Such a motive is easily discovered in his helplessness and his dependence on other people, and it can best be designated as fear of loss of love. If he loses the love of another person upon whom he is dependent, he also ceases to be protected from a variety of dangers. Above all, he is exposed to the danger that this stronger person will show his superiority in the form of punishment. At the beginning, therefore, what is bad is whatever causes one to be threatened with loss of love. For fear of that loss, one must avoid it. (p. 124, italics Freud's)

As to a sense of guilt, we must admit that it is in existence before the super-ego, and therefore before conscience, too. At that time it is the immediate expression of fear of the external authority, a recognition of the tension between the ego and the authority. It is the direct derivative of the conflict between the need for the authority's love and the urge toward instinctual satisfaction, whose inhibition produces the inclination to aggression. The superimposition of these two strata of the sense of guilt—one coming from fear of the *external* authority, the other from fear of the *internal* authority—has hampered our insight into the position of conscience in a number of ways. (1930, pp. 136–137, italics Freud's)

Freud, in the passages quoted above, assumed that guilt arises from a particular kind of disruption in the child's relationships to his parents: a disruption that arises from behavior that the child experiences as provoking punishment or rejection. Perhaps just as important, however, in the production of guilt is the disruption that arises from behavior that the child experiences as worrying, saddening, hindering, draining, or humiliating a parent, or expressing disloyalty to the parent. Indeed, the most profound and powerful feelings of guilt (as Michael Friedman of our research group has emphasized) may be rooted in a person's pathogenic belief that he has, in one way or another, hurt a parent (Friedman, 1985).

The intense wish of the child to maintain his ties to his parents, which, according to Freud, is the motive for the child's development of conscience, is, in the theory that Freud presented in the *Outline* (1940a), an ego wish. The child's motive for maintaining his ties to his parents, as described in the *Outline*, is not for gratification but for self-preservation, security, and safety. Furthermore, the preservation of the self—of safety and security, as Freud tells us—is the task of the ego, which "the id appears to neglect" (p. 199).

The ego wish of the child to retain his parents as protectors is much stronger than are his libidinal attachments to them. That Freud believed this is evident from his observation that the child may repress his sexual interest in the parent of the opposite sex in order to retain the protection and good will of both parents.

GUILT ABOUT REASONABLE EGO GOALS

Since a child must condemn in himself any motive or behavior that seriously threatens his all-important ties to his parents, he may condemn in himself not simply those motives ordinarily thought to be reprehensible, such as the Oedipal motives of murder and incest, but any motives that he infers may threaten his ties to his parents. There is no *a priori* moral principle to guide the child in the development of his conscience. He learns his morality from his particular experiences with his particular parents. He must condemn in himself those impulses, behaviors, and goals that he infers threaten his ties to them. Thus, his particular morality depends not only on his impulses and behaviors, but also on the way, as he experiences it, his particular (and perhaps perverse or foolish) parents react to them.

Therefore, two children who are endowed with identical motives but who grow up in different families should develop different ideas of good and bad. Furthermore, a child may condemn in himself motives not generally considered bad if he infers, correctly or not, that his ties to his parents would be threatened by his expression of such motives. The influence of the child's experiences with his particular parents was stressed by Freud (1940a) in the following words:

Throughout later life it [the superego] represents the influence of a person's childhood, and of the care and education given him by his parents and of his dependence on them—a childhood which is prolonged so greatly in human beings by a family life in common. And in all of this it is not only the personal qualities of these parents that is making itself felt, but also everything that had a determining effect on them themselves, the tastes and standards of the social class in which they lived. (p. 206)

Since a child's unconscious morality depends very much on the special characteristics of his parents, he may develop unconventional unconscious moral ideas. For example, he may not necessarily assume that the punishment fits the crime. A child who was never gluttonous or greedy, or even tempted to be these things, may develop a fear of starvation if he is exposed by his parents or by fate to the danger of starvation. He may link the danger of starvation as a punishment with any of a number of impulses, attitudes, or goals. He may, for example, come to believe that if he is confident of the future, he may be punished by being deprived of food. Nor does the child's morality necessarily correspond to the law of the talion (an eye for an eye) unless his particular experiences with his parents induce him to assume this principle.

A child may come to condemn himself for what is generally thought of as a normal acceptable wish or developmental goal if he infers, whether or not correctly, that by attempting to satisfy this wish or reach this goal he may threaten his all-important ties to his parents. This point has been made by Leo Rangell, who assumed that a patient may feel guilty about an ego interest or goal such as the acquisition of autonomy or independence. "Heretofore, the impulses about which guilt or anxiety are felt come from the id, from instinctual drives, impulses which in their origins are a part of the inborn equipment of man. But man in the modern world is seen in copious examples, from analysis and from life, to be driven by and often guilty about ego forces, ego interests, ego drives if you will" (1975, p. 94).

SEPARATION GUILT

I shall now focus on two kinds of guilt that may be developed in pursuit of reasonable ego goals and that, in my opinion, are as widespread as Oedipal guilt and in some patients more important. These are separation guilt and survivor guilt. Separation guilt may develop in a child who wishes to become more independent of a parent but who infers that were he to do so, he would hurt the parent. This kind of guilt has been described by Modell (1965, 1971). Separation guilt, like castration anxiety, is rooted in a belief. This is the child's belief, which he infers from his experienes, that if he becomes more independent of the parent he will hurt the parent. Modell (1965) wrote:

Certain forms of the negative therapeutic reaction can be understood as a manifestation of a more basic feeling of not having a right to a life; that is, not having a right to a separate existence. . . . Separation from the maternal object in these people is unconsciously *perceived* as causing the death of the mother. To attain something for oneself, to lead a separate existence, is *perceived* as depriving the mother of her basic substance. (p. 330, italics mine)

(I have italicized the word "perceived" to emphasize that Modell implied that separation guilt develops from a belief inferred from experience, rather than from automatic processes.)

The child's acquisition of separation guilt depends on both internal and external factors. It may depend on the strength of his wish to become more independent, his infantile tendency to exaggerate his effect on his parents, his projections onto his parents of his dependency, and his parents' real reactions to his attempts to become more independent of them.

As regards the part played by real experiences in the acquisition of separation guilt, a child whose mother appears to be deeply upset by his attempts to become more independent of her is, all else being equal, more likely to develop separation guilt than a child whose mother is unhurt by his attempts to become more independent of her or is proud of his capacity to be independent.

Modell's concept of separation guilt is akin to Loewald's (1979) idea that as the child matures he may become guilty about assuming a sense of responsibility for his own life. This is because the child experiences his taking such responsibility for himself as at the expense of his parents, who once took such responsibility for him. Loewald considered this form of guilt to be connected both with Oedipal conflict and conflict about separation and individuation, and he considers it universal. Loewald (1979) stated:

It is no exaggeration to say that the assumption of responsibility for one's own life and its conduct is a psychic reality tantamount to the murder of the parents; that is, to the crime of parricide, and it involves dealing with the guilt incurred thereby. . . . A parricide, that is, one who commits an act of parricide, is defined as follows: one who murders a person to whom one stands in an especially sacred relation, as a father, mother, or other near relative, or (in a wider sense) a ruler. Sometimes one guilty of treason (Webster, Second Edition). (p. 755)

Modell assumed that separation guilt is universal. He wrote, "Since I have reported my observations in 1965, I have become increasingly convinced that the issue is not confined to a particular diagnostic group but that it represents a fundamental human conflict" (1971, p. 340).

Asch (1976) has also written about separation guilt. He, too, emphasized the part played by the child's experiences with his parents in his acquisition of separation guilt. In several of Asch's cases, the child developed an exaggerated sense of responsibility for his mother's happiness as a result of his mother's demands that he take a great deal of responsibility for her happiness. In other words, a child, according to Asch, may develop the beliefs underlying separation guilt directly by instruction from his mother. That is, a child whose mother tells him that he must sacrifice for her (even though he consciously repudiates the idea) may come to believe unconsciously that he should sacrifice for her. Moreover, he may behave in accordance with that belief.

A person who suffers from separation guilt may attempt to overcome the guilt by inflicting certain kinds of punishment on himself. He may, in particular, punish himself by intensifying in a self-tormenting way his ties to the parent whom he believes he has hurt by his independence. He may, by identifying with the parent toward whom he feels separation guilt, acquire certain of that parent's most self-destructive behaviors or traits. He may, for example, ruin his marriage by raging at his wife as his father ruined his marriage by such raging. Indeed, he may develop any kind of maladaptive behavior similar to that of the parent whom he believes he damaged by becoming independent, for example, excessive timidity, alcoholism, overeating, or impulsiveness. Alternatively, a person who would like to mollify his conscience so as to reduce his separation guilt may punish himself, not by identifying with the parent from whom he has separated, but by complying in a self-tormenting way with that parent. That is, he may adopt some foolish or maladaptive behaviors such as he unconsciously believes the parent wanted him to adopt. If he infers that his mother wanted him to remain dependent on her, he may become sick and hence dependent on her, or he may develop some crippling symptom that prevents him from becoming independent. One patient I studied, who suffered from separation guilt, developed in childhood an intense fear of using any toilet outside the home, and thus kept himself close to his mother. Another patient in childhood developed such a bad temper that he made himself unpopular with the other children in school. Since he couldn't get along well with his peers, he felt forced to come home and be with his mother, who, as he experienced it, was tolerant of his bad temper and seemed amused by his rages.

SURVIVOR GUILT

Another kind of guilt that plays a part in the psychopathology of many patients has been referred to by Modell as "survivor guilt." This term was used originally to describe the guilt suffered by persons whose parents or siblings had died. However, its meaning has been widened by Modell (1971) to include the guilt of persons who assume they have fared better than their parents or siblings. Survivor guilt, too, is based on a belief. It is a person's belief that by acquiring more of the good things of life than his parents or siblings, he has betrayed them. The person believes that his acquisitions have been obtained at the expense of his parents and siblings. According to Modell (1971):

There is a type of guilt which one can observe in psychoanalysis that may exist independently of the Oedipus complex and probably has its origin in an earlier period of development, although in mental life the contents of both earlier and later periods can be confused and condensed. . . . I am referring to a sense of guilt that is the response to the awareness that one has something more than someone else. This sense of guilt is invariably accompanied by a *thought* which may remain unconscious that what one has obtained has been obtained at the expense of taking something away from somebody else. The matter is further complicated by the fact that the sense of guilt itself may be unconscious and may be noticed only through its derivatives which may appear as self-negating or self-destructive behavior. (p. 339, italics mine)

Survivor guilt, according to Modell, depends on the *thought* (belief) that in a particular family there is only a certain amount of the good things of life to go around. Therefore, a person assumes that the good things (such as success, money, fame, and happiness) he acquires are acquired at the expense of his parents and siblings.

The development of survivor guilt depends on internal and external factors—that is, on motivations and experiences. According to Modell (1971):

The intensity of the guilt may be understood as the consequence of two complementary factors—one is a quantitative instinctual element . . . but there are others in whom the instinctual element does not seem to play a prominent part—guilt of this sort is a consequence, as it were, of environmental accident, i.e. it is a question of the evaluation of the actual fate of other individuals in the nuclear family. . . . If fate has dealt harshly with other members of the family, the survivor may experience guilt, as he has obtained more than his share of the "good." (p. 340)

Since all varieties of guilt (not just separation guilt) arise from the child's fear of disrupting his ties to his parents and siblings (by hurting them, being hurt by them, or losing their love), a person may attempt to avoid guilt of any kind by intensifying his ties to his parents. He may, as in the case of separation guilt, develop a tormenting identification with a parent (or sibling), or a tormenting compliance with a parent (or sibling). Such compliances and identifications are illustrated in both Modell's and Asch's clinical examples. A patient who torments himself by developing the worst traits of a parent or sibling, or by living in the unsatisfactory manner of a parent or sibling, is, in Asch's phrase, "identifying with the victim." Modell, in his paper "On Having the Right to a Life" (1965), illustrated such identification with the victim in two cases, a man and a woman. The man's life was dominated by the urge to destroy all accomplishment. He could only enjoy pleasure under conditions of self-abasement. He had, in childhood, felt fused with his mother, for whom he had contempt. Also, he had failed to identify with his father, who, as the patient experienced it, had abandoned him to his mother. The man identified with his contemptible mother and provoked in his father contempt for him such as he had felt toward his mother. The patient consciously experienced no guilt; however, his life was under the complete domination of unconscious guilt. The woman was "compelled to negate whatever she possessed. She dispelled the pleasure in her marriage by increasing provocations." This patient, too, had failed to identify with her father. She had felt abandoned by him to her mother and could not bear having a better life than her mother, whose life she perceived as one of hardship and degradation. In her treatment, she made a massive unconscious effort to convince Modell that she was bizarre or psychotic and thus that she was not suitable for analysis. The patient, the oldest of three children, "was *convinced* that she had taken for herself the best that there was of her mother's love (i.e., milk), and in fact drained her and robbed her siblings of their birthrights" (Modell, 1965, p. 326, italics mine). (I have emphasized "convinced" to point out Modell's implication that survivor guilt is rooted in a belief.)

Another of Modell's cases (1971) was a wealthy, successful man who suffered from survivor guilt. He assumed that he had obtained his success at his sister's expense. He deadened himself by drinking so as to be no better off than his sister, whose severe psychopathology left her feeling dead. This patient identified with the victim.

Asch's discussion of separation guilt (1976) emphasizes the patient's unconscious belief that he is responsible for his mother. This belief, in several of Asch's cases, was engendered to some extent by the mother's complaints. In one case, the mother, who was long-suffering, told the child (and future patient) that it was his duty to take care of her. He became self-sacrificing. His two marriages were to demanding and ungiving women. In his career he worked hard for little pay. In analysis he was at first unaware that he was complying with his mother, and he was resistant to Asch's attempts to make him aware of it.

In another of Asch's cases, the mother accused the patient of hurting her. She told him that his birth almost killed her and that he had prevented her from having more children. This patient led the life of self-sacrifice that he believed his mother wanted him to live (Asch, 1976).

THE PERIOD OF LIFE IN WHICH A PERSON DEVELOPS SEPARATION GUILT AND SURVIVOR GUILT

The question of at what age is a child prone to develop separation guilt or survivor guilt can be answered only by observation. Asch (1976) has assumed that both kinds of guilt are pregenital, developing before the resolution of the Oedipus complex. Modell (1965, 1971) originally reached the same conclusion. However, in a recent paper (1983), he assumed that separation guilt and survivor guilt may develop independently of the Oedipus complex, before, during, or after it. My own findings, which are based on reconstructions from the analyses of adults, are in accord with Modell's recent article. Judging from my patients, a child may develop separation guilt or survivor guilt relatively early in childhood or as late as adolescence.

My findings are supported by Niederland's study of the survivors of the Holocaust (1981). A number of the survivors whom Niederland studied developed survivor guilt long after the Oedipal period. This suggests that the kind of guilt a child develops depends on the *kind* of trauma he suffers, not just upon *when* in his development he suffers it. A child, of course, may be more prone to developing certain kinds of trauma (and hence certain kinds of guilt) at some periods than at others.

OTHER KINDS OF GUILT

As previously indicated, a child may develop not only Oedipal guilt, separation guilt, and survivor guilt, but guilt about any motive or behavior. This is because he may infer (correctly or not) that any motive or behavior may threaten his all-important ties to his parents. One child may infer that if he is clinging and dependent on his parents he will please them; another child, that if he is clinging and dependent on his parents he will drain them; or the same child may infer both ideas. Another child may infer that he must be a bad boy in order to make his parents feel morally superior, or he may assume that he must be bad to protect an unhappy sibling whom the parents, because of worry, wish to perceive as good. As another example, a child may infer that by competing with a parent he will provoke the parent into a dangerous competition with him. Another child may infer that by competing with a parent he will provoke the parent to reject him, whereas still another child may infer that he must be competitive with his worried parents to assure them that they have not crushed his independence.

SOME CASE ILLUSTRATIONS

As I pointed out earlier, a person who suffers from separation guilt may, in his symptoms or in the course of his life, find a way of being tortured as he believes he tortured the parent about whom he developed guilt. The following clinical example illustrates a common manifestation of this phenomenon.

THE CASE OF MR. M

Mr. M, a patient in his 30s, tormented himself by an obsessive rumination about a high-school girlfriend whom he glamorized and who ultimately rejected him. He would long for the girl and tell himself that by losing her he had lost a great opportunity for happiness. It turned out that Mr. M had felt quite guilty about leaving his mother, whom he perceived as possessive and as having lived mainly for him. In his high-school romance he had unconsciously been identified with his mother. He had experienced the girl's rejection of him as he believed his mother had experienced his rejection of her. He unconsciously experienced the girl's rejection of him (which in retrospect he seemed to have provoked) as a fitting punishment for his rejection of his mother. During treatment, as he made progress in his efforts to free himself from his mother, Mr. M would punish himself by ruminating about his girlfriend's rejection of him.

The patient's sadness at the loss of his girlfriend might, at first glance, appear to have been merely a normal reaction to an unfortunate event, rather than a tormenting symptom nourished by unconscious guilt. The fact that the patient's ruminations about his former girlfriend was a symptom was apparent from the fact that he was tormented by it, as well as from his reactions to my interpretations: He understood them readily. Indeed, he drew a number of parallels between his sadness at losing his girlfriend and his mother's sadness at losing him. Moreover, his insight into the meaning of his preoccupation with his girlfriend enabled him eventually to relinquish it.

A certain kind of patient, as Modell (1965) pointed out, experiences separation guilt during the terminal phase of his analysis (also see Chapter 20). He unconsciously worries about the analyst, whom he believes would feel lost without him. In some patients an intensification of symptoms during the terminal phase has the unconscious purpose of making the analyst feel needed.

Several of my patients, during the terminal phase of their analyses, dreamt of losing a loved one. A woman patient dreamt about the death of a child; a man about the loss of a childhood companion. In both instances the patient was identifying with the victim, that is, with the analyst. In their dreams these patients were attempting to alleviate their feelings of guilt about leaving the analyst by picturing themselves suffering the same kind of torment they believed they were causing the analyst to suffer.

A patient who presents himself as intensely in need of the analyst may be identifying with a possessive parent to whom he felt separation guilt. He may behave toward the analyst in the same possessive, demanding way that, as he experienced it, the parent had behaved toward him. He may be exaggeratedly hurt, for example, when the analyst takes a vacation or cancels an appointment, just as, in his opinion, a parent was hurt by his departures. Such a patient may be helped when the analyst makes him aware that in his behavior, he is not expressing a primary dependency on the analyst but, as consequence of an identification with a parent, behaving as though dependent on the analyst.

THE CASE OF MISS W

The patient presented in the case below suffered from both Oedipal guilt and separation guilt, which she dealt with by tormenting herself as, in her opinion, her mother wanted her to torment herself. She retained a certain type of infantile behavior into adulthood because, although she found it unpleasurable and disadvantageous, she assumed unconsciously that it would please her mother.

Miss W, in childhood, believed herself more attractive than her petulant mother. She had competed with her mother for her father's love and, as she had experienced it, defeated her. She felt responsible for her mother's unhappiness and became guilty. Indeed, she believed that by having had so much more fun with her father than her mother had had with him, she was devastating her mother. Miss W was plagued with worry about her mother until she found a way of restoring her—namely, by having temper tantrums. She assumed, whether or not correctly, that by her temper tantrums she was enabling her mother both to feel morally superior to her and to defeat her in their competition for her father. Her mother, who was usually somewhat depressed, would become lively and indignant when the patient had a tantrum. Moreover, her mother would induce her father to punish her. The mother thereby demonstrated to her daughter that her claims on the father took precedence over her daughter's. Miss W may have had occasional childhood tantrums that were not connected in her mind with the wish to restore her mother. However, after she came to believe that she could use tantrums for that purpose, they became compulsive and remained so for many years.

Miss W's rage satisfied both her separation guilt and her Oedipal guilt. This case shows how behavior that, according to the automatic functioning hypothesis, is thought to be the direct expression of primary infantile rage, may, according to the higher mental functioning hypothesis, be viewed as regulated by a primitive conscience for the purpose of self-punishment. Miss W was guided unconsciously by the belief, which she developed in childhood, that when she was pleasant and successful with a man she was defying her mother and destroying her. She was also guided by the related belief that when she displayed her temper and thereby provoked the man, she was complying with her mother and so restoring her. In other words, the symptom in this case is intended to protect the patient against the danger of losing her mother's love and of destroying her.

THE CASE OF MISS D

This case is interesting because it describes an experiment in nature. The patient, Miss D, made little or no progress during the first 18 months of her treatment. Her analyst, during this period, did not recognize the importance to her psychopathology of her separation guilt. The analyst sought help from a supervisor, who pointed to the great part played by Miss D's separation guilt in her psychopathology. The analyst changed his technique in accord with his new conception of the case and, as will be seen, had dramatically good results.

Miss D, an articulate woman of 28, sought analysis because of bouts of depression and a sense of purposelessness. She derived little pleasure from her career and was unhappy in her personal life. She wished to marry and have children but had not been able to find a husband.

She described herself, in childhood, as having been dependent on her mother and as having had little to do with her father. Her mother, she remembered, had often been exasperated with her for being clingy and had tried to force her to become independent by sending her off to camp. However, Miss D, as she remembered it, had clung to her mother despite her mother's disapproval. The patient was becoming more independent when, at 15, her father died. In reaction to his death, she strengthened her ties to her mother.

In her analysis, Miss D developed a mother transference. She became dependent and clingy toward the analyst as she had been to her mother. The analyst, a senior candidate, interpreted her behavior as the expression of a primary dependence on him. He told her that she was repeating with him her childhood dependence on her mother. The patient, over a period of time, was made worse rather than better by such interpretations.

As Miss D failed to improve, the analyst became disgusted and frustrated. He continued, however, to interpret her dependency in much the same way for about 18 months, then sought help from a supervisor. The supervisor suggested that the patient suffered from separation guilt. Miss D, according to this formulation, had maintained her attachment to her mother and to the analyst for fear that if she were to run her own life, she would hurt them.

In view of the patient's memory of her mother urging her to be independent, this formulation seemed unlikely at first glance. Nonetheless, it proved correct and helped Miss D to break the stalemate that had existed for so long. The patient began to do more things on her own, to feel less draggy, and to retrieve a number of new childhood memories about her mother. She remembered that, although her mother had complained about her clinginess, she had subtly encouraged her to be clingy: She failed to praise her daughter when she did things on her own, nor had she even noticed how capable the patient was of taking care of herself. Also, although Miss D's mother had sent her daughter off to camp to teach her independence, she had seemed unhappy about her going. She had wept at the railroad station and had embarrassed her by calling her every other day on the camp's only telephone.

Miss D inferred that her mother, while berating her for her dependency, was secretly pleased by it. She assumed that her mother had urged her to be independent to assure herself that despite her urgings, the patient was unable to separate herself from her.

Miss D also remembered that she had worried about her mother, who seemed draggy and listless. She would examine her mother carefully when she returned from school to see whether her mother was depressed, and if she was, the child would try to cheer her up. Miss D unconsciously experienced her analyst in the same way she had experienced her mother; she assumed that the analyst's telling her that she was dependent on him reflected his wish that she be dependent on him.

As the patient became aware of these ideas, she began to free herself from their hold on her. She did more things with her friends and went out more with men. Some time later, after Miss D had become considerably more capable of running her own life, she began spontaneously to realize that she had been attached to her mother not only because of separation guilt but also because she had needed her and had been fond of her. Miss D spoke with nostalgia of her mother and herself cooking and taking walks together. She also became more aware of her fondness for the analyst.

The case of Miss D illustrates an observation I have made about a number of patients: that a child may develop a pathogenic belief by inferring parental attitudes exactly opposite to those the parents tell him they have. Miss D's mother told her repeatedly that she wished her to become more independent. Yet Miss D, from her own observations of her mother, inferred that her mother wanted her to be dependent on her.

Another patient I analyzed was, in childhood, frequently punished by his mother for being messy and, in particular, for failing to keep his room neat and tidy. The patient had observed that his mother, who was often depressed, seemed to enjoy punishing him. He inferred that his mother wanted him to be messy so that she could have the pleasure of punishing him. In the analysis, the patient's provocative messiness seemed at first glance to express his defiance of his mother. However, in fact, it much more directly expressed a powerful wish to make her happy by complying with her.

THE CASE OF MRS. A

This case illustrates the importance of unconscious separation guilt and unconscious survivor guilt in the production of certain profound disturbances. The patient, a 36-year-old lawyer, allowed herself to be influenced by other people's wishes, feelings, opinions, and expectations to such an extreme degree that she feared she would lose her sense of self in any close relationship, including her relationship with the analyst. As a consequence of her tendency to take on other people's affects and ideas against her own will, Mrs. A developed intense anxiety about being possessed by the analyst. This anxiety manifested itself in a refusal, during the first few years of analysis, to experience transference feelings or to be swayed by anything that the analyst told her.

Mrs. A's extreme submissiveness stemmed from her repressed pathogenic belief that if she were independent of others or demonstrated superiority to them, she would damage or torment them. This pathogenic belief was engendered by certain traumatic childhood circumstances from which Mrs. A inferred that by becoming separate from her mother and succeeding on her own, she had caused her mother's somatic symptoms, depressions, and paranoid rages.

Mrs. A was quite disturbed about her lifelong history of extreme compliance. She felt that because she had always done what she was supposed to do, she had never been happy. As a child she had done exactly as her mother wished without even being asked. She complained to her mother about this only once: She told her mother that she would like to be asked to do things, rather than being expected to anticipate her mother's wishes.

Her parents, according to Mrs. A, enjoyed telling stories about her childhood that she found horrifying. They bragged that, at age 3, she would sit motionless through long church services, and that by an early age she had learned to keep her room in perfect order. She wondered how her parents had made her so abnormally well-behaved. Her explanation was that she had an inordinate need for approval, was terrified of criticism, and expected to be rejected if she did not submit to other people's wishes. She consciously believed that people remained involved with her only because she did what they wanted. She assumed that they had no interest in her as a separate person.

Mrs. A was unaware of the extent of her compliance with her mother, and of its origins in repressed worry about her mother and pity for her. Her worry and pity for her mother were rooted in a pathogenic belief that she had caused her mother's psychological problems and had the power to cure them.

Mrs. A's mother was, according to Mrs. A, an extremely disturbed, self-destructive, and volatile woman who was symbiotically attached to her daughter. She had chronic emphysema, that she neglected. She displayed a paranoid hypersensitivity to rejection and suffered intensely from envy, insecurity, and low self-esteem. She had no friends, occupation, or interests. She often said that she lived only for her two children—the patient and a defective younger sister—and that she expected them to live only for her. Mrs. A saw her sister as her mother's chief burden and herself as her mother's only source of pleasure and emotional support.

Since early childhood Mrs. A had been aware of her mother's need for her. She believed that her mother yearned to be close to her, to live through her, and to share her life. She felt that her mother identified with her to the extent of losing the distinction between herself and her daughter: She wanted to run her daughter's life and she wanted her daughter to run her life. Sometimes her mother asked Mrs. A directly how she should think or feel. When Mrs. A told her mother she would like to become a lawyer, her mother answered that she would like to do the same thing. Mrs. A pictured herself as having done whatever she could to rescue her mother and to make her feel loved, and important.

Throughout her childhood the patient observed her mother in states of morbid depression, frantic worry, and paranoid rage. Her mother was openly angry at her husband and bitter about her life. She frequently created embarrassing public scenes by inappropriate outbursts. She would complain about her husband and demand that her daughter take her mother's side in arguments with him. If Mrs. A tried to remain neutral, her mother would feel betrayed.

Mrs. A's efforts to fulfill her mother's ambitions for her usually ended badly for both. If the patient was unsuccessful at something, she felt guilty about disappointing her mother. But if she was successful she worried that she would make her mother envious. Her mother would make inordinate demands to be included in whatever her daughter did, until she could no longer meet the demands. Then her mother would feel rejected. She would become withdrawn or enraged and vituperative.

Mrs. A was burdened by her mother's seeming inability to tolerate exclusion. In childhood she would sometimes become quiet and withdrawn without knowing why. Her mother would frantically accuse her of withholding her thoughts and would be enraged that the patient could not explain what was troubling her. The mother would nurse a grudge for years if the patient failed to inform her of a significant event or consult her about an important decision. While at a religious retreat one summer Mrs. A accidentally became pregnant. She felt obligated to get married. After having planned the wedding, she informed her parents of the pregnancy. Her mother reprimanded her for not telling her immediately about the pregnancy, and denounced her sexual immorality. After the delivery her mother took over the care of the infant. The patient felt compelled to turn the baby over to her mother to relieve her mother's chronic depression. Unconsciously, she believed that her marriage and pregnancy had made her mother envious and assumed, therefore, that giving up the care of her baby was both a just punishment and a necessary act of restitution.

To restore her mother, Mrs. A gave up other important activities, accomplishments, and relationships as well. She was usually not aware of making sacrifices; she would simply lose interest in relationships or accomplishments that she had valued previously. For example, in high school she became part of a popular group of girls whom she greatly enjoyed. One day she invited this group to her house and had a wonderful time with them. Her mother eavesdropped on their conversation and later commented on how left out and uncomfortable her daughter had seemed with these girls. Although Mrs. A knew her mother's assessment was false, she nevertheless lost interest in these friends and aligned herself with a less-popular group. She had unconsciously interpreted her mother's remarks as expressing her mother's sense of being excluded by the patient and her friends. To undo the pain she imagined she had caused her mother she sacrificed the friendships.

Out of guilt toward her mother, Mrs. A gave up her first boyfriend at age 18. She was not aware that she had acted out of guilt; she simply assumed that in breaking up with him she had made a bad mistake for which she blamed herself. This boyfriend was the first and only man she had ever loved. Her relationship with him had made her happy and brought her out of a protracted depression. Mrs. A had felt that her mother's chronic depression was growing worse as her own happiness with her boyfriend increased. After a while her mother demanded that she break off with her boyfriend because, according to her mother, he was disloyal to her. The mother's emphysema then flared up, following which the patient lost interest in her boyfriend and terminated the relationship. Unconsciously Mrs. A believed that her mother experienced her involvement with her boyfriend as an act of disloyalty.

As a consequence of her childhood experiences, Mrs. A developed an unconscious belief that her involvements with men, her social successes, her academic accomplishments, and her feelings of pride and happiness made other people feel excluded, envious, and depressed. Even when away from her family, she could not sustain pleasure in her accomplishments. After being elected president of the college debating club, she lost interest in the position, felt fraudulent, became alienated from the group, and resigned. She could not enjoy her academic success because she assumed that her intelligence made others feel stupid. She took no pleasure in her studies and after exams could not retain what she had learned. Moreover, she believed herself uncreative and unintelligent and that she did well in school out of compliance.

As an adult, Mrs. A often felt endangered because she could not separate her feelings and thoughts from those of her mother; she could not decide whether she was acting for herself or for her mother. To protect herself from being too greatly influenced by her mother, she developed an artificial way of relating to her parents. She behaved in a cheerful and self-assured manner whenever she was around them. She never told them about serious problems or about feelings of unhappiness or happiness. She assumed that if she exposed problems or even feelings of uncertainty, her mother would deluge her with unwanted advice that she would feel compelled to follow. If she was unhappy or depressed she expected her mother to feel blamed for not being a good mother. On the other hand, if she told her mother about her happiness she expected her to feel envious and rejected or to demand inclusion in some inappropriate way.

Although Mrs. A's artificial manner with her parents protected her autonomy to some degree, it left her feeling guilty about depriving her mother of a close relationship with her. Mrs. A came to believe that her strained relationship with her parents was the result of her inability to be open with them.

At the beginning of her analysis Mrs. A dealt with her worry about her mother and the survivor guilt she felt in relation to her by denying her mother's severe problems. She blamed herself for their poor relationship, stating that her mother was a loving, supportive parent with whom she (Mrs. A) could have a good relationship if she (Mrs. A) were less guarded and defensive. As a child Mrs. A had denied her intense worry that her mother would become seriously ill. As soon as her mother would recover from an episode of illness, the patient would repress her worry and convince herself that her mother was healthy and happy. Mrs. A also used denial to control her guilt about being better off than her friends or acquaintances. She would minimize either her own strengths or other people's weaknesses to avoid feeling better off than they. Whenever she recognized someone's deficiencies, she would adopt an unrealistically hopeful attitude about his capacity to overcome them.

The patient initially described herself as markedly inferior to her women friends. She wondered why intelligent, competent, and successful women would want to maintain relationships with her. It eventually became clear that her glowing idealizations of her friends protected her from feeling better off than they. The friends she consciously admired the most turned out to be extremely disturbed, unhappy women.

Since early childhood Mrs. A had unconsciously assumed that she was better off than either her mother or her younger sister. Until she was 8 years old her parents lived with her paternal grandfather, who adored the patient while ignoring her mother and sister. Mrs. A noticed that her mother resented this special relationship and felt excluded by the grandfather. She unconsciously inferred that her mother's sensitivity to rejection stemmed from feeling unloved by Mrs. A, and that her mother's sense of inadequacy stemmed from her feeling less attractive and intelligent than she.

Mrs. A's sister was born when she was 5. She suffered from a speech defect that led the parents to assume that she was retarded and to treat her cruelly. After several years of analysis the patient began to recall the sadistic things her mother had done to her sister in an attempt to shame her out of her symptoms. Mrs. A believed that if she had not been bright, well behaved, and attractive her sister would not have seemed defective to her parents and would not have been mistreated by them. She developed a protective relationship with her sister. To alleviate her guilt about being better off than her sister, she began to envy the special attention her sister received because of her disability. She was the only person who had faith that someday her sister would be normal. The gradual amelioration of her sister's speech problem reinforced Mrs. A's existing magical idea that she could cure damaged people by having blind faith in them.

When Mrs. A was 10 years old her parents, as a consequence of her father's unsuccessful career as a library consultant, began a series of moves. These moves were an early indication of her father's deterioration. He developed a serious drinking problem, could not support the family, and began to have numerous affairs. Mrs. A saw him as an irresponsible, vulnerable man who could not protect himself or his children from his wife's sadistic assaults. Nor, in Mrs. A's eyes, could her father help his wife with her increasingly severe psychological problems. Whenever he was away from home, as he usually was, he left his wife in his older daughter's care.

Mrs. A had felt sorry for her father because he received so much verbal abuse from her mother. She felt that her mother did not appreciate her husband and that she rejected his love. Mrs. A maintained a fairly distant relationship with her father in childhood partly because she assumed that her mother could not tolerate the idea of her loving him and partly because she herself found him weak and unreliable. As an adolescent she acquired an additional motive for keeping her distance from her father: He began to behave seductively toward her. After a few drinks he would become physically affectionate, and tell her that he was in love with her. Also, he was possessive; he was competitive with her boyfriends and like her mother seemed to feel rejected by her involvements with men.

The patient unconsciously believed that her father desperately needed to feel intellectually superior to everyone, including his wife and children. Her father, the patient reported, had contempt for his wife, and for other women as well. He seized every opportunity to demonstrate how intelligent he was. The patient complied with her father's need to show off by letting him do her homework for her, by considering him the most intelligent man she knew, and by belittling her own intelligence. However, she unconsciously felt contempt toward her father for his need to belittle women, and she felt guilty for her contempt. She felt guilty, too, that she had made her father feel rejected first by having boyfriends and then by getting married.

Mrs. A was the only member of her family who was able to adjust success-fully to the frequent moves of her childhood. She made friends easily, was well liked by her teachers, and was academically successful. She enjoyed school and had good times with her friends. Her mother, by contrast, was unable to make friends and relied on her daughter to meet her needs. She considered her reward-ing life outside the home as an expression of disloyalty to the family. Her mother told her that she was uncaring and selfish for going off with her friends while the rest of the family suffered.

Mrs. A's sister was quite seriously upset by the repeated family moves. She was frequently in trouble in school and at home.

Mrs. A sought analysis upon the advice of a colleague in her law firm. She was well liked there and was considered one of the most competent members of the staff. She had confessed to the colleague that she experienced an irresistable sexual attraction to a sociopathic financial adviser who was trying to seduce her. She felt herself losing her ability to resist this man's advances.

Mrs. A's stated goal in seeking analysis was to develop the capacity to have a good love relationship with a man. She had recently been divorced after spending 8 years in a joyless and largely asexual marriage. In the end, her husband in-formed her that he did not love her and that he had been having affairs for a number of years. She blamed herself for the failure of the marriage and assumed there was something wrong with her sexually. She doubted her capacity to enjoy sex or to love a man, and she did not believe that a man could love her.

During the first few interviews with her analyst, Mrs. A carried out a major test pertaining to her problems with separation guilt and survivor guilt: She attempted to convince the analyst that she was undeserving of psychoanalysis and unsuitable for it, stating that she lacked the motivation for analysis and that she

was too distrustful to free associate. In the second interview she reported that she
had become sexually involved with the financial adviser who had been pursuing
her. She stated that he had come to her house and that she did not want to turn
him away. She also reported quitting her job and taking up residence with this
man against everyone's advice. She was, she stated, sure that the analyst would be
critical of her for forming a relationshp with this man and that he would never
understand its positive meaning to her. She claimed to love him and to believe
that by her relationship with him she would cure him of his problems, which
included drug abuse, violence, and paranoid rages.

A few sessions later Mrs. A announced that she had decided not to pursue
treatment then. She believed she did not have any problems. She had neither
motivation for analysis nor faith in the analytic process. The analyst inferred that
the patient was unconsciously testing him to assure herself that she would not
hurt him if she rejected him. When he responded by telling her that she should
continue in analysis, Mrs. A was quite relieved, and she quickly decided that she
would like to continue after all.

Once she began treatment, Mrs. A became worried that the treatment would
become of overriding importance to her. She consciously feared that she would
come to depend on the analyst to meet all of her needs, and that after she had
become dependent on him he would reject her. He would, she assumed, discover
that she was too empty, needy, and guarded to free-associate in a meaningful way.
During the opening phase of her treatment, Mrs. A felt weak in relation to the
analyst, whom she experienced as powerful. Unconsciously she expected the
analyst to punish her for having abandoned her mother. She assumed that he
would reject her for being inadequate and dependent, just as she had rejected her
mother for being inadequate and dependent. Mrs. A was even more afraid unconsciously that she would let the analyst dominate her as she had let her mother
dominate her. She was afraid that she would become the analyst's puppet, lose her
sense of self, and feel compelled to accept and act on his interpretations.

Before Mrs. A could permit herself to be influenced by the analyst, she had to
acquire confidence in her capacity to resist being influenced by him. She worked
unconsciously to achieve this goal by repeatedly testing the analyst to disconfirm
her pathogenic belief that she would hurt him if she remained psychologically
separate from him. Thus, she tested the analyst by conspicuously resisting the
analytic process. For example, she would be silent, then provocatively announce
that there were things on her mind that she would never talk about in analysis.
She typically told the analyst about important decisions only after she had acted
upon them. She refused to talk to him about a problem while uncertain about
how to resolve it, because she feared she would be unduly influenced by him.

Her most positive response to an interpretation was to state that it sounded
right but did not carry conviction. She was suspicious about transference interpretations. She took them as attempts on the analyst's part to intrude into her
emotional life. Furthermore, she maintained that she had no feelings about the

analyst, and she experienced resistance interpretations as attempts to manipulate her into disclosing her secrets.

Mrs. A was reluctant to discuss her relationship with her new boyfriend. She continued to believe that her love for him would magically transform him. Their relationship was stormy from the outset. He repeatedly left her only to return after getting into some kind of trouble. Mrs. A assumed responsibility for his well-being. She was unable to reject him despite the fact that he was not only untrustworthy but also violent and menacing. Mrs. A felt guilty about her sexual involvement with him and ashamed of her masochistic behavior toward him. The analyst's attempts to confront her with the self-destructive nature of the relationship were met with impenetrable resistance. She insisted that the analyst could not be objective about her boyfriend because he did not consider him an ideal mate.

The analyst's primary response to the patient's refusal either to free-associate or to express transferences was to remain unprovoked. He attempted systematically to analyze the patient's fear that by maintaining her distance from him she would upset him. Mrs. A responded to this approach by becoming increasingly aware of her belief that the analyst wished her to confide in him, consider him important, be his ideal patient, and, indeed, fall in love with him. As the patient made progress in disconfirming her unconscious belief in her power to hurt the analyst, she gained confidence in her ability to resist being influenced by him against her will. Her confidence that she could oppose the analyst enabled her to safely begin discussing certain distressing preoccupations and to start letting herself be influenced by his interpretations.

By the end of the second year of analysis the patient's conscious experience of the analyst had markedly changed. Rather than being concerned with the analyst's power to hurt her, Mrs. A now worried about her power to hurt him. Mrs. A had developed a strong mother transference to the analyst, in which she unconsciously feared that he was symbiotically attached to her. She feared that if she were forcefully to express her own opinions about his interpretations, the analyst would feel compelled to agree with her. Now the patient felt reassured rather than threatened by the analyst's capacity to confront her resistances and to insist on the validity of his interpretations. She had acquired considerable confidence in her ability independently to assess the correctness of the analyst's interpretations and to reject those she considered false. She also felt she could now safely let herself experience positive transference feelings. She knew she could protect herself from the analyst if he tried to exploit these feelings.

During the third year of analysis Mrs. A announced her intention to marry her boyfriend, who was by this time bankrupt and in the throes of a severe drug addiction. She warned the analyst not to try to stop her, but he confronted her forcefully with the self-destructive nature of her relationship with her boyfriend. He told her that her hopes for a happy life with him were unrealistic, and indeed that she could maintain these hopes only by denying the serious nature of his problems. The analyst told her, too, that she was prepared to sacrifice her happiness in an attempt to rescue her boyfriend, that she had assumed responsibility for his happiness, and that she believed that by her love she could make him happy.

Mrs. A's reaction to this confrontation was dramatic: she experienced great relief, and she undertook a serious analysis of the survivor guilt and separation guilt that she had suffered in relation to her boyfriend. She became able then permanently to extricate herself from her relationship with him and to resist his repeated attempts to manipulate her into taking him back. She began to date other men. However, she also began to contemplate doing certain self-destructive things. For example, she considered giving up a rewarding job that she liked in exchange for one she would have disliked. In each instance Mrs. A would respond with relief when the analyst confronted her with the self-punitive meaning of the action she was contemplating. She also used the analyst's interpretations to acquire further insight into her unconscious guilt and need for punishment.

By the end of the third year of treatment Mrs. A was deeply involved in her analysis. She thought of the analyst as important in her life and she hoped for a favorable outcome to her treatment. She also permitted herself to form strong convictions about the correctness or incorrectness of the analyst's interpretations. She developed a wide range of transference feelings and spoke more freely than ever about certain sources, in childhood, of ambivalence, confusion, shame, anxiety, and despair.

During the next 3 years of analysis Mrs. A overcame her sexual inhibitions, worked out a good relationship with her son, achieved considerable professional success, and developed a satisfactory relationship with a man whom she eventually married.

In this chapter I have attempted to show how prominent a part unconscious guilt plays in neuroses and in all aspects of life. Unconscious guilt and unconscious moral ideas are universal. The child develops them in relation to his parents. He develops his particular unconscious morality from his experiences with his parents and from their teachings. If a child infers and so comes to believe that his attempts to gratify certain crucially important impulses or to reach certain vital developmental goals will threaten his all-important ties to his parents, he may decide to repress or inhibit these impulses or goals. Thus he may seriously damage himself in order to maintain his ties to his parents. He may also develop symptoms that are intended to maintain these ties. The child's wish to maintain his ties to his parents is his most powerful motivation. Much of the adult's psychopathology expresses the wish to maintain such ties.

4

UNCONSCIOUS PATHOGENIC BELIEFS

JOSEPH WEISS

According to the main thrust of Freud's early theory, the unconscious mind contains no beliefs of any kind, including pathogenic beliefs. However, according to the part of Freud's ego psychology that is based on the higher mental functioning hypothesis, and to the views expressed here, the unconscious mind does contain pathogenic beliefs. Pathogenic beliefs are an important part of the unconscious mind, for they play a crucial part in the development and maintenance of all psychopathology. Pathogenic beliefs and the fear, anxiety, shame, and guilt to which they give rise provide the primary motives for the development and maintenance of repressions, inhibitions, and symptoms. Pathogenic beliefs weaken a person's control over certain kinds of behavior. A person may be prevented unconsciously by his pathogenic beliefs from doing certain things that he consciously wants to do, or he may be induced unconsciously to do certain things that consciously he does not want to do. For example, a person who suffers unconsciously from the belief that castration may be used as a punishment for sex may be prevented by this belief from having sexual relations. Or a person whose unconscious pathogenic beliefs give rise to severe survivor guilt may be induced to lead a life of privation despite contrary conscious wishes.

While Freud's theory of superego development suggests that a person may develop a wide variety of pathogenic beliefs, Freud focused mainly on one such belief: the boy's belief that if he pursues his mother sexually he will be punished by castration. However, Freud did refer occasionally to other pathogenic beliefs. He assumed, for example, that the female neurotic's psychopathology is based largely on the pathogenic belief, acquired in childhood, that if she pursues her father sexually she will lose her mother's love. Freud also wrote about the pathogenic belief, which he ascribed to the person's superego, that a person must remain ill because he deserves no better (1940a, p. 180).

As pointed out in Chapter 3, a child may develop a wide variety of pathogenic beliefs other than those described explicitly by Freud. He may, for example, develop the belief underlying separation guilt that if he becomes stronger or more independent he will hurt a parent. Or he may develop the belief underlying survivor guilt that if he acquires some of the good things of life he will betray a parent or a sibling who has not acquired such things. A person, as a consequence of his experiences, may come to believe that almost any impulse, attitude, goal, or affective state is bad or risky, and will, if pursued, endanger him by threatening his ties to his parents.

A pathogenic belief is simple and compelling: It tells the person who adheres to it that if he attempts to gratify a certain impulse or to reach a certain goal or to maintain a certain attitude he will endanger himself. Pathogenic beliefs generally are developed in childhood. However, they may be elaborated in adolescence. Moreover, as Niederland's study (1981) of Holocaust survivors demonstrated, a person in dire circumstances may develop a new pathogenic belief even in adulthood. The pathogenic beliefs developed in childhood are concerned with the major motives of childhood, such as the child's dependency on his parents, his libidinal attachments to his parents, his wish for independence from them, and his wish to compete with them. Pathogenic beliefs tell the person who adheres to them that, by acting on certain major motives, he will disrupt his relations with a parent and so become frightened, guilty, ashamed, worried, and so on. A child must come to fear any motive or behavior that he infers would seriously hurt a parent, provoke severe punishment from a parent, or seriously threaten him with the loss of the parent's love (Freud, 1930, p. 124).

THE PERSISTENCE OF PATHOGENIC BELIEFS

A pathogenic belief, once established, may be difficult to disconfirm. Since it is repressed, the child (and the adult he becomes) cannot consciously work at disconfirming it. He may have no conscious motive for doing so. For example, a child who unconsciously believes that if he becomes more independent of his parents he will damage them may consciously enjoy his dependence on them. He may not be aware that unconsciously he would like to become more independent of them.

A child may have difficulty working unconsciously to disconfirm a pathogenic belief that predicts great danger, for he may unconsciously assume that even testing it is dangerous. Consider, for example, a child who unconsciously believes that if he makes even a slight attempt to become more independent of a parent he will damage the parent. Such a child may be so impaled by this belief that he may delay testing it for many years, until, as a consequence of new experiences, he begins to doubt the belief.

Finally, the child who filters his experiences through the lens of a particular pathogenic belief, like the scientist who perceives his world in terms of a particular theory, may not readily be able to make observations that run counter to the belief, and he may for that reason have trouble disconfirming it. Consider, for example, Miss D, the patient presented in Chapter 3 who unconsciously believed that her mother wanted to possess her. She experienced even her mother's attempts to encourage her independence as evidence of her possessiveness. Miss D assumed that her mother, by encouraging her independence, was attempting to assure herself that her daughter, despite such encouragement, would be unable to grow away from her.

For all these reasons, a particular pathogenic belief may be retained well into adulthood and perhaps for a lifetime. However, certain pathogenic beliefs of childhood are readily disconfirmed by fresh experiences, and so quickly relinquished. The development and rapid disconfirmation of such beliefs are part of the normal growing pains of childhood.

Although pathogenic beliefs are false and maladaptive, they are produced by the child as part of the child's efforts at adaptation. They are attempts by the child (or, in the language of the structural model, of his ego) to understand the dangers of the world, and by understanding them, to avoid them. The id, or the primary process, as Freud described it, cannot produce a pathogenic belief. This is because the id is regulated by the pleasure principle and thus effortlessly (automatically) avoids all painful experiences. It certainly does not form beliefs to explain them.

PATHOGENIC BELIEFS AND PEREMPTORY BEHAVIOR

Pathogenic beliefs and the feelings of fear, anxiety, or guilt that stem from them may limit a person's control over his unconscious mental life. Though neither impulses nor defenses, these beliefs are powerful sources of motivation and may induce the person to behave in certain ways against his conscious will. For example, they may induce the person who is guided by them to carry out peremptory or compulsive behavior. When such behavior becomes persistent and habitual (i.e., when it becomes part of a symptom), it is invariably supported by a pathogenic belief.

An example well known to analysts concerns a person who unconsciously believes that masturbating injures his penis. This person may masturbate, fear that he has injured his penis, and then masturbate again in order to assure himself that he has not injured it. His attempts to reassure himself by masturbation may arouse fresh fears that he has injured his penis, and so induce him still another time, by masturbating, to reassure himself again. He may find some gratification in his masturbation. However, he masturbates compulsively, not to attain gratification, but to reassure himself that he is intact.

Another example concerns a man who overeats compulsively. He overeats not simply to gratify himself but to reassure himself against an anxiety or feeling of guilt that stems from a pathogenic belief. He may, for example, overeat to reassure himself that he will not starve or be deprived of food, or to become unattractive to women and thereby avoid the risk of castration.

THE TWO SEQUENCES BY WHICH A CHILD
MAY DEVELOP A PATHOGENIC BELIEF

A child may develop a pathogenic belief from two different sequences of events. In one sequence, the child first attempts to gratify a certain important impulse or to reach a certain important goal and then discovers that by such attempts he threatens his all-important ties to his parents. The child then develops a pathogenic belief that causally connects his attempts to gratify the impulse or to reach the goal with the threat to the parental ties. As a consequence of the pathogenic belief, the child represses the impulse or the goal in order to retain the parental ties. He fears that if he does not repress these motivations he will act upon them and so endanger himself.

The second sequence begins with the child's experiencing an inherently traumatic event, such as the illness or death of a parent. The child then retrospectively blames himself for the event. He concludes that he brought it about by attempting to gratify a particular impulse or to attain a particular developmental goal. For example, a boy may conclude after his father's death that he caused the death by his hostility to his father or his competitiveness with him. The boy may come to believe that by being hostile or competitive he may bring on another catastrophe analogous to the death of his father. Such a belief may become compelling and persistent, not because of its plausibility but because of the extremely dire consequences the belief foretells. The boy may become afraid to test the belief. In addition, he may be induced by the belief to repress his competitiveness or hostility, for fear that if he does not repress it he will act upon it and so produce a catastrophe.

THE FIRST SEQUENCE AND THE PART PLAYED IN IT BY EXPERIENCE

The sequence in which a child comes to believe that his attempts to gratify an impulse or reach a goal may put him in a situation of danger is exemplified by the boy's acquisition of the belief in castration as a punishment for sexuality. The boy first attempts to gratify his sexuality with his mother, then infers that by doing so he risks castration by his father. The experiences from which the boy infers such a belief, as Freud pointed out, may be distorted. The boy, for example, may greatly overestimate his threat to his father, or he may experience his father as much more punitive than he really is.

However, the boy's tendency to infer a belief in castration may, according to Freud, be powerfully abetted by experiences (such as parental threats of castration or the sight of the female genitalia) that make the belief in castration highly credible (1940a, pp. 189–190). Thus, the intensity of a boy's castration anxiety is not, according to Freud, a simple function of the strength of the boy's Oedipal impulses. It depends on a number of factors, including the reactions of the boy's parents to him. A boy who, like Little Hans, is convincingly threatened with castration, is more likely, all else being equal, to develop greater castration anxiety than a boy whose parents are not threatening.

Similarly, the intensity of the belief underlying a child's guilt about separation from his mother depends not only on the strength of his wish to become more independent of her but on her behavior as well. As Asch has reported, a boy whose mother is possessive and who demands that the boy be devoted to her is (all else being equal) more likely to become convinced of his responsibility for his mother than is a boy whose mother is more matter-of-fact about his attempts to grow away from her. Indeed, a child may develop an exaggerated sense of responsibility for his mother simply because she tells him that he is responsible for her (Asch, 1976, p. 392).

A child's development of the belief underlying survivor guilt (namely, that he has betrayed his parents and siblings by receiving more of the good things of life than they [Modell, 1971]) depends on several factors. A child who is especially acquisitive and greedy and who, motivated by his greed, takes things from his parents and siblings may be more prone to develop this belief than a child who is generous. However, a child who is not especially greedy may develop this belief if fate treats him much better than it treats his parents and siblings.

My formulation about the several factors in the development of pathogenic beliefs is compatible with Freud's formulation about the two factors in the formation of neuroses, namely, the strength of instinct and the strength of trauma (1937, p. 220).

THE SECOND SEQUENCE AND THE PART PLAYED IN IT BY EXPERIENCE

In this sequence the child is first severely traumatized by an experience that is inherently traumatic, such as separation from a parent, parental divorce, or the death or illness of a parent. He then retrospectively assumes that by pursuing some crucial goal or by attempting to satisfy some important impulse (or by maintaining a certain attitude or affective state), he provoked the trauma.

The great part played by such retrospective inference in the lives of many children points to the child's tendency, which stems from the egocentricity of childhood, to take responsibility for whatever happens to him. The child assumes that what his parents or fate mete out to him is what he deserves (Freud, 1930). The child's tendency to comply with the judgments of his parents or of fate makes possible the development of a superego. If the child did not unconsciously assume (although he may consciously not acknowledge it) that what his parents or fate offer him is what he deserves, he would not develop a superego that, as Freud stated, "threatens it [the ego] with punishments exactly like the parents whose place it has taken" (1940a, p. 205). The child learns his morality from his particular experiences with his parents and from the particular way that fate treats him. He has no prior moral principles by which he may judge the merits of the rewards or punishments offered him. Whether or not he has (as Freud sometimes assumed) inherited certain unconscious ideas, he develops his own special morality and indeed his own special pathogenic beliefs from the impact on him (with his various motives) of his particular experiences.

A person's belief that he deserved the childhood traumas he incurred may induce him to repeat these traumas, in various ways, throughout his life. He repeats them because he believes he deserves to experience them. (He may also, as I shall discuss later, repeat them to master them.) A person may repeat his infantile traumas in unexpected ways. For example, a patient who, at age 4, was confined to bed for 6 months for an orthopedic disease, developed the belief that he had better not be too active. Even in his adult life he would punish himself, after being active and successful, by doing nothing for a period of time. Another patient, whose mother died when she was 13, rejected a daughter whom she adored, because she had acquired from her mother's death the pathogenic belief that she did not deserve to enjoy a good mother–daughter relationship.

The idea that the child believes himself responsible for what happens to him is supported by an empirical study, conducted by David Beres, of the effects on children of separation from their parents. Beres, as advisor to a Jewish child placement agency, accumulated a great deal of data about the effects on children of placement away from parents. In his article "Certain Aspects of Superego Functioning" (1958), Beres observed that the child who is separated from his parents invariably assumes that his parents left him as a punishment for something bad he had done. Beres (1958) wrote:

My observations indicate the extraordinary readiness of the child to *interpret* the experience of separation as an expression of hostility on the part of his parents and to assume that the act was justified by the child's wrongdoing. The child identifies with the hostile, rejecting parent, an example of identification with the aggressor, accepts the fantasy of a crime that deserves punishment, and assumes the guilt which such an act requires. (p. 348, italics mine to indicate the importance of inference and hence belief in the development of psychopathology)

As Beres's discussion makes clear, a child who is separated from his parents comes to believe that he committed a crime, and he assumes the guilt that goes with the crime. The guilt is unearned. Its intensity may depend on a number of factors, including the intensity of the child's hostility toward his parents and the degree of trauma the child experiences by the separation.

A child's belief about how (i.e., by what crime) he induced a parent to leave him depends upon many factors. It depends on the main impulses the child was attempting to satisfy in relation to the parent and the main goals he was trying to attain with him before the parent left him. (A child does not blame himself for weak or trivial motivations.) It depends, too, on the parent's prior attitudes toward the child's main impulses and goals. A child whose mother, before leaving him, complained that his demands on her drained her of her strength, might assume that his mother left him because he had been too demanding. Or, a child whose mother, before leaving him, often appeared upset about his attempts to become more independent of her might experience her leaving him as a punishment for his having attempted to become more independent.

A child who is left by a parent when everything seems to be going well may develop the belief that it is dangerous to assume that all is well. He may come to believe that were he to feel complacent, he would be punished by some event which would show that his complacency was ill-founded.

THE RELATIONSHIP OF GUILT TO HOSTILITY

According to a familiar formulation based on the automatic functioning hypothesis, a child is traumatized by the death of a parent if, before the parent's death, the child had been hostile to the parent and wished to get rid of the parent. (The child, according to this formulation, is traumatized by the parent's death because he automatically [without thought] assumes that the wish magically caused the death.)

According to the views expressed here, a child is severely traumatized by the death of a parent whether or not he had unconsciously been especially hostile to the parent beforehand. For a child the death of a parent is inherently traumatic. The child desperately needs his parents to protect him from a variety of dangers. The child's well-being, and even his survival, may depend on his parents remaining alive and healthy.

A child's having been hostile to a parent may or may not play a part in his developing constricting pathogenic beliefs after the death of the parent. If the child had been especially hostile to the parent before the parent's death, and if the parent had appeared especially vulnerable to the child's hostility, the child might have inferred, and so come to believe, that he had, by his hostility, caused the death of the parent. (The relationship between the child's hostility and his feeling responsible for the parent's death in this case would be mediated, not automatically, but by a theory or belief, inferred from experience.) However, as discussed above, after the death of a parent, a child might retrospectively infer that he had, by various motives other than hostility (e.g., dependence or stubbornness), caused the parent's death.

Niederland's observations about the survivors of the Holocaust (1981) make clear that the intensity of a survivor's hostility to his parents and siblings before they were killed was not the crucial factor in the intensity of the guilt (and the belief underlying it) that the survivor developed. The survivors whom Niederland studied had not been especially hostile to their parents and siblings before they were killed. Probably as a goup they had a normal range of hostility. However, they were all severely traumatized by the deaths of their parents and siblings. Niederland assumed that a survivor's guilt did not depend on his prior hostility to his parents and siblings, but rather on his subsequent belief that he had been disloyal to them. The survivor believed himself disloyal for remaining alive after his parents and siblings had been killed. He believed that, by remaining alive, he had betrayed his loved ones. The survivor's guilt, as Niederland conceptualized it, was more an expression of love than of hostility. Niederland (1981) wrote:

The guilt feelings and guilt anxieties and unresolved grief situations, psychoanalytically speaking, are usually considered as being based on early hostility and death wishes with regard to the family members wiped out in the course of the Holocaust. In the patients under scrutiny (during the past 35 years I observed and studied close to 2,000 survivors of the Holocaust), I cannot accept this explanation. It is true that masochistic tendencies are operative in many of them. But in the great majority it is the survival itself which stands at the core of the survivor's conflict. . . . On the basis of my longstanding research, I have reason to believe that the survival is unconsciously felt as a betrayal of the dead parents, and being alive constitutes an ongoing conflict as well as a source of constant feelings of guilt and anxiety. (p. 419)

As Niederland pointed out, the survivors, by their symptoms, expressed their loyalty to their dead parents and siblings. They often behaved as dead. They were silent, moved slowly, were pallid, and felt dead. By behaving in these ways, the survivor was saying to his dead parents and siblings, "I am like you and I am with you."

CASES ILLUSTRATING THE DEVELOPMENT FROM "SHOCK TRAUMA" OF PATHOGENIC BELIEFS AND PSYCHOPATHOLOGY

In each of the cases presented below, a patient in childhood suffered, in Kris's terms, a severe and sudden "shock trauma" (as opposed to a "strain trauma," which develops gradually as a consequence of a pathogenic relationship to a parent). In each of the cases, the patient, after a shocking event, retrospectively inferred that he had caused it. In addition, each patient retrospectively experienced the traumatic event as a punishment for certain pretraumatic motivations. He had, even before the trauma, disapproved to some degree of these motivations. However, after the trauma he became much more severe in his condemnation of them.

THE CASE OF MR. L

The patient, Mr. L, was traumatized at age 5 when his father became seriously injured in a freak skiing accident. The patient was the only grandchild on both sides of an intact family that had been relatively happy before the accident. Mr. L was fond of both parents, but especially of his father. During the 6-month period preceding the accident, the patient had begun to develop a close relationship with his father. He had begun to fish and sail with him in the summer and to ski with him in the winter. He had experienced his new relationship with his father as helping him to get away from his somewhat dour, possessive mother, who would often complain about being rejected by her son.

Mr. L remembered being shocked at the news of his father's accident. However, the long-term effects of the accident on the entire family were just as traumatic to him as was the initial shock. It was several years before the father could move about, and since he could not work, the mother was forced to take a job as a manager at a nearby ski resort. She felt burdened by her responsibility. She often became tired and irritable, and she complained to her son about her worries.

The accident, which deprived Mr. L and his family of much of their earlier happiness, was retrospectively experienced by the patient as punishment for his having been happy. The patient came to believe that he was not supposed to be happy, relaxed, or self-satisfied. He assumed unconsciously that were he to feel good, he would bring disaster to himself and others. He therefore used a number of techniques to keep himself miserable. For example, he always kept some important task unfinished so that he could feel tied down and tortured with worry about it. He was reluctant to become relaxed, for various reasons. Besides fearing that by relaxing he would precipitate a catastrophe, he feared that if he relaxed he would be unprepared for a catastrophe and hence unable to deal with it. During analysis, Mr. L, after a relaxing day, would dream of disaster. His associations to such a dream would lead him back to the early trauma. He was, as his dreams showed, afraid of being complacent again, as he had been at the time of the trauma (see Freud, 1920, p. 32).

After his father's accident, the child became especially guilty about having attempted to become more independent of his mother. Since the accident deprived him of the opportunity of becoming more independent of her, he assumed retrospectively that he had been wrong to have wanted to become more independent, and he more or less relinquished his attempts to do so. Throughout his school years he stayed close to home. In college, which was nearby, he did not participate much in social life although he was friendly and gregarious. Rather, he came home almost every weekend to be with his family.

In analysis, Mr. L was reluctant at first to feel comfortable with the analyst, for fear that were he to feel comfortable with him some catastrophe would befall the analyst. Later, however, Mr. L became able to maintain a good relationship with the analyst. He attempted then to use the analyst as he had attempted to use his father, that is, as someone to help him to escape both from his mother (who still wanted him to come home) and from being dominated by girlfriends, to whom he tended to become overly obligated.

While Mr. L was struggling, with the analyst's help, to become more independent of women, he continued at times to become afraid that the analyst would suddenly become sick or die. Later, after the patient began to develop a good relationship with a woman, he formed a mother transference. He feared that the analyst would criticize his girlfriends as his mother had criticized the girls he brought home, and that the analyst would want to possess him as (in his opinion) his mother had wanted to possess him.

Later still, Mr. L permitted himself to experience his Oedipal rivalry with the analyst. He had warded off his rivalry with the analyst (as in childhood he had warded off his rivalry with his father) as long as he had needed the analyst as an ally in his struggle to feel independent with women. After he had attained this goal and in addition had developed a good relationship with a woman, he could safely compete with the analyst.

This patient's becoming aware of his Oedipal rivalry during the final phases of his treatment permitted the analyst to explore with him the question of whether, earlier in the treatment, his unconscious rivalry with the analyst had contributed to his becoming worried about the analyst's health. It seemed from this exploration that such was not the case. The patient's experiencing his rivalry with the analyst and remembering his rivalry with his father did not revive his worry about either the analyst's or his father's health. As the patient himself pointed out, he was not, at the time of his father's accident, either feeling or expressing rivalry regarding his father. The patient's main wish at that time had been to enlist his father as an ally in his struggle to get away from his mother. At the time of the accident the patient admired, loved, and needed his father. If he felt hostility or guilt to a parent it was to his mother, who was depressed and who would complain whenever he and his father went off without her. The accident, as the patient experienced it, was a punishment not for his competing with his father but for his using his father as an ally in his struggle to escape from his mother. As the patient experienced it, the punishment fit the crime, for it put him once more under the domination of his mother.

It is interesting that Mr. L's belief that by being complacent or independent he would bring on a catastrophe was so hard to disconfirm. The persistence of this belief may be explained in part by the severity of the trauma which gave rise to it. The patient was slow to test and hence slow to overcome his belief, not because the belief was so convincing but because the consequences it foretold were so dire. Even a person who assumed there was only a slight chance that such a belief represented reality would, because of the dire consequences it foretold, be reluctant to test it.

THE CASE OF MR. S

My next case report concerns a patient who was traumatized by a temporary separation at an early age.

Mr. S, at 2½ years of age was, without warning, sent away for 3 months to stay with his uncle and aunt. He was sent away because his younger brother had developed measles, and the family was afraid that Mr. S would catch the disease. Mr. S, however, did not know why he was being sent away. His father drove him to his uncle's home about 100 miles away and left him there, giving him little explanation. The father, to avoid witnessing his son's distress, left abruptly after a brief goodbye and without offering him an explanation for leaving him.

Mr. S, as we were able to discover in his analysis, was not completely toilet trained when he was sent away. He had, in addition, been provoking his parents by his mischievous, rowdy behavior. He had, therefore, assumed that he was sent away as a punishment for these shortcomings. At his uncle and aunt's, Mr. S soon became toilet trained and, in addition, extremely compliant, neat, and deliberate. He stopped being rowdy and became a model boy. On returning home, he was less playful and outgoing than before and remained so for many years.

Mr. S, who was unmarried, entered analysis in his early 30s. In treatment, he re-enacted some of the elements of his childhood situation. Though he was a model of good behavior early in his treatment, he eventually became rowdy and mischievous. He began to have numerous affairs and to drink and be boisterous at parties. He feared that the analyst would punish him for this behavior by rejecting him.

It was only after Mr. S's fear of provoking the analyst into rejecting him for his rowdiness was analyzed that he began to remember more clearly the childhood situation described earlier, and eventually to confirm his memories by asking his parents about his behavior before, during, and after the separation from them.

Many factors other than those discussed here played a part in the patient's childhood traumas. Among them was his jealousy of his brother, who was allowed to stay home while the patient was sent away, and his anger toward his mother for attempting to toilet train him and to curb his energy. Nonetheless, the central element in his neurosis was the unconscious belief that unless he were good (compliant), he would be punished by rejection.

PATHOGENIC BELIEFS AND PSYCHOPATHOLOGY

As I stated earlier, most, or perhaps all, psychopathology is rooted in pathogenic beliefs. Pathogenic beliefs may induce peremptory or compulsive behavior, such as compulsive masturbation or compulsive eating.

It is in obedience to pathogenic beliefs that a child institutes and maintains his repressions, and thus lays the foundation for future neurotic conflicts. Moreover, a person's neurotic symptoms and inhibitions may express his attempts to avoid the dangers foretold by his pathogenic beliefs. This is demonstrated by the observation that a neurotic person who is prevented forcefully from expressing his symptoms or abiding by his inhibitions may experience himself in great danger and become intensely anxious (Freud, 1926a, p. 144).

In general, the neurotic, in his symptoms and inhibitions, attempts to avoid certain dangers similar to those he first experienced in childhood. These dangers in childhood are connected with his loosening or breaking his ties to his real parents, and in adulthood with his loosening or breaking his ties to his internalized parents. The neurotic attempts to avoid such dangers, either by unconsciously complying with his parents or by unconsciously identifying with them. He carries out certain maladaptive behaviors, such as he unconsciously believed his parents wanted him to carry out, or such as, in his unconscious judgment, they themselves carried out.

Freud pointed out that a particular perversion, namely, fetishism, stems from the pathogenic belief in castration as a punishment for sexuality. The fetishist does not, as does the neurotic, remove himself from the danger of castration. Instead, he denies the danger. He unconsciously perceives the fetish as the woman's penis and so through it reassures himself against the frightening idea that women once possessed penises but lost them by castration. The fetishist, in Freud's words, "holds to the *conviction* that the female genitals contain a penis" (1940a, p. 203, italics mine in order to emphasize the implication of unconscious cognition). By holding to this conviction, he reassures himself that castration is not used as a punishment for sexuality. As he reassures himself against this danger, he permits himself to become sexually excited. Though he appears to be excited by the fetish, he does not love it per se but is simply made to feel safe enough by it to experience sexual feelings that ordinarily would arouse castration anxiety.

Freud's explanation for the fetishist's preoccupation with his fetish may be extended to explain other perverse fantasies and behaviors as well, such as, for example, some masochists' obsessive preoccupation with beating fantasies. The masochist, like the fetishist, is, as a consequence of his unconscious pathogenic beliefs, afraid to experience sexual excitement. The male masochist suffers unconsciously from the pathogenic belief that he is dangerous to women and that by having sexual relations with a woman he would hurt her. He is, however, reassured against this belief by the fantasy that the woman is beating him. He unconsciously subscribes to the magical idea that if he is a victim he is not an offender. As he succeeds by this fantasy in overcoming his fear of hurting women, he permits himself to become sexually excited. The masochist is not directly gratified by being beaten; instead, he is reassured by it against an unconscious anxiety about hurting women. However, he makes such a close connection between the idea of being beaten and the pleasurable sexual excitement that he may consciously experience the beating itself as directly gratifying.

THE CASE OF MR. R

As illustrated in the following case, the patient with bondage fantasies may suffer from the unconscious belief that he is too strong for women, whom he perceives as weak and vulnerable.

Mr. R, a French businessman I analyzed years ago, unconsciously had contempt for his mother, whom, as long as he could remember, he had perceived as unable to control him. He perceived her as fragile and possessive, envious of him, and threatened by his strength and vigor. She was, in his opinion, easily upset. When the patient was very young, he would, as he remembered it, make his mother feel helpless just by running restlessly around their small apartment. Mr. R remembers having been sexually aroused at the age of 3½ when his aunt, his mother's more buoyant younger sister, playfully held him down. Later, he became sexually excited when a friendly woman at Sunday school prepared him for a part in a Bible pageant by darkening his eyebrows with eyebrow pencil. In both episodes, Mr. R felt consciously humiliated by being made to submit to a woman. However, in both episodes, Mr. R felt relieved unconsciously by a woman's domination. He was guided unconsciously in his feelings and behavior by the magical idea that if he was a victim, he was not an offender. Since early childhood he had felt in danger of humiliating his mother and other women, and so could feel strong and sexual with a woman only when she demonstrated a capacity to dominate him.

In adolescence, Mr. R's main masturbation fantasy was of being tied down by a woman. When picturing himself restrained by a woman, he was reassured by the awareness that he could not hurt or humiliate her, and this reassurance enabled him to feel strong and sexually excited.

In his adult life certain of Mr. R's symptoms were connected with his bondage fantasies. After a period of vigor and success in his business he would feel an overwhelming, unnatural sense of fatigue, which, as he came to realize, was intended to placate his mother by making him manageable by her.

Mr. R's perception of his mother as vulnerable to him (though no doubt subjective and exaggerated) did not stem primarily from his hostility toward her.

Rather, his hostility stemmed from his perception of her as vulnerable. He felt burdened and angered by his mother's weakness and the worry about her that this caused him. (As I have pointed out, a number of writers, including Asch, have written about the readiness of the young child to accept his mother's claim that he is responsible for her happiness.)

THE CASE OF MISS T

In this instance, a patient who believed she was too strong for her mother demonstrated a mild, common perverse reaction.

Miss T, a black woman, was the daughter of a religious leader who became severely depressed and helpless after the death, in a drowning accident, of the patient's twin sister. Miss T's mother, who was not close to her husband, turned to her surviving daughter for affection and support. The mother slept with the child and seemed to need her desperately. Yet she could not make many of her wishes known directly to her daughter, for fear of imposing on her. The mother would hint to the child what she wanted her to do, and she would comply with what she inferred were her mother's wishes. If, however, she guessed wrong, her mother would pout and even weep. When Miss T was in her late teens, she double-dated with her mother. She attracted men, and then her mother would seduce them.

Miss T felt that she could easily destroy her mother. She felt responsible for her life. Once, during her analysis, she dreamt that she was keeping her mother alive by praying in front of her and that if she stopped praying her mother would die.

When Miss T was 12, she had the following experience, which is the subject of this report: She was at camp. One day the head counselor (a man), who periodically visited each bunk and enforced the camp rules rigidly, told her, firmly but without anger, that she had not made her bed properly. He insisted that she immediately remake it. At that moment Miss T had her first orgasm.

According to my explanation (which was amply confirmed by the patient's productions), Miss T was reassured by the counselor's firmness. She assumed that the counselor was someone she could neither dominate nor destroy. She could therefore permit herself in fantasy to feel strong and close to him, which included becoming sexually aroused by him.

Before ending this chapter, I shall discuss the relationship between the concept that certain kinds of psychopathology reflect a personality deficit and the concept that these kinds of psychopathology are rooted in pathogenic beliefs. The two concepts, which are not antithetical, both assume that poor parental care or what is experienced as such may result in psychopathology. According to the first concept, the child who does not receive adequate parental care, love, or attention, is unable to develop well and so retains a personality deficit. According to the other concept, the child who does not receive adequate parental care, love, or attention develops a particular pathogenic belief, namely, that he does not deserve to be noticed, cared for, or loved. He assumes that he deserved this deprivation.

Both concepts are pertinent. The child who is ignored or rejected does not obtain in his relationship with his parents the experiences he needs to mature. He may become withdrawn and narcissistic. However, unless he had inferred from his early experiences with his parents that he would endanger himself if he attempted to develop a reasonable relationship, either with them or with someone else, he would not retain his psychopathology even after growing away from his parents. He would seize the first opportunity available (e.g., at school) to form a good relationship.

A child such as described above may retain his psychopathology for a long time if, in early childhood, he acquired the belief that he does not deserve to be noticed, cared for, or loved. He may manifest this belief in various ways. He may, to protect himself from rejection, remain unaware of his need for love. He may, from compliance with rejecting parents, feel extremely insignificant. He may identify with unloving parents and be himself unloving. He may be quite withdrawn, or he may permit weak and shallow relationships with others. He may, as he improves, become aware of his need for love, but because of his fear of rejection he may refuse to ask for love. Or he may ask for love in a provocative way, so as to make it unlikely that he will receive it. He may, to avoid the experience of rejection or of not being noticed, become self-centered. Or as he improves, he may display his neediness and sadness.

The concept that such a patient's psychopathology is maintained by the pathogenic belief that he does not deserve to be loved (or perhaps even noticed) is supported by the following observation: A patient in therapy may make rapid progress in overcoming his difficulties once he becomes conscious of this belief, perceives its irrationality, and begins to change it. If the patient's psychopathology simply reflected a continuing deficit, such rapid progress would not be possible. He would be able to change only slowly as he gradually accumulated the experiences he needed to overcome the deficit.

5

THE PATIENT'S PLANS, PURPOSES, AND GOALS

JOSEPH WEISS

In this chapter I shall attempt to show that the psychoanalytic process is regulated to a considerable extent by the patient, through use of his higher mental functions. According to my thesis, therapeutic processes are in essence processes by which the patient works with the analyst to disconfirm his pathogenic beliefs. A patient is strongly motivated unconsciously to work at disconfirming these beliefs. He wishes unconsciously to disconfirm them because they are a source of inhibition, fear, shame, anxiety, guilt, and remorse. He also wishes to disconfirm them because they limit his control over certain impulses, which they warn him not to express, and goals, which they warn him not to seek. This is because a person cannot truly control the expression of an impulse (or the seeking of a goal) if he believes his expressing it will put him in a situation of great danger.

A patient works to disconfirm a pathogenic belief by testing it unconsciously in relation to the analyst and by assimilating insight into it conveyed by the analyst's interpretations. Typically the patient first unconsciously tests the belief, begins to disconfirm it, becomes less anxious about it, and so brings it closer to the surface. Then the analyst interprets it, and the patient makes it conscious and perceives its irrationality. However, a patient may, by unconscious testing alone, gradually disconfirm a pathogenic belief and make it conscious. He also may gradually disconfirm a belief and move forward in his analysis without making it conscious. Or, he may, by the assimilation of insight alone, make a pathogenic belief conscious and disconfirm it.

The patient, according to my thesis, works to disconfirm his pathogenic beliefs (and thus to solve his problems) in an orderly way. He does this work in accordance with unconscious plans, which tell him, for example, what problems he will work to solve at a particular time and what problems he will defer working on until later.

THE BACKGROUND IN FREUD'S WRITINGS OF
THE PLAN CONCEPT: A BRIEF HISTORY

My thesis, that the patient works unconsciously to solve his problems in accordance with his own plans, derives from Freud's writings, in particular from his ego psychology. Freud's early concept of the unconscious mind, to the extent that it is based on the automatic functioning hypothesis, cannot accommodate any kind of unconscious plan. Indeed, the idea that there is no unconscious planning but only impersonal unconscious forces is an essential part of the automatic functioning hypothesis. However, the higher mental functioning hypothesis implies unconscious planning. Such higher mental functions as thinking, anticipating, testing, and deciding imply goals. They also imply attempts to attain such goals. In other words, they imply planning.

The concept I shall propose, that the patient makes and carries out plans for solving his problems (by disconfirming his pathogenic beliefs) derives most directly from Freud's ideas about the patient's control of his unconscious mental life and about the patient's unconscious wish to increase his control of it or, in other words, to master it.

THE CONCEPT OF MASTERY AS DEVELOPED BY FREUD

The concept that the patient wishes unconsciously to solve (master) his problems is not compatible with the theory of the mind presented in the *Papers on Technique* (1911–1915). Indeed, in this theory, which assumes that unconscious mental life is regulated by the pleasure principle, the patient would have no motive for solving problems. This is because, according to this theory, a patient's symptoms are the expression of certain unconscious gratifications, which the patient is strongly motivated unconsciously to retain. If, however, as Freud in his ego psychology sometimes assumed (and as the theory proposed here assumes), a patient's problems stem in part from repellent grim unconscious beliefs and from the distressing affects that derive from such beliefs, the patient will have an unconscious wish to overcome his problems. At the very least, he will wish to change those beliefs that cause him to be frightened, inhibited, or weighed down with guilt.

Freud introduced the concept of an unconscious wish for mastery in *Beyond the Pleasure Principle* (1920) about the time he was developing his ego psychology. He introduced this idea to explain his observation that a patient with a traumatic neurosis repeats his traumatic experiences in his dreams. This observation interested Freud and seemed to him to require explanation because it did not fit his earlier idea that unconscious mental life is dominated by the search for pleasure. The traumatic experiences that the dreamer suffers are not pleasurable. Therefore, their repetition in dreams cannot be explained as a search for pleasure. Why, then, asked Freud (1920), does the dreamer repeat them?

We may assume, rather, that dreams are here helping to carry out another task, which must be accomplished before the dominance of the pleasure principle can even begin. These dreams are endeavoring to master the stimulus retrospectively, by developing the anxiety whose omission was the cause of the traumatic neuroses. They thus afford us a view of the function of the mental apparatus which, though it does not contradict the pleasure principle, is nevertheless independent of it and seems to be more primitive than the purpose of gaining pleasure and avoiding unpleasure. (p. 32)

A few pages after he wrote the above, Freud discussed, in a more general context, the ego's task of binding (mastering) instinctual excitation, which, he stated, must be accomplished before the pleasure principle can be established:

Only after the binding has been accomplished would it be possible for the dominance of the pleasure principle (and of its modification, the reality principle) to proceed unhindered. Until then the other task of the mental apparatus, the task of mastering or binding excitations, would have precedence—not, indeed, in *opposition* to the pleasure principle, but independently of it and to some extent in disregard of it. (p. 35)

Freud then proceeded to discuss the observation that children repeat unpleasurable experiences in play to master them. He pointed out that "they [children] can master a powerful impression far more thoroughly by being active than they could by merely experiencing it passively" (1920, p. 35).

Freud returned to the idea of repetition for mastery in *Inhibitions, Symptoms and Anxiety* (1926a), where he wrote that signal anxiety is the result of the ego's repeating its original reaction to a situation of helplessness in order to master it: "The ego, which experienced the trauma passively, now repeats it actively in a weakened version, in the hope of being able itself to direct its course" (p. 167).

In *An Outline of Psychoanalysis* (1940a), Freud conceived of the ego's working for mastery both of external and internal stimuli, as part of its task of self-preservation (see p. 146). In both *Analysis Terminable and*

Interminable and in the *Outline*, Freud implied that the patient works unconsciously with the analyst to overcome his difficulties. For example, "The analytic situation consists of our allying ourselves with the ego of the person under treatment in order to subdue portions of the id which are uncontrolled—that is to say, to include them in the synthesis of his ego" (1937, p. 235).

THE CONCEPT OF UNCONSCIOUS CONTROL AS DEVELOPED BY FREUD

In his early theorizing Freud assumed that a person exerts little or no control over his unconscious mental life. Thus, a person should be generally unable to bring a repressed mental content to consciousness without it being interpreted. If a repressed mental content that has not been interpreted does come forth, it generally does so automatically, propelled by its own thrust. It may come forth as part of a symptom, that is, in a compromise formation, in which the repressed impulse and the forces opposing it find an element that satisfies both. A good example of such a compromise formation is hysterical vomiting in a woman in whom this symptom expresses both her wish to be pregnant and her disgust at the sexual acts she would have to perform in order to satisfy this wish.

However even in his early writings Freud sometimes assumed that the ego may unconsciously regulate the coming forth of warded-off impulses and that it may do so in accordance with the criteria of danger and safety. For example, he assumed in *The Interpretation of Dreams* (1900) that the censor may permit repressed impulses to find expression in dreams because it has shut down the power of movement and thus can safely permit such impulses to come forth (pp. 567–568). In *Inhibitions, Symptoms and Anxiety* (1926a), Freud stated both explicitly and in general terms that the ego may regulate the coming forth of warded-off impulses and that in doing so it may be guided by the criteria of danger and safety. He developed this idea more fully in the *New Introductory Lectures on Psychoanalysis* (1933) and even more fully in the *Outline* (1940a). He said here that after the ego begins unconsciously to consider a particular course of action it delays carrying out this action until it anticipates the consequences of its carrying it out. The ego attempts in several different ways to gauge the probable effects of an action it would like to perform. It calls on its previous experiences and assesses their pertinence to its current situation. Also, it makes use of "experimental actions," that is, of tests (1940a, p. 199). These are actions that, because they are experimental, are not likely to endanger the ego but instead are likely to provide it with information concerning the consequences of the course of action it wants to carry out.

In the *New Introductory Lectures* (1933), Freud stated explicitly (and with expressions of astonishment) that the thinking that a person carries out in deciding whether to bring a repressed mental content to consciousness is unconscious. In the *Outline*, Freud continued to assume that such thinking may take place far from consciousness. However, he assumed in the *Outline* that everything the ego does, including thinking, while sometimes "phenomenologically unconscious" (i.e., incapable of being made conscious) is, by definition, preconscious (1940a, p. 150).

Though Freud did not write about the ego's unconscious planning explicitly, he did describe a number of unconscious ego activities that assume unconscious planning. For example, in the *Outline* he wrote of the ego as "proposing a course of action" (1940a, p. 199), an activity that is almost synonymous with planning. He also wrote of the ego as "mediating" (1940a, p. 145), as "learning" (p. 145), as "deciding" (p. 199), and as "gaining control of the instincts" (p. 146). Moreover, he stated explicitly that the ego "sets itself the task of self-preservation" (p. 145).

The concept of unconscious planning, which I shall develop later in this chapter, is supported by the concept of the ego that Freud developed in the *Outline*. There Freud assumed both that the ego exerts considerable control over unconscious mental life and that it has a powerful wish to master it. In the *Outline* Freud emphasized the ego's wish for mastery by endowing the ego with the crucial purpose of self-preservation. He assumed, too, that much of the ego's activities are carried out as part of its efforts to realize this purpose. For example, Freud derived two important ego activities from the ego's performing the task of self-preservation: the ego's regulation of behavior in terms of safety and danger, and the ego's gaining control of the demands of the instincts. By deriving these two activities from the ego's crucial task of self-preservation, Freud underlined their centrality and urgency. He assumed, too, that the ego carries out its testing (its use of experimental actions) as part of its task of avoiding danger and thus of performing its task of self-preservation. According to Freud, the ego's use of experimental actions before carrying out a proposed course of action is crucial to its efforts to avoid danger.

If, as Freud wrote in the *Outline*, the ego works unconsciously to gain control of the demands made on it by the instincts, and if it works unconsciously to gain such control without putting itself in a situation of danger, it may also make plans unconsciously to guide it in this work. In order to do such work it would need plans to tell it which impulses it might safely attempt to master at any one time and which impulses it should defer attempting to master until later. Moreover, without such plans the ego would have to rethink its priorities whenever it was challenged by a new demand from the instincts or from conscience. Were it unprepared by prior thought it could not deal effectively with emergencies, either from within or from without, and so would be seriously endangered by them.

Many, perhaps most, analysts seem to have ignored Freud's formulations about the ego's unconscious thinking, believing, testing, and by implication, planning. These formulations are easily ignored because they are stated by Freud only in a few brief, concise paragraphs here and there in his late works. However, certain observations, such as of the phenomenon of crying at the happy ending (which supports the concept of unconscious control in accordance with the criteria of danger and safety), are not easily ignored. Nor are observations such as those from the analysis of Miss P (see Chapter 1) that support the concepts of unconscious testing and unconscious control. It is observations such as these that have inspired certain analysts to write about the ego's unconscious thinking, decision making, testing, and planning.

THE BACKGROUND OF THE PLAN CONCEPT IN RECENT ANALYTIC WRITINGS

Rangell, whose position in many ways is close to my own, has written cogently about the ego's decision making and testing as well as about its control of the analytic process. In his paper "Choice, Conflict, and the Decision-Making Function of the Ego" (1969b), he stated that he wished "to establish the centrality of the decision-making function in psychic life" (p. 599). Rangell also wrote (1968) that the ego tests and scans both the internal and external environment before deciding whether or not it may safely bring a particular impulse to consciousness. He stated that the ego's testing may include the testing of the analyst. He added that the analyst may either pass or fail the patient's tests.

In a later paper (1981), Rangell stated that a person's ego routinely tests every intended instinctual discharge, incoming perception, or unconscious fantasy before it is admitted to consciousness or executed in action. The ego carries out such tests to determine from preliminary reactions what would happen either in the person's mind or in his environment if the perception, impulse, or fantasy is admitted to consciousness or executed in action. He added, "The testing is active. The whole process is unconscious" (p. 120). He stated too that concepts such as those he has derived from Freud's theory of signal anxiety are of great importance and should be used to guide technique and to assess analytic progress.

Rangell has stressed (more than most contemporary analysts) the ego's control of the analytic process. He has written: "Regression in the service of the ego is more than a catchy phrase and in my opinion expresses a core dynamism of the 'process' of analysis" (1968, p. 23). Rangell also wrote, but not extensively, about the ego's unconscious planning (1971).

Rapaport's discussion of the ego's decision-making function (1953) is parallel to Rangell's. Sandler has taken a similar position, stating that the ego may respond not only to signals of anxiety by instituting repressions, but also to signals of safety by lifting repressions (1960).

Loewald has not written explicitly about the patient's unconscious testing of the analyst. However, he assumed that the patient unconsciously perceives the analyst not simply as the reincarnation of a parent (or sibling), but as someone with whom he may develop a new, better, and more secure relationship than those he had with the parent or sibling (1960, pp. 17–19). Loewald's conception that the patient wishes to develop a more secure relationship with the analyst than he had with a parent is compatible with the concept of testing, which I shall discuss in detail later. According to this concept, one of the patient's purposes in testing the analyst is to assure himself that he will not be endangered in his relationship with the analyst as, in his opinion, he had been endangered in his relationship to a parent. Like Rapaport, Loewald assumed that the patient does exert some control over the analytic process. Also, he assumed that the security the patient attains by the prospect of developing a new and better relationship with the analyst enables him to permit a controlled regression, which he carries out as a step to further ego development (1960, p. 17).

Kris has tied his theoretical formulations about the ego's control of the analytic process closely to observation. He wrote that the patient may do considerable work outside his awareness and that he may thereby acquire insight. "The very fact that in the good analytic hour the material comes forth as if 'prepared' or better 'actually prepared' but prepared outside of awareness seems only a confirmation of the view that perhaps all significant intellectual achievements are products or at least derivatives of preconscious mentation" (1956a, p. 447).

Kris, in this passage, assumed both a preconscious wish to solve problems and a capacity to work preconsciously at solving them. As evidence of the ego's preconscious wish for mastery, Kris stated that a patient who brings a repressed mental content to consciousness may feel the same way as someone who has just solved a puzzle or done a problem. Further evidence, according to Kris, of the ego's preconscious capacity to solve problems is his observation that new memories may come forth unobtrusively and without conflict because the patient, before bringing them forth, has performed the work that permits him to tolerate them (1956b).

THE PATIENT'S PLANS, PURPOSES, AND GOALS

It is useful, when thinking about the patient's unconscious plans, purposes, and goals, to keep in mind the distinction Freud made in his tripartite model between unconscious ego motives, superego motives, and id motives. These distinctions, as Freud himself was aware, are not completely satisfactory. They are crude,[1] and they risk the reification of parts of the personality. However, they make a point that some analysts tend to overlook. It is that there *are* powerful unconscious motives, namely, ego motives, which cannot be described as impulses, defenses, or products of conscience. Ego motives, as Freud described them, are shaped by the reality principle, and therefore are in various degrees fitted to reality. They are directed to the solving of problems. (In the *Outline* [1940a], Freud described the ego's motives in terms of its "task" of self-preservation.) Since the ego's motives are directed to the solving of problems, they may seek long-term goals as opposed to immediate gratifications. They tend to reflect thought, to take obstacles into account, and to be reasonable, moderate, and adaptive. The motives of the id and superego are more likely to be unreasonable and extreme. They may include the wish to murder, to commit incest, to merge with another person, or to destroy oneself. The ego of the adult generally abjures such unacceptable or dangerous motives. It may occasionally, as Freud tells us, feel forced to accede in varying degrees to them, but generally it does not make them wholeheartedly its own.

The ego motives with which I shall be concerned are those evolved

---

1. Consider, for example, Oedipal motivations, which are generally thought of as id motives. Yet, a good case could be made for the thesis that the boy's wish to kill his father (which, no doubt, expresses intense hostility) is an adaptive plan developed by the boy's immature ego. The boy, according to this thesis, thinks about his situation, realizes that his access to his mother is impeded by his father, and so concludes that it would be a good idea to kill his father.

by the analytic patient and directed to the solution of his problems. The analytic patient evolves such motives unconsciously, much as a person evolves certain motives consciously. The patient thinks about his problems. He takes account of various stringencies imposed on him by, for example, his impulses, his conscience, his anxieties, his abilities, his current reality, and his assessment of the analyst. He sets himself goals, and he makes and carries out plans for reaching these goals. Such plans, purposes, and goals are relatively simple. *They are nothing like blueprints. They may simply point the patient, during a period of his treatment, in a particular direction.*

A good example of an unconscious plan is that carried out by Mrs. G, the patient presented in Chapter 1 who spontaneously brought forth a previously repressed fantasy of being beaten by the analyst. She was guided before the emergence of this fantasy by her goal of becoming conscious of and overcoming her fear of hurting the analyst, to whom she had developed a father transference. By overcoming this fear she hoped to acquire the capacity both to disagree with the analyst and to cooperate with him.

During these sessions Mrs. G worked steadily towards her goal by unconsciously testing the analyst. She tested him by criticizing him, at first timidly and then more and more directly. As she succeeded by such testing in becoming conscious of and overcoming her fear of hurting the analyst, she became able to cooperate with him and even to submit to him. She could cooperate and even submit, knowing that she had acquired the capacity to stop cooperating or submitting whenever she felt endangered by doing so.

During these sessions Mrs. G's goal was to overcome certain pathogenic beliefs that she acquired in childhood in her relationship with her father and which she subsequently generalized to all men. These were the belief that if she criticized a man she would hurt him and the related belief that if she felt close to a man she would become trapped in a masochistic relationship with him.

Mrs. G was unconsciously powerfully motivated to bring forth and change her pathogenic belief that if she differed with a man she would hurt him. This belief caused her considerable unconscious anxiety and guilt. It kept her from feeling close to her husband because she feared that if she became close to him she would have to agree with him in everything, and so be dominated by him.

Mrs. G's goals (or plans) illustrate the following points: A patient's goals are simple, they are directed to overcoming pathogenic beliefs, and they require the patient to test the analyst. They are reasonable ego goals fitted to reality. Mrs. G's goal was to acquire the capacity to be herself in a relationship with a man, that is, to feel able to disagree with him and to feel comfortable being close to him.

EVIDENCE FOR THE CONCEPT OF UNCONSCIOUS PLAN

At this point I shall support the concept of an unconscious plan by an observation which I have made clinically and which our research group has demonstrated by formal research methods (see Chapters 19, 20, and 22). This observation is that there is a high correlation between (1) the analyst's making interpretations that he (or, in our research, a group of independent judges) infers should help the patient carry out his unconscious plans, and (2) the patient's using the interpretations to gain insight and to make analytic progress. Thus, a suitable patient is likely to gain insight and to make progress (although not necessarily without at times experiencing considerable anxiety and conflict), as long as the analyst consistently makes interpretations that the patient can use in his struggle to carry out his plans. However, a patient is likely neither to gain insight nor to make progress when the analyst consistently makes interpretations that the patient unconsciously experiences as hindering him in his struggle to carry out his plans.

When the analyst helps the patient to go where he unconsciously wants to go, the analyst feels as though he is pushing a large round rock down a gentle but perhaps bumpy slope. The rock may have its jolts, its stops, and its starts, but it moves forward. When the analyst hinders the patient from going where he unconsciously wants to go, the analyst feels as though he is pushing the rock uphill. It is hard work, and once the pressure on the rock is removed, it may roll backwards; the ground that had been won with such difficulty may be quickly lost.

SOME CASE ILLUSTRATIONS OF THE PLAN CONCEPT

THE CASE OF MR. B

My first illustration of the plan concept is a case studied by our research group in which the analyst, by his inaccurate interpretations, hindered the patient from carrying out his plan. The analyst misled the patient into believing that he suffered from a primary homosexual attachment to him (the analyst), whereas in fact the patient suffered from unconscious worry about him. He worried that if he were successful he would hurt the analyst. His homosexual attachment to the analyst was not the expression of a primary impulse but rather an attempt to placate the analyst and so to protect himself from his worry about him.

The analyst's interpretations not only misled the patient, they made him worse. The patient unconsciously inferred from them that his pathogenic belief about the danger of hurting the analyst was correct. He assumed that the analyst focused on his homosexuality because he felt challenged by him. As he became more worried about the analyst than before, the patient unconsciously experienced a greater need to restore him, and so intensified his homosexual attachment to him.

Mr. B, a young man with an obsessive–compulsive character (who aspired to be an architect) sought help for inhibitions both in his work and in his love life. Mr. B, in his childhood, had been highly competitive with his father and three older brothers. He had, moreover, perceived them as highly competitive with him. He had also perceived them as envious of him and highly vulnerable to his challenges. Therefore he had kept himself from being too successful in order both to placate them and to prevent them from becoming hurt, envious, or punitive.

Mr. B's behavior from the beginning of therapy was guided by a particular plan. It was to become conscious of and to disconfirm the pathogenic belief that if he were to permit himself to feel strong and successful, especially with women, he would challenge other men and provoke them to envy and retaliation. Mr. B tested this pathogenic belief in relation to the analyst, toward whom he rapidly developed a father transference. He would offer the analyst what could aptly be called multiple-choice tests. He would provide the analyst with considerable evidence of his successes with women. He would suggest that he felt comfortable with women and attracted to them, that he could enjoy sexual relations with them, and that he had recently had several satisfying affairs. However, he would also hint that he was struggling with powerful homosexual impulses. He hoped by such multiple-choice tests to discover whether or not the analyst was (as in his opinion his father had been) competitive with him and so inclined to put him down. He assumed unconsciously that if the analyst wanted him to succeed with women, he would not feel challenged by his successes with them and would acknowledge the successes which he was reporting. He assumed, too, that if the analyst were envious of him he would minimize his successes and focus on his homosexuality.

During the first 10 sessions the analyst remained relatively inactive, and the patient became more relaxed, more outspoken about his successes with women, and more aware that he felt capable of succeeding with women. He inferred that since the analyst did not, by referring to homosexuality, seize the opportunity of humiliating him, the analyst wanted him to succeed.

However, beginning around session 10, the analyst (who believed that the patient was bragging about his heterosexuality primarily to undo his shame about his homosexual impulses) began to focus his analytic attention on the patient's homosexuality. Mr. B, out of compliance with the analyst, accepted the analyst's interpretations. Moreover, he produced new material, including previously repressed childhood memories, which confirmed the analyst's ideas. However, he became progressively more anxious, depressed, resistant, and inhibited. He stopped going out with women. He unconsciously inferred from the analyst's interpretations that the analyst felt challenged by his successes. He therefore weakened himself in order to placate the analyst.

As our study of his analysis revealed, Mr. B (despite his transient insights into his homosexuality) gradually became less insightful than before during the first year of analysis. Then the analyst, apparently alarmed by the patient's unfavorable course, consulted several experienced colleagues. As a result of these consultations, he perceived his error, changed his technique, and began to focus in his interpretations not on Mr. B's homosexuality but on his Oedipal fear that by his heterosexual successes he would incur the envy and vengeance of the analyst. Mr. B began almost immediately to do better and continued to do so. He made good use of the analyst's interpretations, which he amply confirmed. He had a long analysis (7 years), which on the whole was successful. He began a serious study of architecture, was admitted to graduate school, and did well there. He also made a satisfactory marriage.

THE CASE OF MISS D

Another patient who was temporarily set back by a series of incorrect interpretations has already been discussed (Chapter 3).

Miss D was an articulate woman who was guided unconsciously by her wish, and the plans she made to carry it out, to overcome her separation guilt. She had been unable psychologically to free herself from her mother and to develop a life of her own. She had in childhood been convinced that were she to become more independent of her mother she would hurt her mother. Moreover, she had experienced her mother's encouraging her to become more independent as motivated by her mother's wish to assure herself that Miss D, despite her mother's encouragement, would be unable to grow away from her.

Miss D developed a mother transference. She experienced the analyst's interpretations of her dependency on him as she had experienced her mother's complaints about her dependency: She assumed that the analyst secretly wanted her to need him. She reacted to the analyst's interpretations (which ran counter to her plans) by becoming worried about him and more dependent on him.

Miss D, however, responded quite well when the analyst, in the 18th month of the treatment, changed his interpretations. He began then to make interpretations that helped the patient to carry out her plans. He told her that she was remaining dependent on him because she feared that were she to become more independent of him she would hurt him. Then, for over a year, Miss D worked with the analyst to overcome her separation guilt and became conscious of many new memories of her childhood worry about her mother. She remembered her childhood impression that her mother needed the patient to need her. Moreover, she remembered that when her mother had sent her off to camp to encourage her independence, her mother wept at the train station, then called her frequently on the camp's only telephone.

During the last part of her analysis, after Miss D had overcome her separation guilt, she faced Oedipal problems, and, in addition, became able to tolerate her genuine fondness both for her mother and for the analyst. For this patient, the development of "the right to her own life" (to use Ella Sharpe's phrase [1950]) was a precondition for her facing both her Oedipal problems and her genuine dependency on the analyst.

Miss D, at the beginning of her analysis, reacted unfavorably to the interpretation of her infantile dependency because this interpretation was not accurate. At best it took account of certain repressed impulses that she had expressed in her relationship with her mother and was later expressing in relation to the analyst. However, it did not take account of her wish to relinquish these impulses. Moreover, it took account neither of her goal of becoming independent, nor of her guilt about this goal, nor of her unconscious pathogenic belief that were she to become independent she would upset the analyst as she believed she had upset her mother.

It is worth pointing out here that not all patients who suffer from separation guilt react as Miss D did to the analyst's interpretations of her dependency. Miss D was somewhat unusual in that she had concluded quite early in life that her mother's complaints about her dependency were evidence that her mother wished her to be dependent. Also, she had experienced the analyst's interpretations of her dependency in the same way as she had experienced her mother's complaints about it. Another patient with separation guilt might have assumed that the analyst's interpretations of her dependency were intended to help her to become more independent. Another patient might have been relieved by such interpretations and used them in her struggle to become more independent. In general, as pointed out earlier, some patients are more flexible than others. They are more able than others to extract from the analyst's interpretations those ideas that they need to disconfirm their pathogenic beliefs. Such patients may be able to make use of a wide variety of analytic approaches, and within certain limits may be able to change their plans so as to make their plans congruent with the analyst's.

I shall now present a familiar observation that provides strong support for the idea that a patient regulates his treatment in accordance with certain unconscious plans, purposes, and goals. It is that a patient may work for a long time to solve a certain problem or to reach a particular goal, and then after he has solved the problem or reached the goal, set himself another goal. A good example of this observation concerns a patient, Mr. N, who for the first 3 years of his analysis focused almost entirely on his career, and during the last year and a half on his relations with women.

THE CASE OF MR. N

This patient scarely mentioned his sex life during the first 3 years of his treatment. Yet his sex life was not deeply warded off. He would on a few occasions casually refer to an affair, or he would, in his associations to a dream, remember some recent sexual experience. However, his sex life, during the first 3 years, was not the focus of his analytic attention. Then, after the patient became secure in his career, he turned seriously to the problem of finding a suitable wife. He spoke then a great deal about his relationships with women, including his sexual relationships. Toward the end of his analysis, while looking back on its course, Mr. N told the analyst, "I could never have thought of marriage until I had developed a good grip on my professional life." He would be comfortable with women, as he explained, only if he could approach them "from a position of strength."

The automatic functioning hypothesis, which assumes that a patient's productions are determined solely by the dynamic interplay of impulse and defense, cannot account easily for the course of Mr. N's analysis. The patient's sexual impulses, which presumably were of roughly the same intensity throughout his treatment, were not deeply repressed. According to the automatic functioning hypothesis, Mr. N should have been concerned with his sexuality to more or less the same degree throughout his treatment. However, the fact that he was scarcely at all concerned with it at first but quite concerned with it later is readily explained by the assumption that he unconsciously decided first to work at establishing his career, then to look for a wife.

THE RELATIONSHIP BETWEEN A PATIENT'S UNCONSCIOUS PLANS AND HIS UNCONSCIOUS ASSESSMENTS OF SAFETY

A patient in making his plans is unconsciously guided by many considerations, especially by his assessments of what he may do safely. Unless he is under considerable pressure (from the analyst, from his conscience, from his life situation, or from his wishes), he does not face his central unconscious conflicts until he has acquired the strength and the confidence in the analyst to deal with them safely. Therefore, at the beginning of treatment he generally does not attempt to face his central conflicts, but rather he attempts to find a way of working that will protect him from such conflicts while enabling him to gain the strength to deal with them later. For example, Mrs. G could not safely tackle her Oedipal problems (she could not safely fall in love) until she knew that she could maintain herself with a man without falling into a masochistic relationship with him. Miss P, the lawyer presented in Chapter 1, did not feel safe in forming a relationship with a man until she had assured herself that she did not deserve to be rejected by men.

As my examples have shown and as illustrated below, a patient, while working to reach a particular goal, assesses all of the analyst's comments for their pertinence to that goal.

THE CASE OF MR. O

Mr. O, who suffered from castration anxiety, unconsciously feared that by masturbating (and by other behaviors), he would challenge the authority of the analyst and so provoke the analyst to punish him. As the patient later revealed, he was afraid to masturbate and seldom did so. When he did masturbate, he used isolation to make his masturbation unreal to him. After masturbating he would tend to forget (or isolate) the entire experience. During the several months in which he struggled unconsciously to bring his masturbation into the open, Mr. O listened unconsciously to every comment the analyst made to infer how the analyst would react to his talking about his masturbation. He would unconsciously ask himself, "Would the analyst feel challenged by my discussing masturbation and so be tempted to punish me for it, or would he be tolerant of my masturbation?" If Mr. O inferred that the analyst would not be punitive, he would move closer to discussing his masturbation. If he inferred that the analyst would be punitive, he would move further from discussing it. The patient remained unconsciously concerned with inferring how the analyst would react to his discussing masturbation until the analyst helped him to make it conscious by interpreting his fear of being punished for it.

During this period the patient unconsciously tested the analyst by making veiled references to masturbation, in order to determine, before discussing it, how the analyst would react to his bringing it forth. By such testing of the analyst the patient worked steadily, in accordance with an unconscious plan, until he accomplished his goal.

In general, as I have illustrated by the examples presented above, a patient, during each part of his treatment, works in accordance with a particular unconscious plan toward the attainment of a particular unconscious goal. In working to attain such a goal, the patient unconsciously tests the analyst. He attempts by such testing to disconfirm a certain pathogenic belief (or family of beliefs) and by doing so to make himself more secure in his relationship with the analyst. The patient's overcoming his pathogenic beliefs and his becoming more secure with the analyst are both part of the same process. This is because the patient's pathogenic beliefs warn him not to rely on the analyst and prevent him from feeling secure with him.

A patient (as demonstrated by research that will be presented in Chapters 19, 20, and 22) who is struggling to disconfirm a particular pathogenic belief is especially helped by an interpretation if he can use it in his struggle to disconfirm the belief. The patient is relieved by such an interpretation, comes to feel more confidence in the analyst, and becomes less afraid of those mental contents he has been warding off in obedience to the belief. He becomes bolder, more insightful, more outgoing, and clearer in his thinking. In addition, he may react to the interpretation by producing confirmatory material. (Alternatively, a patient who has unconsciously been encouraged by a helpful interpretation, instead of bringing forth new material, may present the analyst with a bolder and more direct test of the pathogenic belief he is working to disconfirm.)

A patient may make good use unconsciously of an interpretation with which he does not consciously agree. He may unconsciously gain relief from the interpretation but not experience the relief. An example of this occurred in the analysis of Miss P (Chapter 1). She unconsciously believed that she was a drain on the analyst and so deserved to be rejected by him. She worked unconsciously by testing the analyst to disconfirm this belief. She tested the analyst by telling him that she had received maximum benefit from treatment and so was planning to stop. The analyst reacted by pointing out that her wish to stop was the expression of certain resistances, including resistances stemming from her fear that the analyst would reject her. The patient consciously dismissed the analyst's interpretations and persisted in her determination to stop. However, while consciously opposing the interpretations, she unconsciously revealed that she was relieved by them; she became less tense and anxious and friendlier to the analyst.

Just as a patient may be helped by an interpretation that he can use in his struggle to disconfirm a pathogenic belief, he may, as in the case of Mr. B, be set back by an interpretation that he experiences as confirming this belief. He may then become more anxious and defensive, less bold, less insightful, less clear in his thinking, and less confident of the analyst. In addition, a patient may, out of compliance to the analyst, consciously agree with a poor interpretation, yet reveal by his unconscious reactions to it that he has experienced it as hindering him in his progress.

6

THE PATIENT'S UNCONSCIOUS WORK

JOSEPH WEISS

I shall here develop the idea, introduced in the last chapter, that the psychoanalytic process is in essence a process by which the patient works with the analyst, both consciously and unconsciously, to disconfirm his pathogenic beliefs. He does this by unconsciously testing his beliefs in relation to the analyst and by assimilating insight into them conveyed by the analyst's interpretations. (Research on the patient's unconscious testing of his pathogenic beliefs is presented in Chapters 17 and 18. Research on the effects of interpretation is presented in Chapters 19, 20, and 22. Interpretation is discussed in Chapter 21.)

TESTING

Throughout his treatment, the patient tests his pathogenic beliefs in his relationship to the analyst. Indeed, the various repetitions during analysis of his early childhood experiences, while serving the patient in various ways, generally serve him as tests both of his pathogenic beliefs and of the analyst. He may test both the pathogenic beliefs and the analyst at the same time, because by the same tests he may learn something about both.

One well-known form of testing is the unconscious testing of limits. A patient who is testing limits hopes unconsciously that the analyst will maintain limits and thus help the patient to disconfirm the pathogenic belief that he can make the analyst lose his authority as, in his experience, he made a parent lose his authority.

The patient tests the analyst not only to determine whether the analyst can maintain limits, but also to assess the analyst in other ways. The patient tests the analyst not only at the beginning of analysis but throughout the treatment. Freud observed that the patient in analysis never stops repeating his past. He wrote, "As long as a patient is in the treatment, he cannot escape from the compulsion to repeat" (1914, p. 150). Such repetitions often serve, among other functions, the function of testing.

In testing a pathogenic belief, a patient makes use unconsciously of what Freud described as "experimental actions" (1940a, p. 199). A patient may test a pathogenic belief by doing certain things in relation to the analyst (he may express certain impulses or seek certain goals) which, according to the belief, should threaten his ties to the analyst and so put him in a situation of danger. If the patient infers from such trial actions that he does not affect the analyst as the belief predicts, he may become less anxious and take a step toward disconfirming the belief. He may bring the belief closer to consciousness and begin to overcome certain inhibitions and to lift certain repressions that he had maintained in obedience to the belief. If, on the other hand, the patient infers that he does affect the analyst as the belief predicts, he may temporarily become more anxious, defensive, or inhibited than he was before, and he may intensify the repression of the belief.

The patient, while testing a pathogenic belief, defies it. Therefore, while testing it he is likely to feel fear, anxiety, or guilt. These feelings are a major source of resistance to treatment.

A patient's testing is like thinking in that it is a means by which a patient, through a relatively small expenditure of effort and at low risk, determines whether he may safely carry out a particular proposed course of action. The patient's unconscious testing of the analyst is also an example of reality testing as Freud described it in the *Outline* (1940a). Freud stated there that since memories may become conscious, a person is in danger of confusing memories and current perceptions. The ego, according to Freud, "guards against this possibility by the institution of reality testing" (p. 199). The patient's unconscious testing of the analyst is a kind of reality testing in that, by testing the analyst, the patient attempts to find out whether his impressions of the analyst are based on memories or on accurate current impressions, that is, on transferences or on the analyst's current behavior.

Before carrying out a major new initiative, a patient attempts, both by thought and by trial actions, to anticipate how the analyst is likely to react (Freud, 1940a). He attempts to infer how the analyst will behave, by reviewing those of the analyst's previous remarks and attitudes that bear on his concerns about the analyst. After he has taken his investigation as far as he can by thought alone, he may continue it by trial actions.

The patient's testing of the analyst is in some ways similar to the testing by which a person in everyday life may attempt to learn about someone who is important to him. Any person may be reluctant to carry out a potentially dangerous piece of behavior before he has made himself reasonably sure, by use of trial actions, that he will not put himself in a situation of danger. For example, a man may keep himself from falling in love with a woman until he has tested her, consciously or unconsciously, to determine how she is likely to react to his loving her.

A person in everyday life may be conscious of his testing, but the analytic patient generally is not. He cannot be conscious of testing a belief which is itself unconscious. Nor can he be conscious that by his testing he is working to bring forth a particular mental content if the content itself is unconscious.

A person is especially prone to test someone if he would like to change his relationship to him. For example, he may be especially prone to test someone either if he would like to form a new relationship with him or to put an old relationship on a new basis. A person who has formed a stable and satisfactory relationship with another person may not frequently need to present him with significant tests. The same, however, does not hold for the analytic patient. The patient in analysis attempts throughout treatment to change his relationship to the analyst by changing his pathogenic beliefs. He therefore tests the analyst throughout treatment. This unconscious testing of the analyst is a crucial part of his working to solve his problems.

Testing by trial actions is a fundamental human activity. It is a basic means by which a person may attempt to understand someone who is important to him, and thus is a crucial part of his reality testing. The patient evaluates the analyst's reactions to his tests against the background of the analyst's usual analytic stance. The patient in general unconsciously wants the analyst to react to his tests by maintaining his usual stance. He does not want the analyst, for example, to be seduced by his sexual interest, hurt by his hostility, or humiliated by his contempt. If a patient perceives the analyst as reacting in one of these ways, he experiences him as failing his tests. The patient may then become anxious.

If a patient in pursuit of a particular goal tests the analyst, and if the analyst fails the test, the patient may pursue the same goal by a more pointed test, which he assumes the analyst is likely to pass.

A patient who was working to disconfirm the pathogenic belief that he could force others to do whatever he wanted them to do asked the analyst to change his appointment to an earlier time, which he assumed would be inconvenient. The patient became anxious when the analyst acceded. The patient sometime later asked the analyst to reduce his fee, and was relieved when the analyst did not.

If, while testing the analyst, the patient becomes afraid that the analyst will fail the test, the patient may coach him on how to pass it.

A patient who feared that the analyst would reject him tempted the analyst to do just that by announcing abruptly that he had decided to discontinue the treatment. When the analyst remained silent, the patient became increasingly anxious. He feared that the analyst would permit him to terminate, and so he coached him by saying, "Whenever I do something impulsive, I regret it later."

WAYS IN WHICH THE PATIENT TESTS THE ANALYST

Remembering, Repeating and Working-Through (1914) is one of Freud's fundamental articles on technique. It is, of course, based mainly on the automatic functioning hypothesis. Freud began it by contrasting his original technique with his current technique. He wrote: "In its first phase—that of Breuer's catharsis—analytic technique consisted of bringing directly into focus the moment at which the symptom was formed and in persistently endeavoring to reproduce the mental processes involved in that situation, in order to direct their discharge along the path of conscious activity" (p. 147).

From the original technique Freud evolved a new technique, in which the patient is asked not to remember a particular moment but to report whatever is on the surface of his mind, that is, to free-associate. The analyst then "employs the art of interpretation mainly for the purpose of recognizing the resistances which appear there and making them conscious to the patient" (p. 147). The purpose of the new technique remained the same: "Descriptively speaking, it is to fill in the gaps in memory" (p. 148).

Under the new technique, there are some cases which behave like those under the hypnotic technique up to a point and only later cease to do so; but others behave differently from the beginning—if we confine ourselves to the second type in order to bring out the difference, we may say that the patient does not *remember* anything that was forgotten and repressed but acts it out. He reproduces it, not as a memory but as an action; he repeats it, without, of course, knowing that he is repeating it.

For instance, the patient does not say that he remembers that he used to be defiant and critical towards a parent's authority; instead he behaves in that way to the doctor. . . . as long as a patient is in the treatment, he cannot escape from the compulsion to repeat; and in the end we understand that this is his way of remembering. (p. 150)

The patient's repeating rather than remembering is, according to Freud, related to his transferring and resisting, as follows: "The transference is itself only a piece of repetition." Moreover, "the greater the resistance the more extensively will acting out (repetition) replace remembering" (p. 151).

The task of the physician who employs the new technique is to analyze the patient's repetitions, his transferring, and his acting out by tracing them back into the past.

These views marked a great advance in the understanding of human behavior. In *Remembering, Repeating and Working-Through* Freud made clear that there is a powerful relationship between repeating and remembering. He showed that repeating often precedes remembering, and that it may be converted to remembering through the art of interpretation.

These basic observations have stood the test of time. However, the theory Freud used to account for them, in the light of the higher mental functioning hypothesis he introduced in certain of his later works, is no longer completely adequate. It is, as I shall later discuss, unable to account completely for certain readily made observations about the relationship between repeating and remembering.

The views I shall develop below (which are based on the higher mental functioning hypothesis) are related to those presented by Freud as follows: In *Remembering, Repeating and Working-Through*, the patient's repetitions are carried out automatically as a consequence of the patient's compulsion to repeat. In my account, they are to some degree controlled unconsciously by the patient, and they are carried out for various purposes, including that of testing the analyst. According to *Remembering, Repeating and Working-Through*, the patient's repetitions are carried out in the service of his resistances. In my view, such repetitions, while serving a defensive function, may also test the analyst and hence may be part of the patient's preparation for remembering. In *Remembering, Repeating and Working-Through*, the patient repeats (rather than remembers) in basically one way, that is, by transferring. According to my view, the patient repeats rather than remembers in basically two ways, which are equally important: by turning passive into active and by transferring.

As I have already pointed out, a patient who, as in Freud's example, defies the analyst instead of remembering his defiance of a parent may be testing the analyst. The evidence that the patient may be testing the analyst is straightforward. It is the observation (which we have demonstrated in the formal research presented in Chapter 18) that if the patient unconsciously expresses a powerful transference to the analyst and if the analyst retains his neutrality in the face of the patient's transferring, the patient may become unconsciously less anxious and more relaxed than he had been. He may, moreover, while relaxed, become more insightful. He may, for example, bring forth a previously repressed memory. If, for example, a patient has been transferring by expressing a hostile defiance of the analyst, he may remember an occasion in childhood when he had expressed hostile defiance of a parent. He may, in addition, keep the memory in consciousness without coming into conflict with it and use the insight he gained from it to attain a better understanding of his problems.

The theory Freud presented in *Remembering, Repeating and Working-Through* cannot explain this observation. If the patient's transferring of, say, his defiance, were the automatic and uncontrolled expression of impulse and defense, he should be unconsciously frustrated by the analyst's neutrality. That is, he should be frustrated in his wish to gratify the hostile defiance by hurting the analyst. The defiance therefore should become intensified, and the patient should be more in unconscious conflict with it than before. In other words, the patient should become unconsciously more tense rather than more relaxed. Moreover, he should not ordinarily become conscious of a repressed memory without interpretation. He might become conscious of such a memory if, as a consequence of the frustration of the transference, the libido, which had sought gratification in the transference, flowed back to a repressed memory of gratification (e.g., a gratifying memory of defiance). However, were the patient, as a consequence, to become conscious of such a memory, he would not be able both to remain calm about it and to use his insight into it to advance the cause of his analysis. If the memory became so intense that it came forth more or less unopposed by defenses, the patient should become anxious about it, come into conflict with it, and attempt to re-repress it. If it came forth more or less opposed by defenses (e.g., if it were isolated), the patient should remain calm about it, but he should not be able to use it to advance the cause of his analysis.

However, the hypothesis that a patient, by transferring, may be testing the analyst and that this testing may be planned and carried out unconsciously by the ego can readily explain the patient's reacting to the analyst's neutrality by becoming more relaxed and also by bringing forth a new memory. According to this hypothesis, the patient may be attempting by his transferring to test a pathogenic belief in the hope of disconfirming it. For example, he may be attempting to test the belief that by defying the analyst he will provoke punishment from him, as, in his experience, he had, by defying his father, provoked punishment from him.

If the patient who is testing the analyst by repeatedly defying him infers from the analyst's neutral reaction to his defiance that he has not provoked the analyst, he may take a step toward overcoming his pathogenic belief about the dangers connected with expressing defiance. He may become less anxious than he had been about defying the analyst and therefore calmer in relation to him. Also, feeling less endangered by his defiance, he may permit himself to become more conscious of it. He may in addition begin to question his belief that he deserved the punishments he received from his father for defying him. Having become less guilty about his childhood defiance of his father, he may unconsciously decide that he can safely remember it and so bring it to consciousness. Moreover, since he may overcome his guilt and anxiety about the memories before bringing them forth, he may make them conscious in relatively undisguised form, keep them in consciousness, and use them to advance the cause of his analysis.

TURNING PASSIVE INTO ACTIVE AND TRANSFERRING

As I have already stated, the analytic patient may, according to our observations, unconsciously test the analyst by repeating the past (rather than by remembering it) in two different ways: by turning passive into active and by transferring. In turning passive into active the patient behaves as in his experience a parent had behaved toward him. In transferring he behaves as in his experience he had behaved toward a parent. Both turning passive into active and transferring may be defined more specifically in terms of the patient's infantile traumas and the pathogenic beliefs to which these traumas gave rise. The patient who turns passive into active reproduces in his relationship with the analyst parental behavior that he had experienced as traumatic; that is, he identifies with a parent and does to the analyst those traumatizing things a parent had previously done to him. A patient who transfers reproduces behaviors such as those by which, in his opinion, he had provoked the traumatic parental behavior.

Turning passive into active and transferring are similar in certain important ways. They are both carried out by all patients. In carrying them out, the patient repeats the infantile situation with his parents which, as the patient experienced it, had led to his being traumatized. In turning passive into active he repeats it with the roles reversed; in transferring he repeats it directly. Both turning passive into active and transferring may be used as defenses to ward off memories of trauma. A patient who is turning passive into active may be unconsciously using the defense of identification with the aggressor to ward off memories of trauma experienced at the hands of a parent whom he perceived as an aggressor. A patient who is transferring and thus unconsciously repeating with the analyst those motives and behaviors by which (in his opinion) he had provoked the traumatic parental actions may be doing so to avoid remembering the childhood motives and behaviors and the traumatic parental reactions to them. Both turning passive into active and transferring may be used as vehicles for the expression of powerful affects and impulses. Finally, both forms of repetition may be used by the patient as tests the patient performs in his struggle to master his infantile traumas and to disconfirm the pathogenic beliefs which stem from them.

In turning passive into active the patient attempts, by reproducing them actively, to master traumas (and to overcome the beliefs inferred from them) that he once experienced passively. The idea that a patient may actively repeat traumatic impressions in order to master them was introduced by Freud in *Beyond the Pleasure Principle* (1920, p. 35) and developed further by him in *Inhibitions, Symptoms and Anxiety* (1926a). A number of other analysts have since discussed the part played by turning passive into active both in children's play (A. Freud, 1936) and in the analysis of adult patients (Klein, 1976).

A patient who tests the analyst by turning passive into active hopes to demonstrate that the analyst will not be upset by him as, in his opinion, he had been upset (traumatized) by a parent. That is, the patient hopes unconsciously that the analyst will retain his analytic stance. For example, the patient who believes he deserved the rejections he received from a parent, and thus that he deserves to be rejected by the analyst, may test the analyst by being cold to him. He hopes that the analyst will retain his analytic stance and give no evidence of feeling that he (the analyst) deserves the patient's rejections.

A patient, while testing the analyst, observes him carefully. If a patient who is turning passive into active repeatedly observes that the analyst does not react to him as (in his opinion) he had reacted to a parent, he may be relieved. He may tentatively decide that the analyst is not vulnerable to trauma in the same way that he (the patient) had been vulnerable to it. In addition, he may (as described by Gitelson, 1962) temporarily identify with the analyst and so become less vulnerable to trauma. He may, moreover, manifest his decreased vulnerability and his increased sense of safety by changing his behavior or by developing new insights. For instance, if the patient in the above example infers that the analyst does not react to his indifference by believing himself a bad person who deserves to be rejected, the patient may temporarily identify with the analyst. He may take a step toward overcoming the pathogenic belief that he deserves to be rejected by the analyst and that he deserved the rejection he received from his parents. He may become more friendly to the analyst and more aware of his fear of rejection by him, or he may retrieve childhood memories of having been rejected by his parents.

By temporarily identifying with the analyst, a patient, as illustrated above, may begin to question his pathogenic beliefs. He may feel safe enough to bring them closer to consciousness. He may overcome certain of the inhibitions or lift some of the repressions he maintained in obedience to the beliefs. He may (if earlier he had been afraid to transfer) begin to feel strong enough safely to transfer, and thus to test his pathogenic beliefs by transferring. (In general, as I shall discuss later, it is safer to turn passive into active than to transfer.) Or he may, as in the example presented below, go directly from turning passive into active to remembering. He may retrieve, in more vivid meaningful detail, the experiences from which he had acquired his pathogenic beliefs.

THE CASE OF DR. Z

Dr. Z had been working unconsciously for several days to retrieve certain childhood memories of parental intercourse. Then in the middle of an analytic session, he picked up a ceramic ashtray from a table beside the couch and played with it carelessly, balancing it precariously on his fingertips.

After a while the analyst asked him, "How do you imagine I feel watching you?" "Impaled," the patient replied. "You are afraid to move or talk, because you are afraid you would disturb me and make me drop the ashtray. You are afraid to watch me, yet you are afraid to stop watching." A few minutes later Dr. Z remembered more clearly than before his feelings while witnessing parental intercourse. He had felt impaled, afraid of disturbing his parents, afraid to look, and afraid to look away. He had pretended to be asleep but had, in fact, been tense and excited.

Dr. Z, by playing with the ashtray, was turning passive into active, for he was creating a situation calculated to arouse in the analyst affects and ideas similar to those connected with his traumatic memories. He wanted to find out whether the analyst would be anxious and afraid of disturbing him as he had been anxious and afraid of disturbing his parents. As he observed that the analyst felt neither anxious about him nor afraid of disturbing him, he temporarily identified with the analyst. He began to feel less anxious about the parental intercourse which he had observed, and so could risk remembering it. He acquired insight into his early primal scene experience without its being interpreted.

A patient, by transferring, tests his pathogenic beliefs more directly than by turning passive into active. He reproduces with the analyst behavior similar to that by which, in his opinion, he had provoked the parental behavior he had experienced as traumatic. He hopes that the analyst will not react to such behavior as, in his experience, a parent had reacted to it. He hopes, for example, that he will not hurt the analyst by his defiance, as, in his opinion, he had hurt a parent, or that he will not humiliate the analyst by his contempt, or seduce him by his admiration. If, over a period of time, the patient infers, from observing the analyst, that he does not affect the analyst as his pathogenic beliefs predict, he may temporarily take another step toward loosening the hold of these beliefs on him. That is, he may become less convinced that he was responsible for the traumatic parental reactions of his childhood. He may, therefore, come to feel less guilty, ashamed, or anxious about his childhood traumas. He may (as illustrated in Chapter 1 by the case of Miss P) make changes both in his behavior and in his level of insight. He may become more conscious both of repressed childhood traumatic experiences and of repressed pathogenic beliefs. He may also bring forth and gain control of the impulses and the developmental goals that, in childhood, he had repressed in obedience to such beliefs.

THE CASE OF PROFESSOR T

In the following presentation, a patient first worked to overcome certain pathogenic beliefs by testing them through turning passive into active. He succeeded by such testing in loosening the hold on him of the beliefs. He thereby became strong enough both to test the beliefs by transferring and to remember some of the traumatic experiences from which the beliefs arose.

Professor T, who taught history in a local university, suffered from a profound lack of initiative or enthusiasm. In early childhood he had been traumatized by his inhibited, insipid mother whom he described as "very blah." His relationship with her had been especially important to him because his father had been away from home when the patient was 2 to 6 years old.

Professor T reported that his mother did little herself and that she discouraged him from doing anything. If, for example, the patient told his mother that he would like to play on a nearby beach, she generally found some specific reason why he should not, such as, "It's too cold" or "It's too hot" or "It's too windy." If his mother could not find a good reason for discouraging him from doing a particular thing, she would simply ask him in a weary, whiny voice, "Are you sure you would like to do that?" Moreover, if the patient were to defy his mother and, for example, go to the beach, she would complain on his return that she had been worried about him the whole time he was gone.

In addition to the above, she would disappoint him by promising to do certain things with him but then not do them. Then, when he complained about her neglect she would turn him away in an insipid weary manner, with a patently flimsy excuse.

Professor T developed the unconscious pathogenic belief (which he repressed) that to please his mother he had to renounce his sense of adventure and stop taking initiative. Although at the beginning of treatment he was aware of his lack of initiative, he was not then aware that in renouncing his initiative he was complying with his mother. He was unable then to retrieve his disappointment in his mother, nor could he remember affectively those rare occasions on which he had felt relaxed and adventurous.

Professor T, during the second year of his analysis, began a kind of testing which he continued from time to time over the next year. He would turn passive into active by reacting to the analyst's comments or interpretations in an insipid, weary manner, especially if the analyst made his comments enthusiastically. He would question the value of the analyst's comments and indeed of the entire analysis, and hint that he might find it too much trouble to continue the treatment. If the analyst did not permit the patient's attitude to discourage him, the patient in the next session would sometimes be more cheerful and take more initiative in the analysis. The patient's reactions to the analyst's remaining undiscouraged (and so passing the patient's tests) was strikingly illustrated by the following: On five occasions after the patient had been particularly insipid and the analyst undeterred, the patient reported a dream of adventure. In one such dream he was on a safari in Africa. In associating to this dream, the patient remembered the sense of adventure he sometimes felt when he did manage to leave home and explore the neighborhood beach and its tidepools.

My explanation of this sequence is as follows: Professor T observed that the analyst, when confronted by the patient's whiny behavior, did not feel obliged to become that way himself. The patient observed that the analyst retained his usual degree of initiative and enthusiasm in the face of his discouraging insipidity. The patient then temporarily identified with the analyst and began to realize that he too could retain his initiative and even be adventurous in the face of his (internalized) mother's discouragement.

In one session, about 6 months after the adventure dreams, Professor T was especially insipid and whiny. The analyst, again undeterred, told him that he was being insipid like his mother and that by being insipid he feared he would discourage the analyst as his mother had discouraged him. During the next session, the patient permitted himself, for the first time, to experience intense disappointment. He complained bitterly about a publishing house that was delaying delivery of some books he needed for his class. He was on the verge of tears. He then began to talk about his mother's having repeatedly disappointed him. He wept openly and repeated a number of times, "It's sad, it's very sad."

Professor T was able to remember his feeling of disappointment in his mother after he had again demonstrated to himself that the analyst could retain his usual initiative and optimism in the face of his whiny, discouraging tone. The patient had identified temporarily with the analyst's capacity not to feel discouraged and had realized more fully that he himself did not have to feel discouraged, either by his mother or by the publishing company. It was this realization that enabled him to face his disappointment. He could face it, knowing that he would not have to be overwhelmed by it.

Since the sessions described above, Professor T has become even more convinced that he may take initiative without risk of being traumatized. He has taken more initiative both in his everyday life and in his analysis. In taking such initiative, the patient has been transferring. He has, in relation to the analyst, been doing the very thing that provoked his mother to whine and to worry about him. Thus he has been risking the possibility that he will be traumatized by the analyst as, in his opinion, he had been traumatized by his mother.

The distinction between turning passive into active and transferring may be blurred in the analysis of certain patients. This is because a patient, in childhood, may identify with a parental attitude that he finds upsetting and treat the parent as, in his experience, the parent treated him. A mother who whines at her daughter may raise a daughter who whines at her. However, the distinction between turning passive into active and transferring may be relatively clear in the analysis of a patient who, in childhood, suffered a discrete shocking trauma.

This distinction was sharp in the analysis of a patient whose parents had both died in a plane crash when she was 13½ and who was subsequently cared for by wealthy relatives. This patient, during the first part of her analysis, mainly turned passive into active. She made frequent attempts to leave the analyst, not only as a defense against the transference, but to assure herself that the analyst would not be devastated by her leaving him, as she had been devastated at her parents' leaving her by dying. As she observed that the analyst could tolerate the possibility of her leaving him, she identified with him and temporarily became more able to think about the loss of her parents. She became able to use the analyst's interpretations about her grieving for them. In the second part of her analysis the patient transferred more and more directly. She eventually permitted herself to love the analyst and thus to run the risk that she would be traumatized by losing him as she had been traumatized when she lost her parents. Moreover, since the patient's loving the analyst did not bring about her losing him, the patient became less convinced of the pathogenic belief that she would inevitably lose whatever she loved and valued. She became fully conscious of this belief and of its derivation from the loss of her parents.

As is illustrated by the above schematic presentation, a patient may work throughout an entire analysis to master just one kind of trauma and the pathogenic belief (or family of beliefs) that arose from it.

HOW THE PATIENT REGULATES THE COURSE OF AN ANALYSIS

The patient regulates the course of his treatment by considerations of safety. He is reluctant at each stage of the treatment to endanger himself by unconsciously expressing certain impulses, by attempting unconsciously to reach certain goals, or by becoming conscious of certain previously repressed mental contents before he is ready to tolerate them. He may in some instances be able to pace himself so that he proceeds through the entire analysis without putting himself in danger. Or he may for various reasons be unable to protect himself from certain dangers. He may endanger himself (as did Mr. B) by complying with an analyst who is pressuring him in a direction contrary to his unconscious plans. Or, he may endanger himself by complying with a demanding conscience that, for example, pressures him to make certain confessions before he is comfortable making them. Or, he may feel forced by the circumstances of his everyday life to take up certain topics before he is able to deal with them safely. Or, he may, as is well known, feel forced by the intensity of his wishes to put himself in danger.

In many but not all instances, a patient may work more safely by turning passive into active than by transferring. This is because a patient while turning passive into active is maintaining a relatively safe position. He is maintaining a strong defense which may be conceptualized in various ways: as identification with the aggressor, as a defense against the transference, or as a narcissistic defense (see the case of Professor T).

A patient generally both transfers and turns passive into active throughout his analysis. If he has not been especially traumatized, he may begin the analysis by developing strong transferences. However, a patient who has been especially traumatized is likely (because it is usually safer) to work at the beginning of treatment mainly by turning passive into active. If he transfers at the beginning, he is likely to do so in a controlled and limited way so as to avoid trauma. A patient who, at the beginning of his analysis, works mainly by turning passive into active, may, as a consequence of such work, develop the strength to work later in the treatment by developing powerful transferences.

Consider, for example, a patient who suffered from the pathogenic belief that his possessive and rejecting mother needed him to love her. He did not attempt during the first part of his treatment to become conscious of his love for the analyst (with whom he had developed a mother transference). Were he to have brought it forth then, he would have risked feeling possessed and seduced by the analyst as, in his opinion, he had been possessed and seduced by his mother. During the first year of his treatment, this patient tested the analyst mainly by complaining that the analyst was selfish, ungiving, and of little or no help to him. On several occasions he threatened to quit. By such testing he succeeded in demonstrating to himself that his not loving the analyst would not hurt the analyst. After he had assured himself that he could safely reject the analyst, he permitted himself, over a period of time, to experience his transference love for him. He could safely love the analyst once he knew that he could, by rejecting him, extricate himself from his relationship with him.

In general, a patient tackles less dangerous problems before more dangerous ones. As he solves the less dangerous problems and so makes headway in changing his pathogenic beliefs, he becomes stronger and more secure, and he develops certain new capacities. These accomplishments permit him safely to tackle problems that earlier he would have been unable to face. As he tackles and solves the new problems, he becomes able to face and solve still newer problems. (For a discussion of various topics in the theory of therapy such as interpretation and the patient's experiences with the analyst, see Chapter 21.)

THERAPEUTIC VERSUS NEUROTIC PROCESSES

The concept of therapy as a process in which a patient gradually disconfirms his pathogenic beliefs permits us to make a distinction between therapeutic and neurotic processes. A therapeutic process is one in which the patient disconfirms certain pathogenic beliefs, becomes more conscious of them, and so gains control over the affects, impulses, ideas, and developmental goals he was warding off in obedience to these beliefs. It is a process in which the patient becomes more insightful and less anxious, guilty, and defensive. A neurotic process is the opposite of a therapeutic process. In a neurotic process a patient finds his pathogenic beliefs confirmed by his experiences so that he becomes more frightened, anxious, guilty, or ashamed. He intensifies his repressions and therefore becomes less conscious of his pathogenic beliefs and of the various motives, affects, and ideas that he was warding off in obedience to them. He becomes less insightful and more defensive.

THE CASE OF MR. Y

In the following example, a patient was traumatized during his analysis when he experienced certain of the analyst's interpretations as confirming a pathogenic belief. He temporarily became worse. However, after several months during which the patient accomplished very little, he began to work well again, and he eventually succeeded in completing his treatment.

The patient, Mr. Y, was a 30-year-old literary agent. According to him, his mother was flamboyant, hysterical, possessive, and sexually seductive. His father was a staid businessman who was more or less under his mother's thumb. In childhood, the patient had been tied to his mother by his worry about her. He had wanted to break away from her but was afraid that were he to do so, he would hurt her. In his attempts to break away from his mother, he had received little or no help from his father. On those few occasions when the child had stood up to his mother, his father had taken her side and forced him to apologize.

Mr. Y, during the first two years of treatment, regulated his relationship to the analyst in accordance with his wish for the analyst to help him become more independent. He struggled to become successful in his work but felt anxious, knowing that, by attaining success at work, he would be in a position to escape his mother's domination. The analyst, who perceived the patient's motivations primarily in Oedipal terms, interpreted his anxiety about becoming independent as based on "guilt about success." Mr. Y experienced this interpretation as in accordance with his plans and so responded well to it. He became conscious that he had been holding himself back to protect his parents. He worked hard and did well.

After attaining success in work, Mr. Y began to focus on his relationships with women. Because of his unconscious fear of being trapped by women, he had tended to treat them casually. He would maintain a relationship with a woman for a while, then pull away from her just as she was becoming interested in him. After leaving the woman, he would become depressed. Although he was consciously casual in his relations with women, Mr. Y suffered unconsciously from guilt about rejecting them. Indeed, he wished unconsciously for the analyst to help him to overcome the feelings of guilt and depression he experienced after rejecting them. The analyst, however, did not understand Mr. Y's motivations.

From the analyst's point of view, the patient's problem with women was similar to his earlier problem about work; that is, it reflected an Oedipal conflict that made him afraid of success.

The analyst, therefore, interpreted the patient's ambivalence to a particular girlfriend in Oedipal terms. He suggested to the patient that he liked the girl, but was afraid to let things work out for fear of hurting him (the analyst). The patient, after the hour in which the analyst offered this interpretation, went to his girlfriend's apartment and had intercourse with her. After that he had a frightening and unpleasant experience: He found himself remembering with unusual vividness the smell of his mother's nude body. He became anxious and broke away from his girlfriend. He also became discouraged with the analysis, and was tempted to stop it. However, instead of stopping, he withdrew emotionally for several months, during which he attempted to hide his discouragement by a cheerful display of pseudonormal behavior.

As Mr. Y later became aware, he had been traumatized by the analyst's Oedipal interpretation about his girlfriend. He had experienced the interpretation as implying that he was fond of his girlfriend and as suggesting to him that he should remain attached to her. Indeed, he had experienced this interpretation as, in childhood, he had experienced his father's insistence that he remain attached to his mother. Moreover, he had experienced it as confirming the pathogenic idea that he would not be able—and should not attempt—to become independent of women.

Mr. Y's recovery from the analyst's error is instructive. After marking time for about 3 months, Mr. Y began once more to become involved with women. He treated them as before, rejecting a woman as soon as she became interested in him. The analyst, who had become aware of his error, now attempted to demonstrate to the patient that, though he was consciously comfortable about rejecting women, he was warding off considerable unconscious worry about them. According to the analyst's interpretations, Mr. Y suffered unconsciously from an exaggerated worry about women. This worry was based on the omnipotent idea, which the patient had acquired in his childhood relation to his mother, that if he were at all independent with a woman he would hurt her.

Mr. Y reacted favorably to the analyst's interpretations, and he became more trusting of the analyst. He became more conscious of his previously repressed worry about women and less worried about them. He became conscious, too, of his intense childhood sense of responsibility for his mother. As Mr. Y became less worried about women, he developed a good relationship with a woman. He then began to face his Oedipal conflicts.

7

DREAMS AND THEIR VARIOUS PURPOSES

JOSEPH WEISS

In this chapter I shall present observations about dreams that support the theory of the mind proposed in this book. This theory was developed mainly from observations of the behavior of the analytic patient. However, a theory of the mind would rest on a weak foundation unless it could account for important phenomena, such as dreams, which are different from the phenomena it was developed to explain. Moreover, a theory of the mind that did not account well for dreams would be of little or no interest to analysts. As stated in Chapter 1, an investigator, in developing a theory, should cast a wide net; he should use whatever evidence is pertinent, including informal observations as well as observations obtained in rigorous research.

In the present chapter I shall attempt to show that dreams reflect the same processes as those underlying the behavior of the patient during analytic treatment. They are products of the dreamer's thoughts (his higher mental functions), and they reflect the dreamer's unconscious concerns, as well as his plans and policies for dealing with these concerns. Moreover, the dreamer exerts control over his unconscious mental life. He regulates the production of dreams in accordance with the criteria of safety and danger.

My thesis may be put in the language of Freud's tripartite model as follows: The ego produces dreams in an attempt to deal adaptively with its problems, including those that arise from the demands on it of the instincts, of conscience, and of current reality. It produces dreams as part of its task of self-preservation.

My conception of dream formation rests ultimately on observation. However, this conception is compatible with certain ideas that Freud stated, but did not develop fully, in certain of his late works and that have subsequently been discussed by other writers.

A BRIEF HISTORY OF FREUD'S IDEAS
ABOUT DREAM FORMATION

Freud based his original theory of dream formation on the automatic functioning hypothesis. In *The Interpretation of Dreams* (1900), in which Freud presented his original theory in considerable detail, he assigned the ego a relatively small part in the formation of dreams. He assumed here that dreams express a primitive mental process (the primary process) in which unconscious wishes seek gratification by cathecting memories of gratification (p. 566); for example, the hungry infant hallucinates the image of the mother's breast.

In the primary process as Freud defined it, infantile wishes seek gratification in hallucinatory images in which they are depicted as fulfilled. This process is regulated by the pleasure principle and is carried out automatically without regard for thought, belief, or assessment of current reality. Freud stated explicitly in *The Interpretation of Dreams* that although dreams may contain judgments, criticisms, appreciations, explanations, or arguments, the thought processes which produce them are not an essential part of the formation of dreams. Thus, Freud wrote: *"Everything that appears in dreams as the ostensible activity of the function of judgment is to be regarded not as an intellectual achievement of dream work, but as belonging to the material of the dream-thoughts and as having been lifted from them into the manifest content of the dreams as a ready-made structure"* (1900, p. 445, italics Freud's).

Freud, however, assumed here that the production of dreams is regulated to a certain extent by considerations of danger and safety. He argued that the censor (he later assigned the censor's task to the ego) may permit repressed impulses to find expression in dreams because it has turned off the power of motility so that impulses unable to find expression in action may be allowed to become conscious without danger to the dreamer.

In discussing particular dreams (1900), Freud was not confined by his theory of dream formation. He implied, but did not state explicitly, that certain dreams are formed not automatically but by unconscious thought and that their purpose is not wish fulfillment but preparation for action. For example, in his discussion of examination dreams, Freud assumed that the dreamer unconsciously anticipates a certain task (similar to the examination) that he fears he will not be able to carry out successfully. In the dream he remembers that sometime in the past he had worried about a similar task but had carried it out successfully. He thereby reassures himself about the impending task. In Freud's words: "It would seem then that anxious examination dreams (which, as has been confirmed over and over again, appear when the dreamer has some responsible activity ahead of him next day and is afraid there may be a fiasco) search for some occasion in the past in which great anxiety has turned out to be unjustified and has been contradicted by the event" (1900, p. 274).

Examination dreams are intended not to fulfill an infantile wish but to reduce anxiety about an impending task. They are therefore oriented to reality and are a preparation for real action. The dreamer, in creating an examination dream, makes prominent use of a kind of thought process that the id is unable to carry out. The dreamer anticipates the impending task and, in the light of certain past achievements, assesses his capacity to carry it out. The dreamer's purpose is to prepare himself for the upcoming task by offering himself encouragement. Thus the dreamer, in producing an examination dream, does something that in the *Outline* Freud assumed is done by the ego.

Freud's discussion of examination dreams anticipated developments in the theory of dreams that he did not make explicit and general until the *Outline*. Freud changed his theory of dream formation gradually. His first change, a relatively modest one, concerned the production of punishment dreams. Such dreams are challenges to Freud's earlier view, because in both their manifest and latent contents they are so unpleasant. If a dream is so unpleasant, how can it be regarded as the fulfillment of an infantile libidinal wish? Freud solved this problem by maintaining that punishment dreams are wish fulfillments, but that they fulfill wishes derived not from the system Unconscious, but from the unconscious ego (in particular from the part of the ego that Freud was later to refer to as the superego). Punishment dreams, according to Freud, suggest that the ego may contribute more to the formation of dreams than heretofore recognized.

It must be admitted that their recognition means in a certain sense a new addition to the theory of dreams. What is fulfilled in them is equally an unconscious wish, namely a wish that the dreamer may be punished for a repressed and forbidden wishful impulse. To that extent dreams of this kind fall in with the condition that has been laid down here that the motive force for constructing a dream must be provided by a wish belonging to the unconscious. A closer psychological analysis, however, shows how they differ from other wishful dreams. In the cases forming Group B [dreams in which distressing dream-thoughts make their way into the manifest content of the dreams] the dream-constructing wish is an unconscious one and belongs to the repressed, while in punishment-dreams, though it is equally an unconscious one, it must be reckoned as belonging not to the repressed but to the "ego." Thus, punishment-dreams indicate the possibility that the ego may have a greater share than was supposed in the construction of the dreams. . . . The essential characteristic of punishment-dreams would thus be that in their case the dream-constructing wish is not an unconscious wish derived from the repressed (from the system *Ucs.*), but a punitive one reacting against it and belonging to the ego, though at the same time an unconscious (that is to say, preconscious) one. (added to *The Interpretation of Dreams* [1900] in 1919, pp. 556–558)

The next change Freud made in his theory of dreams was more fundamental. It was inspired by certain dreams of patients suffering from traumatic neuroses, who in these dreams relived the painful and frightening traumatic experiences from which their neuroses arose. Such dreams, Freud wrote, inevitably lead the dreamer back to the situation in which the trauma occurred (1920). Such dreams are concerned with experiences which, as Freud pointed out, are not and could never have been pleasurable. They cannot be conceptualized as regulated by the pleasure principle, as expressing an infantile wish arising in the unconscious, or as the expression of an unconscious wish for punishment. They are, Freud concluded, motivated by a wish for mastery, a wish Freud was later to assign to the ego. Indeed, Freud was later to emphasize the importance of the task of mastering external and internal stimuli by considering it among those things the ego does in the interest of self-preservation (1940a, pp. 145–146).

Freud, in 1920, stated directly that traumatic dreams are an exception to the proposition that dreams are wish fulfillments: "It is impossible to classify as wish-fulfillments the dreams we have been discussing which occur in traumatic neuroses or the dreams, during psychoanalysis, which bring back to memory the psychical traumas of childhood" (p. 32).

Freud stated directly, too, that traumatic dreams are not produced in accordance with the pleasure principle: "We may assume, rather, that dreams are here helping to carry out another task which must be accomplished before the dominance of the pleasure principle can even begin. These dreams are endeavoring to master the stimulus retrospectively, by developing the anxiety whose omission was the cause of the traumatic neuroses" (1920, p. 22).

In the *Outline* Freud presented his entire theory of dream formation in a mere seven pages and he discussed the ego's part in the formation of dreams in just two or three paragraphs. About the ego's role, he wrote that though the motive for the formation of dreams may originate in the id or in the ego, it is the ego that produces dreams. He maintained his earlier view that dreams are wish fulfillments, but offered a new explanation of how in a dream a wish becomes fulfilled. In *The Interpretation of Dreams* Freud had assumed that infantile wishes, as a consequence of automatic processes, may be depicted as fulfilled. In the *Outline*, however, Freud stated that certain wishes (which may or may not be infantile), as a consequence of a decision made by the ego, may be depicted as fulfilled.

As regards the ego's part in the formation of dreams, Freud wrote in the *Outline* (1940a):

It remains for us to give a dynamic explanation of why the sleeping ego takes on the task of the dream-work at all. The explanation is fortunately easy to find. With the help of the unconscious, every dream that is in process of formation makes a demand upon the ego—for the satisfaction of an instinct, if the dream originates from the id; for the solution of a conflict, the removal of a doubt or the forming of an intention, if the dream originates from a residue of preconscious activity in waking life. The sleeping ego, however, is focused on the wish to maintain sleep; it feels this demand as a disturbance and seeks to get rid of the disturbance. The ego succeeds in doing this by what appears to be an act of compliance: it meets the demand with what is in the circumstances a harmless *fulfilment of a wish* and so gets rid of it. (pp. 169-170)

Freud illustrated this ego activity by three examples, one of which was: "A need for food makes itself felt in a dreamer during his sleep: he has a dream of a delicious meal and sleeps on. The choice, of course, is open to him either of waking up and eating something or continuing to sleep. He *decided* in favor of the latter and satisfied his hunger by means of the dream" (1940a, p. 170, italics mine).

Since Freud, other analysts have written that the ego plays a central part in the formation of dreams. For example, according to Arlow and Brenner, "It [the structural theory] postulates that ego functions, in this case defenses and integrative functions, participate in the dream work throughout its course" (1964, p. 135). Moreover, "We expect to learn from the analysis of our patient's dreams about the nature of the fears associated with their instinctual wishes, about their unconscious need to punish themselves, and even about the defenses which at the moment they are unconsciously employing in their struggles against their wishes" (p. 141). I shall add that we also expect to learn about the patient's pathogenic beliefs, his unconscious plans, policies, purposes, and goals.

Thomas French went even further than Arlow and Brenner. He emphasized the problem-solving function of dreams: "We have postulated that the dream work, like the thought processes directing our ordinary waking activity, is dominated by the need to find a solution for a problem" (1954, p. 15).

DREAMS OF PRISONERS OF WAR AND THEIR ADAPTIVE FUNCTIONS

The pertinence of the concept that the ego produces dreams and that it does so for certain vitally important adaptive purposes (such as warning, consoling, or working for mastery) is evident from the study of persons who are under great stress or who have undergone great stress. It was from his observations of patients with traumatic neuroses that Freud discovered that dreams may be produced by the ego as part of its task of mastering excitation. Extreme situations are, in general, likely to reveal factors that may not be obvious under normal circumstances. In situations where survival is at stake, the great part played in the production of dreams by the ego (which Freud tells us in the *Outline* is responsible for self-preservation) is particularly clear.

The part played by the ego in the production of dreams may be illustrated by dreams of former prisoners of war. My account here of such dreams is based on a study carried out by Dr. Paul Balson while he was Director of Psychiatric Research at Letterman Army Hospital (1975). Balson studied the dreams of five former prisoners of war, each of whom was interviewed intensively and three of whom received psychotherapy. Balson's procedure of studying the veterans' dreams years after they were produced seems justified for the following reasons: The dreams had been especially vivid in their imagery, and had made such powerful impressions on the veterans that they were confident that they remembered their dreams fairly accurately. In addition, the dreams were typical; all five tended to produce the same kinds of dreams. It seems highly unlikely that the five veterans would distort their memories of their dreams in the same ways.

The veterans produced a variety of dreams. However, I shall confine my discussion to three kinds, each of which was both typical and adaptive. (Each veteran, of course, did not necessarily produce all three kinds of dreams.) The three kinds of dreams corresponded, respectively, to three quite different (and, in each case, stressful) situations in which the veterans found themselves. These were the situations of the soldiers (1) before their capture, (2) during prolonged imprisonment in which they were mistreated, and (3) after their release from prison camp. The fact that in each of these situations the soldiers produced typical dreams suggests that each situation was so compelling that the feelings it mobilized (and the tasks it required the soldiers to perform) more or less overrode individual differences.

In Balson's opinion, each of the three kinds of dreams that the veterans produced was adaptive: "In all of these subjects these distinctive dream styles and patterns clearly enabled each individual prisoner to adapt to each successive stage of this prolonged and multifaceted psychological and physical trauma. The value of these dreams and their sequential patterning before, during, and immediately following the captivity appeared beyond objective or subjective refutation" (1975, p. 21).

WARNING DREAMS OF PRISONERS OF WAR

Before he was captured, a soldier who was exposed to the danger of capture typically produced frightening dreams that he was being captured. This kind of dream may be described as a warning dream. It performs in sleep the same function as, according to Sharpe (1950), certain fantasies foretelling danger perform in waking life. In warning dreams, the dreamer, to use Sharpe's phrase, is producing a "cautionary tale." The dreamer tells himself, "If I am not careful, I will be captured." The dream, as Freud told us in *The Interpretation of Dreams* (1900), has no way of representing such conjunctions as "if" in pictorial form. The best the dream can do to represent the possibility of capture is to depict the situation of capture.

The soldier's warning dream is adaptive. It orients him throughout the night to the grave danger he is facing, and it thereby prepares him for it. In Balson's (1975) words:

It can reasonably be assumed that the dream patterns from the period of time prior to capture . . . provided evidence of ego adaptive maneuvers directed towards enabling the individual to prepare for anticipated major environmental alterations, e.g., "I kept dreaming of death . . . being trapped in a burning helicopter . . . when I actually was burned and captured it seemed almost familiar somehow . . . almost expected." (p. 18)

The warning dream performs its function whether or not it is interpreted or the dreamer is able to explain its meaning. (In Balson's examples, the soldiers understood the meaning of their warning dreams.) It keeps the dreamer aware of the possibility of capture and, by preventing him from sleeping too soundly, may make him more able to react adaptively to the danger of capture and therefore be less vulnerable to capture.

A soldier's dream of being captured cannot readily be explained as the direct expression of an infantile wish. This is because the possibility of capture is, to the soldier, terrifying. He could, if captured, be killed. A dream of being captured could, of course, be explained as the direct expression of an unconscious wish for punishment. However, such an explanation is implausible. It either fails to connect the soldier's dangerous situation with his dreams, or it assumes that soldiers in danger of capture typically develop a wish to be punished by being captured. Moreover, a much more compelling explanation is at hand, which assumes that the dream is produced by the ego as a warning to the dreamer. According to this assumption, the ego, in producing a warning dream, is carrying out the same vital function that it carries out in waking life when it produces an anxiety signal. It carries out this function, as Freud tells us in the *Outline* (1940a), as part of its task of self-preservation.

BLISSFUL DREAMS OF PRISONERS OF WAR

Immediately after capture a soldier typically produced traumatic dreams in which he relived the circumstances of his capture. However, after prolonged internment (in which the soldiers were treated badly) he produced blissful dreams of gratification, of power, or of being serene.

The theory presented in *The Interpretation of Dreams* is able to some extent to explain the captured soldier's production of blissful dreams, but it cannot explain it completely. The theory of *The Interpretation of Dreams* assumes that dreams are produced when powerful unconscious wishes that cannot find gratification in action find gratification instead in hallucinatory wish fulfillment. That theory assumes, moreover, that the process by which dreams are formed (the flowback of excitation to perception) is regulated automatically by the pleasure principle without regard for the dreamer's unconscious beliefs or his unconscious assessments of his current reality. That theory accounts well for the content of the captured soldier's blissful dream. A soldier, after a prolonged and tortured stay in prison camp, no doubt felt intensely deprived and frustrated. He no doubt longed to be gratified, powerful, or serene. He could not satisfy this wish in reality. He could satisfy it in his dreams by depicting it as fulfilled.

The theory presented in *The Interpretation of Dreams*, however, cannot account for the observation that a soldier did not produce blissful dreams either before his capture or after he had escaped. The soldier in the field who was in danger of being captured should have had as strong a wish to be gratified, powerful, or serene as the soldier after his capture, yet he produced not blissful dreams but warning dreams.

Moreover, both the content and the timing of the captured soldier's blissful dreams are well explained by the concept that the dreamer (or his ego) regulates the production of dreams and does so for an adaptive purpose. The dreamer, according to my formulation, assesses his situation. He concludes that he cannot change it; his fate has been taken out of his hands, so that he has nothing to lose by temporarily relinquishing any efforts to further his cause. The dreamer then decides to permit a blissful dream. He carries out a policy of denial. By producing such a dream, the dreamer not only denies his present situation, he offers himself consolation and a measure of hope. The decision of the dreamer to produce such a dream is adaptive, and its value does not depend on the dreamer's conscious understanding of it. This is because a blissful dream, by relaxing the dreamer, helps him to indulge in a deep sleep and thus to restore himself. It permits him to relax without putting him in any more danger than he is already facing, and it offers the dreamer a measure of hope during a period of despair.

In Balson's view, too, the soldiers' blissful dreams were adaptive: "The dreams functioned as partial attempts at mastery. When the subject was being severely deprived, propagandized, or physically abused and tortured, the dreams would be seen as an escape and as a means of 'gaining back my strength to go on'" (1975, p. 12). In one dream reported by Balson, a soldier who had been made to feel extremely helpless pictured himself as powerful and able to eat, drink, and have sex according to his wishes. He enjoyed the dream immensely, stating, "I felt so serene and powerful" (p. 12).

TRAUMATIC DREAMS OF PRISONERS OF WAR

After he was released and was out of danger, a soldier typically produced the kind of traumatic dreams that Freud referred to in *Beyond the Pleasure Principle* (1920). In these dreams the soldier repeated the frightening experiences of his life in prison camp. As Freud (1920) has convincingly argued, traumatic dreams of this kind are not produced in accordance with the pleasure principle. They repeat experiences that are not and could never have been pleasurable. Their purpose may be self-punishment; escaped prisoners may suffer from survivor guilt. However, Freud emphasized another function of traumatic dreams, which he considered more fundamental than the attainment of pleasure: It is to master traumatic experiences. This purpose (mastery) is, in the *Outline* (1940a), ascribed to the ego, which, according to Freud, seeks mastery of its inner and outer world as part of its task of self-preservation.

Repetition for mastery, as Freud (1920) pointed out, is a part of children's play. A child who has suffered a trauma passively attempts by repeating it actively to master it. However, an adult's reaction to a trauma is not so different from a child's. An adult who, for example, has been traumatized by an automobile accident may, after the accident, become preoccupied with it. He may spend a great deal of time mentally reviewing the circumstances of the accident. He may even go to the scene of the accident to better understand just how it came about. Moreover, he may develop a neurosis. He may become quite anxious about driving, or he may be temporarily unwilling or unable to drive.

How does the driver develop this problem, and how, by going over it in his mind, does he work to solve it? According to my thesis, an adult driver may react to an accident in much the same way as a child may react to a traumatic experience. Both may develop a neurosis. Moreover, they may develop their neuroses in much the same way: by developing a pathogenic belief. The driver may develop a pathogenic belief about his responsibility for the accident and about the likelihood that he will suffer a similar accident in the future. He may also partially repress the pathogenic belief, as well as the circumstances of the accident and the feelings of horror he was in danger of experiencing at the time of the accident. Thus, after the accident the traumatized driver may not be able to understand just how it happened, not only because he did not have the attention at the time to encompass it, but also because he has repressed his memories of it. A driver who has repressed his traumatic memories of an accident may maintain his repressions for varying lengths of time. He may remain calm and avoid thinking about the accident for just a few hours, until he is in the security of his home, surrounded by his family. He may then begin to lift his repressions and bring forth the circumstances of the accident and the previously repressed feelings of terror and horror. Or he may repress the memories of the accident for a much longer time. Eventually, however, the driver, by repeatedly going over the details of the accident, may permit himself, in a gradual and controlled manner and at his own pace, to face the circumstances of the accident and to remember the terror and horror. He ordinarily permits himself to remember the accident and to face these feelings only as rapidly as he can safely do so. He may, by gradually facing his feelings, become able to lift the repressions warding off the traumatic experience, to become conscious of and master the emotions connected with the experience, and to bring forth and change the pathogenic beliefs derived from it.

The soldier, whose primary task during prolonged internment was to console himself and to keep himself hopeful, faced an entirely different kind of task once he had escaped. His greatly improved situation now gave him the security and strength to face the same kind of task as the driver had faced after the accident, which was to master his traumatic experiences. According to Balson (1975):

The traumatic dreams of reliving which occurred immediately following capture and immediately following release clearly appeared to serve the same adaptive and restorative psychological functions as any dream pattern characteristic of a period of intense stress or trauma. These traumatic dreams of reliving appeared to allow the individual an opportunity for partial psychological mastery and affect expression in relationship to the traumatic events. (p. 19)

The soldier's task was similar to that of the driver, but more difficult. The soldier was more severely traumatized than the driver. He experienced more horror and terror. His repressions were deeper, and his pathogenic beliefs (which, as Balson pointed out, may include the belief that he was captured as a punishment for some wrongdoing) were more dire.

The soldier, like the moviegoer, kept the traumatic experiences repressed until he was out of danger. Then he attempted, by repetitively going over the experiences of his capture and imprisonment, to master them. However, at first he kept the repressions intact during his waking life and began the task of lifting them only in his dreams. The soldier's beginning this crucial task in his dreams is an example of my thesis that in dreams a person expresses his major unconscious plans, purposes, and goals.

Both the soldier's repression of his traumatic experiences while in danger and his attempts to lift his repressions once safe were adaptive. During an emergency it is adaptive for a person to institute repressions to prevent himself from being paralyzed by overwhelming feelings. However, it is equally adaptive for him after an emergency has passed to lift the repressions. It is only by lifting his repressions that a person may gain a clear understanding of the horrifying traumatic events he has experienced. He may then, by understanding these traumas, overcome both the emotions connected with them and the pathogenic beliefs inferred from them.

DREAMS AS THE EXPRESSION OF POLICY

Each of the kinds of dreams discussed above is about the dreamer's major current concerns and each expresses the dreamer's (or his ego's) policy toward these concerns. The chief concern of the soldier before capture was the danger of being captured. His policy toward the danger as he expressed it in his warning dreams was "Be careful!" The chief concern of the soldier after prolonged capture was his despair and hopelessness. His policy toward this despair, as expressed in his blissful dreams, was to offer himself denial, consolation, and hope. (The soldier's blissful dreams should not be regarded simply as a maladaptive turning away from reality. Such dreams do turn the dreamer away from reality. However, in a hopeless situation, denying current concerns and offering oneself a degree of hope may be adaptive.) The chief concern of the escaped soldier was to overcome the effects of the experiences he had been through. In his traumatic dreams he expressed a policy toward these concerns and began to carry it out; he told himself, "Remember the experiences you have been through, understand them, and master the feelings and ideas which they aroused in you." Examination dreams, too, illustrate my thesis that in his dreams a dreamer expresses a policy. In an examination dream the dreamer encourages himself by telling himself, "Don't take your worries so seriously!"

For each of the kinds of dreams discussed above (but not in all kinds of dreams) the plot or story of the dream contributes to its meaning. The story carries the message the dreamer must convey to himself and creates the mood or affect the dreamer needs to experience. Such was the case, too, in the example reported by Freud in the *Outline* of the dreamer who appeased his appetite by dreaming that he was eating a meal. The fact that this dream of eating was in visual imagery and hence closer to experience than verbal thought helped the dream to perform its function of appeasing the dreamer's appetite and enabling him to sleep.

Such was the case, too, in the dreams produced by the former prisoners of war. These, Balson tells us, were depicted in especially vivid visual imagery. The vividness of these dreams may reflect the urgency of the task which the dreams were intended to perform. A vivid realistic dream about being captured may serve as a more effective warning than a pallid and vague dream, and more effective still than the verbal thought "Be careful or you will be captured." Similarly, a vivid realistic dream of a situation in which he is satisfied, powerful, or serene may be a greater balm to a troubled soldier's spirits than a pallid, vague one and a greater balm still than a verbal thought such as, "Console yourself by forgetting your troubles." Indeed, the soldier, during such a dream and even after awakening, may experience some of the relaxation and happiness he would feel if he really were in the situation his dream depicts.

The vividness of the escaped soldier's dreams may also be adaptive. His vivid dreams about the circumstances of his capture and of his life in prison camp may help him to remember and ultimately to master these experiences better than his conscious attempts to remember them.

The dreams discussed above, as already noted, perform their functions whether or not the dreamer is able consciously to interpret them. The soldier who, before capture, dreamed that he was being captured, was reminded in his dreams of his chief danger and indeed his chief concern—capture. He was warned of this danger whether or not he consciously wished to be warned of it, and whether or not he consciously recognized that to be warned of danger was the purpose of the dream. He was, in addition, induced by the dream to sleep lightly and thus to be more alert to danger.

The soldier who, after capture, permitted himself blissful dreams, was offering himself consolation and enabling himself to enjoy a deep and restful sleep. He consoled himself whether or not he consciously wished for consolation, and whether or not he consciously realized that to console himself was the purpose of the dream.

The soldier who, after his escape, dreamed of the circumstances of his capture, was beginning to do the work he needed to do to overcome the effects of his traumatic experiences. He was beginning to do this work whether or not he consciously wanted to do it or consciously realized that he was doing it. Similarly, the person who, according to Freud, dreamed of eating to appease his appetite and so was enabled to remain asleep was helped by his dream to stay asleep whether or not he consciously understood the meaning of the dream.

THE SUBJECT MATTER OF DREAMS

A person's dreams, as I have said, reflect his chief concerns, in particular those concerns that he is unable by conscious thought alone to sort out or put in perspective, or toward which he is unable consciously to develop a policy or plan. A person, for various reasons, may be unable by conscious thought alone to deal successfully with certain problems. The veterans whose dreams I have just described could not by conscious thought alone deal successfully with their problems because their problems were so overwhelming. Likewise, a person may be unable by conscious thought to deal successfully with a problem because, as a result of his repressions, he cannot permit himself consciously to face it. In either case, a person who cannot deal successfully with a crucial problem consciously may attempt to deal with it in his dreams.

The dreams of analytic patients generally reflect problems that the patient cannot face as a consequence of his repressions. Therefore, during a period of his analysis in which he is working unconsciously to solve a particular problem, a patient may produce a particular kind of dream. After he has succeeded in making that problem conscious and has acquired the capacity to deal with it successfully by conscious thought, he may stop producing that kind of dream.

Such was the case in the analysis of Mr. Q, who, for a time during his treatment, was not conscious of his profound distrust of the analyst. During that period, he produced dreams in which he warned himself that, were he to trust the analyst, he would put himself in a situation of danger. After he became conscious of his distrust of the analyst and was able consciously to tolerate not trusting him, he stopped producing such dreams.

Mr. Q was a successful businessman whose childhood problem was similar in certain ways to that of the typical case presented by Freud in the *Outline* (1940a). Mr. Q was the son of young parents and their only son until he was 5 years old, when his younger sister was born. Like the patient described in the *Outline*, Mr. Q in early childhood was close to his mother and interested in her sexually. His mother would take him into her bed when his father, an insurance executive, was away on a business trip. Mr. Q dreaded his father's return, not only because it meant that he had to stop sleeping with his mother, but because he hated and feared his father.

Mr. Q described his father as cruel, punitive, and rejecting. Mr. Q was competitive with his father and assumed that his father was competitive with him. Moreover, he assumed that his father was envious of his close relationship with his mother, for, as he experienced it, his mother preferred him to his father.

In short, Mr. Q developed a typical Oedipal constellation as described by Freud. He also developed typical castration anxiety. He literally (as opposed to metaphorically) believed that he would be castrated for his sexual interest in his mother. He did not remember being threatened with castration by either of his parents, but he did remember that his uncle, a pediatrician, threatened to castrate him if he did not stop squirming during a physical exam.

Mr. Q, during the period of his analysis on which I shall report, repeated with the analyst the childhood conflicts about trust that he had experienced with his father. During this period the patient consciously admired the analyst and wanted to like and trust him. He believed that unless he liked and trusted the analyst he would not be successfully analyzed. He also wanted to experience with the analyst closeness such as he had been unable to experience with his father. Unconsciously, however, Mr. Q was deeply distrustful of the analyst. He felt intensely guilty about his distrust, and was afraid to experience it. He unconsciously feared that were he to experience or express it, he would hurt the analyst and thus provoke punishment and rejection from him.

Although Mr. Q was struggling consciously to like the analyst, he wished unconsciously to overcome his fear of him and his need to placate him by being compliant, noncompetitive, and admiring.

During the period of his analysis described above, Mr. Q would wake up early with frightening dreams on the days he was to see the analyst (two or three times a week). Often he would be unable to get back to sleep. Mr. Q's associations to the dreams made it clear that the dreams were intended to warn him that although the analyst might appear friendly and trustworthy, he was in fact malicious and not to be trusted.

In one such dream the patient depicted the analyst as a friendly, pleasant plantation owner who genially led the patient on a tour of his mansion but who was indifferent to the misery of the slaves, who were being tortured in their quarters. In another dream, the patient depicted himself as a young circus performer and the analyst as an older performer who told the patient about a fantastic stunt. If the patient and the older performer had attempted this stunt, the patient would have been injured or killed and the older performer would have been completely safe.

Mr. Q produced warning dreams of this kind for about two months. As he became able, with the analyst's help, to consciously tolerate both his distrust of the analyst and his contempt for him, he stopped having this kind of dream. He had no need for such dreams after he realized that he was required neither to like the analyst nor to comply with him, and that he could reject any of the analyst's comments with which he did not agree.

During this period of his analysis, Mr. Q prepared himself unconsciously for his analytic sessions by reminding himself in his dreams about his belief that the analyst was not to be trusted.

In the next example, the patient, an analytic candidate, prepared himself in a dream for an analytic session by offering himself reassurance that he could not permit himself consciously to feel. The patient, who had developed a father transference, had been wary about telling the analyst about his successes with women. He feared consciously that by bragging to the analyst he would make him jealous, as he believed he had made his father jealous. He had begun to realize that his conception of the analyst as vulnerable stemmed from a father transference, but he had been unable consciously to retain an image of the analyst as strong and generous.

In his dream the patient was watching in a matter of fact way as one of his own patients, a young PhD student, made love with a girlfriend in a park. As the dreamer's associations made clear, one purpose of the dream was to prepare the dreamer to tell the analyst about his sexual relationship with his own girlfriend. He was enjoying it and feared that in describing it to the analyst, he would make the analyst jealous. In the dream, he told himself, "Since I am not jealous when watching my patient making love, I should assume that my analyst will not be jealous when hearing about my lovemaking."

In the following example, a patient, Mr. K, produced a series of terrifying warning dreams. They all had the same message: that if he were to break away from his mother by dating a woman, he would kill his mother. The patient understood his dreams. He had been conscious of his separation guilt, but not of its intensity. He was made aware by his dreams of the intensity of his guilt. He experienced the dreams as telling him that he was not yet ready to form a heterosexual relationship.

The patient, a professional musician in his 30s, decided during his analysis to struggle against his homosexuality by forcing himself to have sexual relations with women. Early in life, the patient had developed a symbiotic relationship with his mother, whom he described as highly emotional, angry, seductive, and possessive. She would sleep with the patient when his father, a remote figure, was out of town. She would also, at times, punish the patient by beating him.

Mr. K was almost conscious of his belief that, were he to develop a sexual relationship with a woman, he would kill his mother, whom he believed lived primarily for him. He decided, largley out of unconscious compliance to the analyst and despite great anxiety, to date an attractive woman he met at work. Almost immediately after starting to date her, he began to have horrible nightmares of his mother dying. Mr. K visualized his mother, emaciated and pale, lying in her coffin, calling him in a weird voice to return to her. The nightmares were so vivid and frightening that the patient dreaded going to sleep, and they continued until the patient stopped dating the woman. Mr. K was able to interpret his dreams himself; he knew consciously that their message was untrue. Yet his dreams were so vivid, realistic, and terrifying that he could not ignore them.

Punishment dreams, along with warning dreams and encouragement dreams, are relatively common. They are much more common, for example, than blissful dreams, which are relatively rare. (A person, in my experience, may produce a blissful dream in two circumstances: if he is without hope and thus is in no danger of being lulled into a false sense of security, or if he assumes that a certain important person is watching over him and protecting him from danger.)

In the following dream, which is a punishment dream, the dreamer, who felt guilty about defeating his rivals, attempted to relieve himself of his guilt by a dream in which he turned the tables on himself, and so identified with the victim.

An analytic patient in his 20s attained a position that he expected would put him in the center of a number of interesting activities while relegating his rivals to the sidelines. He felt guilty about his rivals. He found relief in a dream in which he depicted himself in the sixth grade, sitting with the girls from his class while watching the popular athletic boys compete in a baseball tournament.

ARE DREAMS FORMED AUTOMATICALLY
OR BY THE EGO? ABSURD DREAMS
AS A CASE IN POINT

In *The Interpretation of Dreams* (1900), Freud stated that two separate functions may be distinguished in mental activity during the construction of a dream: the production of the dream thoughts (day residues), and their transformation by the dream work into the dream. The mind, according to Freud, employs all of its faculties in the production of dream thoughts. These are normal (secondary process) thoughts that are formed in waking life by the preconscious and retain their charge of interest during sleep. These thoughts are concerned with various things, including problem solving and the forming of intentions. However, these thoughts are not an *essential* part of the dream, and the solutions they propose or the intentions they form are not part of the dream's interpretation.

The *essential* part of the dream, according to the theory presented in *The Interpretation of Dreams*, is the dream work. The dream work is not like normal thinking. Rather, it functions automatically in accordance with the laws governing the primary process. "The dream work is not simply less cautious, more careless, more irrational, more frightful, more forgetful, or more incomplete than waking thought: It is different from it qualitatively and for that reason not completely comparable with it. It does not think, calculate, or judge in any way at all; it restricts itself to giving things a new form" (1900, p. 507). The dream work, Freud tells us, is the *essence* of dreaming. "At bottom dreams are nothing more than a particular form of thinking made possible by the conditions of the state of sleep. It is the *dream work* which creates that form and it alone is the essence of dreaming" (1900, footnote, pp. 506–507).

Freud gradually changed his conception of dream formation. In the *Outline* he no longer assumed that dreams are formed automatically by the primary process, but rather that they are formed by the ego, which "takes on the task of the dream work" (1940a, p. 169).

The views proposed here, like Freud's views in the *Outline*, assume that the ego plays a central part in the construction of dreams, and that in forming them it makes use of thought similar to conscious thought. The ego may express its plans, purposes, and goals in dreams, and it may attempt to solve problems. Moreover, the plans, purposes, and goals that the ego expresses and the solutions to problems that it offers are an essential part of the meaning of dreams.

In order to compare Freud's early theory of dream formation with the theory he presented in the *Outline* and on which the views presented here are based, I shall discuss absurd dreams. In *The Interpretation of Dreams*, Freud conceived of the formation of absurd dreams as taking place in two steps: Before going to sleep, the person produces normal thoughts that contain an element of derision or criticism. Then the dream work, which does not function logically but by the primary process, transforms the thought into the dream, using absurdity to express the derision or criticism.

According to the views proposed here (which are compatible with those which Freud presented in the *Outline*), the use of absurdity in dreams is not the result of automatic processes, nor is it qualitatively different from its use in normal conscious thought (i.e., in the exercise of certain higher mental functions) and should be attributed not to the primary process but to the ego. The ego may use absurdity in dreams in a logical and normal way, just as it may in normal conscious argumentation in order to make a point. In some dreams the ego uses absurdity in a way which is akin to the method of logical proof employed by Greek geometers and called "reduction to absurdity." Such dreams have the structure of an argument: A particular premise that the dreamer would like to disprove is shown to lead to an absurd conclusion. This kind of dream may be illustrated by the following example:

Miss F, a woman in her early 20s, had, throughout childhood, been very close to her identical twin sister. She was, however, at the time of the dream, separating herself from her twin and experiencing considerable guilt. She had begun an affair but feared that this would hurt her sister. It was in these circumstances that Miss F produced a dream in which she pictured herself and her sister as married to one another and about to have a baby. She woke up thinking, "How absurd." As her associations made clear, the patient was by this dream telling herself that, however much she loved her sister, she would not be able to have a baby with her, and therefore that her happiness depended on leaving her sister and developing a relationship with a man.

In constructing this dream Miss F began with the premise that she should love her sister, and that she could in a love relationship with her achieve everything that she wanted in any relationship. In the dream, she proceeded to carry this premise to its logical conclusion, by depicting her sister and her having a baby, and she showed herself by the manifestly false conclusion that the premise she began with was false: She could not achieve with her sister everything that she wanted in a relationship. Miss F could not directly disavow her idea that she should seek happiness in her relationship with her sister to the exclusion of other relationships. However, she could reduce this idea to absurdity.

This dream no doubt expresses derision. However, it is best understood not primarily as the expression of an impulse toward derision but as a normal thought about a particular problem and directed to the solution of that problem. The derision is a part of the thought and an inherent part of its logic. Miss F used derision to mock a premise she had held out of guilt. Her purpose was to weaken the hold on her of this premise.

This dream illustrates a fundamental difference between Miss F's experience and the experience of the person who uses irony or reduction to absurdity in waking life: The difference is the dreamer's relative lack of self-observation. The dreamer generally does not know he is being ironic or using reduction to absurdity until after awakening.

A dream that, in my opinion (although not necessarily in the opinion of Dr. Renik) makes use of reduction to absurdity, has been reported by Owen Renik (1981, p. 159). He described a patient who out of guilt would falsely accuse herself of plagiarism. She dreamt that she stole a bicycle, but on waking up she remembered that it belonged to her. She thereby reduced to absurdity her idea that she was a plagiarist.

A young professional man was frequently worried that none of his hopes would be realized. Like his mother, who had often warned him to take advantage of his opportunities, he was afraid to stop worrying for fear that if he did so he would indeed miss some opportunity. In his dream, which he recognized as absurd, he sat down happily to a large, delicious meal, only to be disappointed when it walked away from him.

In this dream, the patient mocked his mother's teaching and, by doing so, reassured himself that he need not be constantly concerned with the possibility of losing his opportunities.

A young businessman, out of compliance to his father, believed that he should do everything scientifically, including choosing a wife. After he fell in love with an attractive woman he was inclined to forget his father's advice, but he could not quite bring himself to do so. However, as he came to understand his spiteful obedience to his father, he eventually became able to forget his father's advice and marry the woman. While he was working on this problem, the patient dreamt that he found himself in a store measuring numerous socks with a ruler to find the pair that fit him perfectly.

In general, a person who uses absurdity in his dreams also uses it in his waking thoughts. A good example of this occurred in the analysis of a young college student who had suffered a severe loss around her 13th year. Afterward, she developed the magical idea that unless she were worried about losing something which she valued, she would, in fact, lose it.

In the first year of her analysis, she began one hour by telling me in a worried voice that she was concerned about the four-month vacation I was about to take. However, after I had questioned her about it she made clear that she knew my vacation was to be only 3 weeks. Later in the same hour, the patient reported a recent dream in which she experienced an intense longing to be accepted at a certain university. After waking up she realized the dream was absurd because she was already in her junior year at that university. In both her dream and her waking thought she showed herself that her fear of loss was absurd.

In the following example, the dreamer reassures himself in a patently false way that his wife is healthy. Since the reassurance is false and indeed absurd, the purpose of the dream is not to reassure the dreamer but to warn him.

The patient, who was not completely aware of his worry about his wife, produced a dream that was simply a vivid image of a woman's torso endowed with large breasts. The patient's first comment on the dream was that he experienced the breasts as overwhelming, as though the woman were an Amazon. Then he thought that the dream image indicated how a woman's torso might have appeared to him when he was a young child.

Next the dreamer commented that his wife has large breasts and is quite proud of them. His wife, he then remembered, has seemed worried about herself lately. She has had a persistent unexplained fever and certain confusing symptoms. The patient then began to realize that he too has been worried about his wife but has been denying his worry about her.

It occurred to him then that the dream might express an attempt to reassure himself about his wife. However, further investigation revealed that it meant just the opposite. That is, it told the dreamer, "Though your wife is proud and sexy, she nonetheless may be ill and should see a doctor. Stop attempting to offer yourself false reassurances about her health!"

As the dreamer became aware of the meaning of the dream, he remembered something that he had not understood earlier; namely, that he had awakened from the dream with a feeling of anxiety appropriate to the dream's message: that he stop denying his worry.

I shall end this chapter with a dream that is akin to the dreams of prisoners of war, in that it occurred under extremely dire circumstances; it was vivid and realistic; its purpose—to offer consolation—was evident; and it offered great consolation and relief both at the time it was dreamt and for quite a while afterward.

The dreamer, a 30-year-old carpenter who was the father of two children, came to therapy after he killed his wife in a shooting accident while unloading a defective gun. The shooting was truly an accident, and the patient's wife died instantly. The patient, at the beginning of his treatment (which was not an analysis), was distraught and indeed suicidal. He felt intense grief and guilt. His therapist focused on the accidental nature of the killing and in various ways supported the patient in his struggle not to think of himself as a murderer. After 8 months of therapy, the patient attained enough relief of guilt to permit himself to produce the following vivid, realistic dream: "I accidentally shot my wife. She staggered to where I was sitting, then lay dying in my arms. As she was dying, she told me that she knew that my shooting her was accidental, and she forgave me for it."

The patient was able in this dream to offer himself much-needed relief and consolation. He kept the dream in mind for a long period of time. He reacted to the dream as though to a real event—that is, as though his wife had in fact forgiven him. He was relieved by the dream despite the fact that he knew it was only a dream and that his wife was dead and could not forgive him.

This dream makes apparent the power of dreams, with their vividness and closeness to experience, to carry a message to the dreamer. The patient could not offer himself comparable relief by simply telling himself, "My wife would surely forgive me." This dream, like the blissful dreams of captured soldiers, offered a desperate dreamer an experience he could remember and use to console himself for a long time after he produced it.

RESEARCH FINDINGS
A: INTRODUCTION

8

INTRODUCTION TO
THE RESEARCH PROBLEM

HAROLD SAMPSON

In Part II of this book we will describe how we tested the higher mental functioning hypothesis presented in Part I by formal empirical research. We will show how we investigated this broad, general hypothesis by testing the explanatory power of two particular hypotheses derived from it, namely, the hypothesis of unconscious control and the plan hypothesis. We tested each of these against a corresponding hypothesis based on the assumption of unconscious automatic functioning. We also tested each in its own right.

In testing a hypothesis against its alternative we asked: Which provides the better fit with observation? In testing a hypothesis in its own right we asked: Does this hypothesis reliably predict empirically observable events?

THE HYPOTHESES WE TESTED

THE HIGHER MENTAL FUNCTIONING HYPOTHESIS OF UNCONSCIOUS CONTROL

According to this hypothesis, a patient may exert some control unconsciously over his repressions. He may institute them, maintain them, or lift them. If he lifts them he may express in behavior the contents he had warded off by them and permit these contents to become conscious. In deciding whether or not to lift his repressions, and to express or experience the contents previously warded off by them, the patient is guided by his unconscious appraisal of whether he may safely do so. (The patient's purpose in deciding to make a content conscious or to express it in his behavior is, in general, to master it.)

Informal evidence was presented in Part I for the idea that a patient may lift the repressions opposing certain mental contents or relax the inhibitions opposing certain behaviors when he considers it safe to do so.

One example concerned Miss P, the lawyer who spontaneously retrieved certain previously repressed memories of parental rejection, after she had assured herself that the analyst would not reject her, as in her opinion her parents had rejected her. Knowing that the analyst would not reject her, she decided that she could safely face the repressed memories. Another example concerned Mrs. G, who criticized the analyst after she assured herself that she would not hurt him by doing so, as in her opinion she had hurt her father by criticizing him.

An alternative to the unconscious control hypothesis, the dynamic hypothesis, assumes unconscious automatic functioning. It provides a different explanation from the unconscious control hypothesis for the patient's experiencing or expressing previously repressed mental contents. According to this hypothesis a patient cannot control his repressions or inhibitions. These are regulated automatically by indications of pleasure and pain. Repressed contents may spontaneously either find expression in behavior or become conscious, as a consequence of shifts in the dynamic equilibrium between repressed and repressing forces. If the repressed forces are strengthened relative to the repressing forces, they may push forth to consciousness propelled by their own thrusts, or they may find expression in behavior in more or less well-disguised compromise formations.

We shall present a number of empirical studies (Chapters 11–14) that test the unconscious control hypothesis against the dynamic hypothesis by examining how well each accounts for an analytic patient spontaneously either becoming conscious of previously warded-off contents or expressing these contents more overtly in his behavior.

THE PLAN HYPOTHESIS

According to this hypothesis, the analytic patient makes and carries out plans (which are largely unconscious) to work in relation to the analyst at the task of solving his problems (Chapters 1, 5, and 6). He works to solve problems by changing pathogenic beliefs. He works to change pathogenic beliefs both by testing them in relation to the analyst and by assimilating insight into them conveyed to him by analytic interpretations.

The plan hypothesis provides a number of testable empirical consequences (Chapter 15). For example, it predicts that the analytic patient, unless pressed off course by the analyst, will work persistently during any given period of his analysis in a particular direction, that is, toward changing certain pathogenic beliefs and thereby attaining certain goals.

It predicts that the patient is likely to test certain pathogenic beliefs in relation to the analyst. It also predicts how the patient is likely to react to the analyst's responses to the tests. It assumes that the patient's reactions depend on whether he can use the analyst's responses (including the analyst's interpretations) in his struggle to move toward his immediate goals, or whether he feels impeded by them in his efforts to move toward these goals.

We will present a number of empirical studies (Chapters 16–20) that bear on the explanatory power of the plan hypothesis. We shall demonstrate (Chapter 16) that qualified judges, working independently of each other, can agree highly on the main features of a patient's unconscious plan. We will test predictions derived from the plan hypothesis about the patient's testing of the analyst (Chapters 17 and 18) and about the patient's responses to the analyst's comments and interpretations (Chapters 19, 20, and 22). Moreover, we will test the explanatory power of the plan hypothesis against the explanatory power of an alternative hypothesis that assumes unconscious automatic functioning (Chapters 18 and 20).

FORMAL RESEARCH METHODS

We tested the unconscious control hypothesis and the plan hypothesis by formal research methods, and thus by more systematic, specialized, and controlled methods of investigation than those used in most psychoanalytic studies. Formal research involves studies planned in advance to answer a particular question or to obtain evidence bearing on the answer. It requires that the data used in the study are public in the sense that they are accessible for review by independent investigators. It requires that classifications and ratings of the data be made reliably by judges working independently of each other. Finally, it requires that data analyses be made by explicit and public procedures. These conditions, in combination with others discussed in the next chapter, allow independent evaluation of the entire research process, and also facilitate attempts to replicate the work.

SIGNIFICANCE OF THE RESEARCH

The research tests the explanatory power of hypotheses that are central to the psychoanalytic theory of therapy and that also, in our opinion, explain the patient's behavior in other psychotherapies. Therefore, research on these hypotheses should be of interest both to psychoanalysts and to other mental health professionals.

The hypotheses we tested have practical as well as theoretical implications. They guide the practitioner's understanding of the patient's behavior in therapy, and they tell him how he may facilitate the patient's progress.

The research goes beyond clinical studies. It subjects psychoanalytic hypotheses about therapy to formal study. In doing so, it suggests that theoretical differences in our field, as in other sciences, may be resolved by rigorous investigations designed to test the explanatory powers of competing psychoanalytic hypotheses.

9

OUR RESEARCH APPROACH

HAROLD SAMPSON
JOSEPH WEISS

TESTING HYPOTHESES

INTRODUCTION

In carrying out our research into the psychoanalytic process we followed a course used successfully by investigators in other scientific fields but seldom by psychoanalytic investigators. This course is to test the power of certain broad hypotheses to explain significant data pertinent to the field.

In testing psychoanalytic hypotheses, we reason from hypotheses to empirical consequences. That is, we make certain predictions from our hypotheses and then devise procedures by which we may reliably determine whether these predictions are borne out by observation. In testing competing psychoanalytic hypotheses against one another, we follow a similar course. We deduce certain situations in which one hypothesis predicts a particular finding and a competing hypothesis predicts a different finding. Then we devise procedures to determine which hypothesis provides the more accurate predictions.

Our research approach grew out of the investigations of the psychoanalytic process that Weiss carried out informally in the studies from process notes, reported in Part I. In those investigations Weiss studied certain clinical phenomena in an attempt to determine how well alternative psychoanalytic hypotheses could explain them. For example, Weiss examined Miss P's spontaneous recovery of memories of parental rejection and showed that her recovery of these memories could be better explained by the assumptions of the higher mental functioning hypothesis than by the assumptions of the automatic functioning hypothesis. In the research reported here we have formalized the methods that Weiss had used informally.

DEDUCING EMPIRICAL CONSEQUENCES
FROM PSYCHOANALYTIC HYPOTHESES

The task of deducing testable consequences from psychoanalytic theory is similar to the task of deducing them from any scientific theory. It may be difficult. In many situations the same body of data may support competing hypotheses. However, it is the task of the psychoanalytic investigator to make such deductions and thus to find those points at which an hypothesis may be tested. Weiss suggested, in Part I, a number of points at which the automatic functioning hypothesis may be tested against the higher mental functioning hypothesis. In Part II, we have specified additional points in which these two hypotheses may be tested against one another, and we have described means of carrying out such tests.

In making deductions from a psychoanalytic hypothesis, it may be necessary to specify not one outcome but a class of outcomes or a series of alternative outcomes. This is because an hypothesized underlying process—for example, "the intensification of libidinal drives"—may be manifested in a number of different behaviors. The specification of outcomes is a less formidable problem than it may seem in the abstract. An underlying process, such as the intensification of libidinal drives, will be manifested in only a limited number of ways, each of which may be specifiable. For example, in the Menninger Psychotherapy Research Project, the following predictions were made: "Patients whose neurotic needs are not gratified within the transference respond to this frustration with regressive and/or resistive reactions and/or painful affects" (Sargent, Horwitz, Wallerstein, & Applebaum, 1968, p. 85).

According to these predictions, the nongratification of a patient's neurotic needs in the transference brings about a state of frustration, which may be expressed in the patient's behavior in just several ways. This prediction, which is based on the automatic functioning hypothesis, can be tested against observation. Indeed, as we shall report later (Chapter 18), we tested a significant part of it against a corresponding prediction of the higher mental functioning hypothesis.

The automatic functioning hypothesis bases its predictions about the nongratification of the patient's neurotic needs on the assumption that the patient, by expressing such needs, is attempting unconsciously to gratify certain unconscious impulses. It assumes therefore that the nongratification of these needs will produce *frustration, tension, and conflict*. The higher mental functioning hypothesis bases its predictions about the nongratification of the patient's neurotic needs on the assumption that the patient, by manifesting such needs, may be testing the analyst. It assumes therefore that in some circumstances the nongratification of a patient's needs may result in the *reduction of his anxiety and tension.* This is because in expressing his needs a patient may be testing the analyst by making unconscious demands on him that he hopes the analyst will not gratify. Thus, the two hypotheses make different predictions, which can be checked and compared by observation.

The investigator, in deducing empirical consequences from psychoanalytic hypotheses, is not following a well-traveled path. There is no strong tradition within psychoanalysis of deducing testable consequences from a particular hypothesis. The investigator, therefore, will not find a consensus among his colleagues about the correctness of his deductions. However, if psychoanalytic theory is meaningful, such deductions are possible, and if psychoanalytic theory is to be tested empirically, such deductions are necessary.

CASE-SPECIFIC METHODS

The hypotheses we are testing were derived by Weiss from numerous case studies, and they have been checked clinically by other members of our group. Although a hypothesis is derived from numerous studies on different kinds of patients, it is tested rigorously on one case at a time. As noted earlier, all of the empirical work in this book was carried out on the psychoanalysis of a single patient, Mrs. C.

Although our hypotheses are general, we test them on particular cases. In testing them on a particular case, we determine how they apply to that case. For example, if we are concerned with investigating how patients work to overcome their pathogenic beliefs, we must, in studying a particular patient, determine *that* patient's pathogenic beliefs, his particular plans for overcoming them, and the various ways he may test his beliefs in relation to the analyst.

The usual method of investigating the value of a particular kind of treatment is to study a large number of cases, some of which have been offered that kind of treatment, others of which have not. The value of the treatment may be determined by correlating the kind of treatment with its outcome. The method of treatment is the independent variable, the outcome the dependent variable, and the N is the number of cases studied. In single-case studies, such as ours, the independent variable and the dependent variable are all within one case. Consider, for example, our studies of the effectiveness of certain kinds of interventions (Chapters 19, 20, and 22). In these studies we tested the hypothesis that certain kinds of interventions by the analyst are more effective than others. We assumed in particular that plan-compatible interventions—that is, interventions which we inferred would help the patient to carry out his plans—would be more effective in giving the patient immediate help than interventions that, we inferred, would not help the patient to carry out his plans or would hinder him in carrying them out. We assumed, too, that the effectiveness of an interpretation could be measured by the degree to which the patient responded to it by tackling his problems and by developing insights into them.

In studying the effectiveness of interventions in the analysis of Mrs. C, a number of judges working independently of each other rated each of the analyst's interventions for its plan compatibility. Then, a second set of judges who were blind to the analyst's interventions studied segments of the patient's speech before and after each intervention. The judges rated a segment of the patient's speech preceding and following each intervention for her boldness in tackling problems and for her insightfulness. We assumed that the change in the patient's boldness and insight between the preintervention segment and the postintervention segment would measure her response to the intervention. By comparing the judges' ratings of the segments of speech (before and after a number of interventions) for their boldness and their insightfulness, we tested whether the patient did indeed make more progress when she was offered plan-compatible interpretations than when she was not.

In this type of single-case research design, each case is its own control; that is, the patient and the analyst are held constant. The unit of study includes the segment of the patient's speech preceding the intervention, the intervention itself, and the segment of the patient's speech after the intervention. The N or sample size for testing our hypothesis is the number of units studied. The independent variable is the degree to which the analyst's interventions are plan compatible, and the dependent variables are the changes in the patient's boldness and insightfulness from before the analyst's interventions to after them. By utilizing this kind of research design, the moment-to-moment shifts in the patient's behavior can be related to specific therapist interventions. The advantage of this research strategy over more traditional designs has been discussed recently by Fiske (1977), Greenberg (1983), and Rice and Greenberg (1984).

In testing alternative hypotheses we carry out a number of related studies on an individual case, each of which bears on the hypotheses. By doing so, we obtain converging lines of evidence bearing on the explanatory power of the different hypotheses. In addition, we avoid *ad hoc* hypotheses, which can account plausibly for a single finding but not for a network of interrelated findings.

CONTROLS AGAINST ERROR AND BIAS

We used a number of controls against potential sources of error or bias.

PUBLIC AND COMPREHENSIVE DATA

We selected for study a patient, Mrs. C, whose analysis was documented by tapes, verbatim transcripts, and process notes, and (with permission of the treating analyst) may be made accessible to other investigators. Thus, our research data may be studied by others.

The psychoanalysis of Mrs. C was, with her permission, audio-recorded in its entirety by the treating analyst for research purposes. We obtained verbatim typewritten transcripts[1] of every session during the period of analysis we chose for our initial study, namely, the first 100 sessions. We obtained in addition a random sample of verbatim transcripts throughout the entire analysis. We also obtained verbatim transcripts of seven blocks of 12 sessions, which were selected arbitrarily at approximately half-year intervals throughout the analysis.

The treating analyst also took notes during each analytic session, from which he dictated after each session a detailed summary of the session. We obtained these summaries—the analyst's process notes—for every session of the entire analysis.

We required and obtained both good process notes and verbatim transcripts. Process notes provide the investigator with an overview of an extended sweep of hours, as well as a relatively convenient guide to critical incidents, recurrent patterns, and significant changes. In previous work we had used process notes successfully to trace subtle changes in two analytic patients' behavior, attitudes, feelings, memories, and so forth, over more than 100 sessions (Sampson, Weiss, Mlodnosky, & Hause, 1972; Wolfson & Sampson, 1976). Moreover, we had verified (Wolfson & Sampson, 1976) the accuracy of findings in a process notes study by demonstrating that these findings were similar to those obtained by working directly from verbatim transcripts.

---

1. The transcripts were coded by the treating analyst to disguise the patient's identity.

Nonetheless, verbatim transcripts were also indispensable for our research. They freed us from the limitations of the analyst's selective perception, recall, and reporting. In many instances they enabled us to carry out a study on process notes, then verify the accuracy of our findings in a sample of verbatim transcripts. They also made it possible for us to carry out a number of studies of patient–analyst interactions directly on verbatim transcripts.

INDEPENDENCE OF THE TREATMENT FROM THE RESEARCH

We required and obtained a case in which the material produced by the patient was not and could not have been influenced by our theoretical expectations. The analysis of Mrs. C was entirely independent of our research. It was carried out in a city distant from our own, and it was completed some time before our research on it began. At the time he carried out this analysis, the analyst was unfamiliar with our ideas. His case formulation (Chapter 10) and his hypotheses about the therapeutic process were derived more or less from the automatic functioning hypothesis. His formulation and his ideas about the analytic process were distinctly different from our own. When the analyst became familiar with our ideas about the case years after the completion of the analysis, he found them novel and did not agree with them. The patient, too, was unfamiliar with our hypotheses about the analytic process. She was not in the mental health field. Moreover, our hypotheses were not published during her analysis.

RELIABLE CODIFICATION OF PATIENT AND ANALYST MATERIAL

In the studies reported in this book, we used 19 different measures of the patient's behavior (of thoughts, ways of working, affects, etc.) and 5 of the analyst's behavior. A list of the measures used is presented in the front of the book. The first time a measure is used, it is described and references concerning it are presented; subsequent instances of its use refer the reader to the chapter in which the measure was described. Measures or scales not in common use are presented in the appendices.

Each measure was scored or rated by two or more judges working independently of each other, and in each instance the degree of agreement between judges was calculated.

"BLIND" JUDGMENTS

It is necessary to limit the information provided raters in order to prevent their possible biases influencing their ratings in favor of or against a particular hypothesis. The raters we used were blind to (i.e., not permitted to see) certain patient or analyst material.

For example, in studies of how the analyst's reactions to the patient's testing may influence the patient's subsequent behavior, judges who rated the analyst's reactions were not permitted to see the patient's subsequent behaviors. Nor were the judges who rated the patient's testing behaviors permitted to see the analyst's reactions to the tests. Also, in our studies of testing we used many separate measures of the patient's immediate responses to the analyst (Chapters 17 and 18). In these studies, a separate group of judges rated each of the measures in order to avoid a halo effect (a positive or negative appraisal of one variable influencing the appraisals of other variables).

In studies of changes in a particular variable over a period of time, the judges who rated instances of the variable were blind to the session from which the segment containing the variable was excerpted. For example, we conducted a study to determine whether Mrs. C became more assertive during the first 100 sessions of her analysis as follows: We excerpted all instances of her assertiveness (or lack thereof) in the transcripts of the first 100 sessions. We typed these on $3'' \times 5''$ cards and presented them in random order to judges who were asked to rate them on an assertiveness scale (Chapter 13).

A NOTE ON REPLICATION

The ultimate guarantee of freedom from both error and research bias is independent replication of research findings. Members of the Mount Zion Psychotherapy Research Group have for some time been replicating various aspects of the work reported in this book (see Chapter 22). Replications by members outside of our research group ultimately will be indispensable to confirming or disconfirming our findings.

To facilitate independent replication, we have tried to make each step in our various studies explicit. One step in our research process, however, cannot be presented in a way that would enable an independent investigator to carry it out adequately: This is the step of assessing, from case material, a patient's unconscious plan to overcome his problems. A plan formulation includes inferences about a patient's pathogenic beliefs, the ways by which he may work to disconfirm these beliefs, and the behaviors and interventions by the analyst that he will perceive as disconfirming his pathogenic beliefs. The assessment of the patient's plan is a crucial step in studies involving hypotheses about plans, tests, and the analyst's interventions. We cannot fully communicate here how to go about formulating a patient's plan. This is because it is not possible to communicate from books or manuals the application of *any* theory to clinical material, especially if that application requires inference.

There are two possible ways to overcome this obstacle to independent replication studies. The first solution would be for the independent investigator who wishes to replicate our studies to visit us and become sufficiently conversant with the clinical application of our theory to apply it himself to a new case. The second solution would be for the investigator to have members of our research group do *blind* formulations (based on the first few sessions of a case) of a patient's plans, goals, tests, and so forth.

MORE ABOUT THE ANALYSIS WE STUDIED

The psychoanalysis we selected for study was carried through to a mutually agreed-upon termination. It was judged to be successful by the analyst, the patient, and a research group (not our own) that evaluated the patient's analytic progress.

We chose a successful case for intensive study because such a case would enable us to test hypotheses concerning how analytic progress takes place. We assumed that even in the most successful analysis there would be a considerable range in the usefulness of the analyst's interventions. There would, we assumed, be enough range to enable us to test hypotheses about the kinds of interventions that may impede or facilitate the patient's progress.

The analyst who treated Mrs. C was a male psychoanalyst who had been trained at a recognized psychoanalytic institute. He had graduated from that institute several years before he undertook the analysis we studied. Because the treating analyst recognized the importance that a recorded analysis might have for research, he chose to be supervised during his treatment of this case. The supervisor, with whom he met weekly, is a well-known senior analyst.

B: THE PATIENT STUDIED

10

MRS. C

JOSEPH WEISS
SUZANNE GASSNER
MARSHALL BUSH

In this chapter we shall introduce the patient, Mrs. C, whose psycho-analysis was the subject of the present research. We shall begin with an account of how she presented herself to her analyst at the beginning of treatment. We shall then present two different psychoanalytic formulations about her, both based on inferences from the material of the early sessions.

The first formulation was prepared by a research group in another city consisting of several senior analysts. This group was not connected to our own, and they prepared their formulation for their own studies. Their formulation, which approximates that of the treating analyst, provides an alternative view of the case to the one to which we subscribe. The second formulation was prepared by our research group. It was based initially on a close study of the analyst's process notes of the first 10 treatment sessions. This initial formulation was enriched subsequently by study of the verbatim transcripts of these sessions.

MRS. C AT THE BEGINNING

At the time she sought treatment, Mrs. C was an attractive 28-year-old social worker in a Catholic agency. She had been married for 2 years to a successful businessman. Her chief complaint concerned her sex life. She did not enjoy sex, did not have orgasms, and indeed was reluctant to have intercourse. She sought treatment at the insistence of her husband, who had threatened to divorce her if she did not overcome her sexual difficulties.

She had other complaints as well: She was unable to relax and enjoy herself. She felt tense and driven at work and at home. She tended to worry about others. She was self-critical. She suffered whenever she made even a minor mistake. She tended to blame herself for problems with her family and others, even when she was clearly not in the wrong. She felt emotionally constricted and inhibited in her behavior. She had trouble disagreeing either with her parents or her husband. With her husband she was afraid of "simply being a nonentity" who would serve him but have no status herself. She was uncomfortable with the other social workers at the agency and with the clients. She was especially uncomfortable in relationships with her male clients. She was overly strict and impatient with them.

Mrs. C implied at the beginning that she would like to become more relaxed, less self-critical, less worried about others, more assertive, and to enjoy herself more.

MRS. C'S BACKGROUND

Mrs. C came from an upper-middle-class midwestern family. Her father was a successful businessman; her mother was a housewife who did volunteer work for charitable agencies. The patient was the second of four children. She had an older sister and a younger sister and brother. According to the patient, her parents were tense and uncomfortable, both with each other and with their children. The father tyrannized the mother with his occasional fits of temper. The mother took his abuse without complaint.

The parents displayed little or no affection toward each other. They were so unresponsive to each other that Mrs. C wondered how she had been conceived. She could not imagine her parents getting close enough to have sex. Indeed, according to Mrs. C, her parents permitted themselves little pleasure of any kind. They were joyless, puritanical, grim, and hard-working. They seemed to believe that it is wrong for a person to enjoy his work. Even their recreational activities with the children were carried out as tasks, dutifully performed for the children's welfare, and brought them no pleasure.

Both parents were reactionary in their political and social views. For example, they opposed government programs intended to help children from poor families to go to college. The patient's mother believed that women on welfare who become pregnant should be sterilized.

Neither parent could see things from another's point of view. If a friend disagreed with one of their opinions, they would shake their heads sadly at the friend's inability to understand. If one of their children disagreed with their values or opinions, both parents, but especially the father, would be quite hurt. The patient's father expected his family to agree with him about even trivial things, such as his taste in movies or automobiles. He was also moved to tears when one of his children freely offered agreement with him. He took such agreement as a sign of loyalty and love. Mrs. C's parents had at one time received a letter from her younger sister telling them what good parents they had been. The father cherished this letter. He referred to it occasionally with tears in his eyes.

Mrs. C perceived both parents, but especially her father, as possessive. Her father, who, she implied, was overly attached to her, had been alarmed about her spending a year after college as an English tutor to a European family. He had feared that she would have an affair with the father of the family. The mother, who, the patient implied, was envious of her daughter's youth and attractiveness, had warned her in high school not to let herself remain alone with a man lest she lose control of her sexual feelings. The patient was amazed that her mother, who seemed so controlled and devoid of sexual feeling herself, could even have imagined that danger.

Mrs. C perceived both her parents as fragile. She could easily upset her father by demonstrating independence or by simply disagreeing with him. She had, on a number of occasions in childhood, provoked him unwittingly into fits of rage, which aroused in her terror, contempt, and worry about him. She perceived her mother as efficient in her housework but as helpless to deal with her family's anger and aggression. The mother could not protect herself from her children, the children from each other, or the children from the father. The children would ridicule and pummel each other in front of the mother, who would stand by helplessly, unable to intervene.

In the following episode, which occurred when Mrs. C was 6, both of her parents behaved characteristically. The patient's sister had hit her in the stomach, and the child had gone weeping and complaining to her mother. When she could not get her mother's attention, she became frustrated and hit her mother in the stomach. Her mother made no attempt to defend herself. She doubled over in pain, wept, and went to her room. Later, when her father heard about what his daughter had done, he became enraged. He punished her immediately, even though she was at the time entertaining a friend from school. He beat her and threw her into a closet. Mrs. C had been horrified at the father's loss of control, and she believed that for a short time her father had wanted to kill her. Not long after the above episode, she became enraged at her younger brother and wanted to kill him.

Mrs. C felt sure of her mother's love but not of her father's. She had in early childhood perceived him as a kind of superman, but now she felt confused about him. She tried to maintain her early image of him as a superman but instead saw him as a pathetic man constantly requiring reassurance and in danger of losing control of himself.

Mrs. C's relations to her siblings were presented in a contradictory way. Sometimes she described vividly how envious she was of them; other times she implied that she felt superior to them. For example, on one occasion she spoke earnestly about how envious she was of her younger sister. She complained that her parents listened respectfully to whatever her sister said but ignored what Mrs. C said or considered it stupid. Some time later, however, she explained that her mother had been disappointed in her sister, who was lazy and did not work, but in order to conceal her disappointment in the sister had been especially attentive to her.

Mrs. C experienced contradictory feelings also in her relationship to her younger brother. Her disregard for him and her feelings of superiority toward him could be inferred from a number of her statements about him. Her envy of him, however, could be established without inference: She suffered consciously throughout childhood from envy of her brother for his possessing a penis. Indeed, her earliest memory connected with sex was of carrying a stick between her legs, which in her mind represented a penis. Her belief in the inferiority of her genitalia was intensified when at age 10 she injured her perineum by falling on a stick and had to have the wound repaired by surgery.

MRS. C'S CONTRADICTORY BEHAVIOR

Mrs. C demonstrated contradictory feelings or behavior in ways other than those described above. She would, as part of her use of the defense of undoing, first explain a certain piece of behavior in one way, then in another. For example, on one occasion she described her reluctance to disagree with others as stemming from her fear of hurting them. A short time later she explained it as stemming from her feeling too weak and helpless to disagree. During one analytic hour, Mrs. C told the analyst that she felt confused and unorganized. Yet, while describing these feelings, she was articulate, clear, and organized. During another hour she reported how retiring she was socially, but later the same hour she described an episode in which she was at a party smoking a cigar and holding center stage. On still another occasion Mrs. C told the analyst that she could not form her own opinions, then unobtrusively offered some perceptive comments about a movie.

MRS. C'S IDEAS ABOUT THE GENESIS OF HER PROBLEMS

Mrs. C offered a number of opinions about how she had developed certain of her problems. She suggested at one point that her fear of intercourse may have stemmed from her childhood injury to her genitals. When she was an adolescent, her mother, in admonishing her to avoid sex, pointed out that because of her old injury she might find intercourse especially painful.

Mrs. C developed the idea that she had felt highly constrained by her loyalty to her parents. She stated that she had wished she wasn't their child so she wouldn't belong to them and wouldn't have to be like them. She made clear that she viewed her parents as leading a joyless and unsatisfactory life, and that she wanted to be different from them. She implied also that she felt superior to them.

Mrs. C suggested that her unwillingness to be intimate with her husband was modeled after her parents, who could not enjoy intimacy with each other. She suggested also that she had acquired certain of her character traits from her parents. She had grown up to be much like her mother: grim, burdened, joyless, inhibited, and worried; she had also, like her father, developed a need for frequent approval and reassurance.

Mrs. C also implied that she had developed certain of her difficulties out of compliance to her parents. She had complied with them by staying close to home, avoiding adventure, and accepting their opinions. She suggested that it was out of compliance to them that she became so inhibited about having her own opinions, making her own decisions, and leading her own life.

Finally, Mrs. C suggested that certain of her difficulties stemmed from her tendency to blame herself for problems for which she was not responsible. She described an episode at the agency that illustrates her tendency to take blame: A fellow social worker became so upset that she had to take a leave of absence. Mrs. C's initial thought was, "I'm glad it's not me." She felt sorry for her colleague, and then began to wonder if she had in some way contributed to this colleague's difficulties.

THE TWO FORMULATIONS

The opening sessions of the analysis, from which the material presented above is summarized, were studied independently by the two research groups described earlier. Each produced a psychoanalytic formulation that attempted both to account for the development of Mrs. C's psycho-pathology and to predict how she would be motivated in her treatment. The two formulations, as will be seen, are quite different.

THE OTHER GROUP'S FORMULATION

According to the group of researchers in another city, Mrs. C's difficulties were crystallized after the birth of her brother when she was 6. After this time Mrs. C noticed a marked change in her father's, and to a lesser extent her mother's, attitude toward her. She felt that her parents valued her brother more than her, and that her father in particular shifted his love from her to her younger brother. She assumed that her father preferred her younger brother because he had a penis and she did not. She assumed, too, that because she lacked a penis she was doomed to an inferior position in life.

Mrs. C's primary unconscious wish was to redress her castrated state. She envied men and longed to have a penis. She attempted, both in analysis and in life, to obtain a penis of her own, as well as to deny the men in her life their pride in their penises by aggressively withholding admiration and sexual response or by criticizing and attacking them.

OUR FORMULATION

According to our formulation, Mrs. C's problems arose primarily not from unconscious envy but from unconscious guilt. She perceived her parents as fragile and vulnerable. She believed they would be severely damaged if she held ideas or values different from theirs, or disagreed with them, or led an independent life that was freer, less burdened, and less joyless than their lives. She also unconsciously felt superior and contemptuous toward her parents and siblings, and unconsciously pictured them as weak and envious. She protected herself from hurting them by making herself weak, constricted, and helpless.

She conceived of her parents as requiring her to be loyal to them: to remain close by, to lead the same kind of life they led, and to have the same kinds of ideas they had. She wished to separate herself from her parents and to develop a life of her own, but held herself back out of fear of hurting them.

Mrs. C's penis envy, which had been completely conscious from her early childhood, was in our view not a primary motive. It was one of a number of means by which she attempted to belittle herself so as to restore others. For example, by envying her brother, she attempted both to placate her conscience and to restore her brother. She used her penis envy, too, to placate her father. Her penis envy implied for her that she admired her father. She would rather envy him than hurt him by becoming independent of him and taking pleasure in her femininity.

She also maintained her envy of her brother to restore her mother. She suffered from Oedipal guilt toward her mother. She unconsciously believed that her mother was tortured by envy of her daughter's attractiveness and youth. She therefore punished herself by making herself experience the same kind of envy in relation to her brother that she believed her mother experienced in relation to her.

Mrs. C's penis envy had the same structure as a beating fantasy (see Chapter 4). (Mrs. C in fact became conscious of previously repressed beating fantasies toward the end of the third year of her analysis.) This structure was based on her primitive idea that if she was a victim, she was not an offender. For example, by picturing herself as victimized by her brother, she could protect herself from her fear of victimizing him.

Mrs. C's envy of her sisters had the same structure as her envy of her brother. She used it to protect them from what she believed to be their envy of her and, in addition, to make amends to them for being more attractive, intelligent, and successful than they.

Mrs. C used a different but related means to protect her parents from her unconscious feelings of superiority and contempt: She identified with them as victims and adopted some of their worst features. For example, she became driven, anxious, grim, joyless, and tense like her mother, and in need of frequent approval and reassurance like her father. She was impatient and severe in her relationships with the male clients at the agency, as her father had been with her. She avoided intimacy with her husband, as, in her opinion, her parents had avoided intimacy with each other.

Mrs. C's conflict was between her wishes to be strong, independent, loving, and uninhibited and her guilt about wanting these things. She wished to become independent and to be able to display her good qualities. However, she feared that were she to do so, she would hurt her parents and siblings.

Mrs. C had an obsessive–compulsive character structure. She used repression, undoing, and isolation as defenses. She would do something which gave her pleasure, then feel guilty about it and undo it. For example, she would undo her feelings of superiority by her feelings of envy. She would undo her feeling that she was a nice person by becoming mean. She would undo her sense of independence and conviction by becoming helpless and unable to make up her mind.

OUR PREDICTIONS

Our predictions about the goals Mrs. C would pursue follow from the above formulation. According to our most general predictions, Mrs. C would work to change her pathogenic beliefs about her exaggerated sense of responsibility for others and about her fear of hurting them. More specifically, she would struggle (especially in relation to the analyst) to change the pathogenic beliefs underlying her separation guilt, survivor guilt, and Oedipal guilt. She would hope thereby to overcome the inhibitions, the repressions, and the need to punish herself that stemmed from these beliefs. She would also hope to enjoy herself more, be more comfortable as an independent person, and be more attractive, capable, and compassionate. She would work to become both independent with her husband and able to enjoy intimacy, including sexual intimacy, with him. Finally, she would struggle to lift the repression of the childhood experiences from which she had inferred her pathogenic beliefs, so that she could better understand the origins of her difficulties.

C: THE UNCONSCIOUS CONTROL HYPOTHESIS

11

INTRODUCTION TO STUDIES ABOUT THE REGULATION OF UNCONSCIOUS MENTAL LIFE

HAROLD SAMPSON

TWO PSYCHOANALYTIC HYPOTHESES

This chapter introduces our first group of empirical studies. These are concerned with the explanatory power of two hypotheses: the unconscious control hypothesis (discussed in Chapter 8) and its alternative, the dynamic hypothesis.

The *dynamic hypothesis* is based on automatic functioning concepts. According to this hypothesis, repressions are regulated by indications of pleasure and pain, and this regulation is automatic. The patient cannot exert control over his repressions. The unconscious becomes conscious, or finds expression in behavior, because of shifts in the dynamic equilibrium between repressed and repressing forces.

The *unconscious control hypothesis* is based on higher mental functioning concepts. According to this hypothesis, repressions are regulated by assessments of danger and safety, and this regulation takes place on the basis of thoughts, anticipations, judgments, and decisions. Thus, the analytic patient may exert unconscious control over his repressions. He may decide unconsciously whether to maintain the repression of an unconscious content or to lift the repression and bring the content forth (express or experience it). In making his decisions, the patient is guided by unconscious appraisals of danger and safety.

The two hypotheses differ in a number of ways. They are based on different fundamental assumptions about unconscious mental functioning (Chapters 1 and 2). They offer different explanations for central and familiar psychoanalytic processes. For example, the dynamic hypothesis assumes that transferences become powerful because they are frustrated or because the defenses against them are undermined. The unconscious control hypothesis assumes that transferences become powerful because the patient, after disconfirming certain pathogenic beliefs, decides unconsciously that he can safely express them (Chapter 21).

The two hypotheses may produce differing clinical intuitions about the analytic patient's behavior. For example, if a patient begins to express strong sexual feelings toward the analyst, an analyst using the dynamic hypothesis may assume either that the patient's sexual impulses have been intensified or that his defenses against them have been weakened. He may assume, in addition, that the patient is expressing these impulses as a gratification and/or a resistance. In contrast, an analyst using the unconscious control hypothesis may infer that the patient has decided unconsciously that he can safely express these impulses. The analyst may assume, in addition, that the patient is expressing these impulses primarily as a step toward making them conscious and gaining control over them.

SOME EVIDENCE FOR THE UNCONSCIOUS CONTROL HYPOTHESIS

I shall now review some evidence, from clinical observations and informal research studies, that lends support to the unconscious control hypothesis and illustrates its explanatory power.

CRYING AT THE HAPPY ENDING

Weiss described in Chapter 1 the phenomenon of crying at a happy ending, in everyday life and in psychoanalysis. In this phenomenon, a person spontaneously and without conflict or tension becomes conscious of a previously repressed sad content after some circumstantial or internal change makes it safe for him to experience it. For example, right after the birth of a son, Dr. N, while rejoicing in his birth, felt sad, wept, and vividly recalled previously forgotten memories of another son who had died years earlier. She remembered her happiness with him and her feelings of devastation when he died. Dr. N experienced the birth of her second son as replacing her earlier loss. Her crying at the happy ending supports the hypothesis that the birth of her second son made it safe for her to experience the repressed memories of her first son. According to this hypothesis, she knew that she would no longer be overwhelmed by these memories so that she lifted her defenses and brought them to consciousness.

The observations that powerful repressed contents may become conscious spontaneously and without conflict and that they may become conscious just when it would seem likely that the person could safely experience them support that idea that the person may recognize unconsciously that it is safe to experience the contents and so may decide to lift his repressions and bring forth the repressed contents.

RECOVERY FROM TRAUMATIC EXPERIENCES

It has been observed frequently that a person recovering from trauma may recall the traumatic experience after a change in his circumstances should make it safe for him to recall it. For example, pilots are more likely to recall flying accidents in dreams after they have been grounded, and coal miners are more likely to recall disasters after they have changed their occupations (Davis, 1958). The dreams of prisoners of war reported by Balson (1975) and summarized in Chapter 7 illustrate the same point. The prisoners dreamt about the suffering of imprisonment only after they were free and out of danger. These observations are analogous to observations of crying at the happy ending and they support the unconscious control hypothesis. The traumatized person is likely to recall the trauma fully only after he is no longer endangered. He can then safely bring the trauma to consciousness.

OBSERVATIONS FROM PSYCHOANALYSIS

The neurotic patient in analysis is rarely overwhelmed or traumatized when he becomes conscious of previously repressed material (Weiss, 1971). This is the case even when the material is intense and affectively powerful, as in the example from Chapter 1 of Miss P, the lawyer who felt intense sadness and wept for some time when she remembered a childhood event that she had experienced as maternal rejection. The observation that the neurotic patient is rarely traumatized by the emergence of repressed material suggests that the patient may be regulating its emergence to consciousness. This observation cannot be explained as due to the *analyst's* regulation of the rate at which the patient becomes conscious of unconscious contents. The analyst cannot always know that unconscious material is about to become conscious; moreover, even if he does know this, he cannot necessarily help the patient to titrate its emergence. Nor can the dynamic hypothesis explain convincingly the observation that a patient may, in the absence of any interpretation, suddenly experience powerful previously repressed mental contents. He may experience them without feeling anxiety or conflict about them, and he may comfortably keep them in consciousness and link them to other contents in an effort to advance the therapy. The dynamic hypothesis could explain the sudden emergence of powerful previously repressed contents by the assumption that they were pushed to consciousness by an intensification of certain impulses that were frustrated in the transference. However, if previously repressed mental contents emerged in this way, their coming forth would be marked by conflict and anxiety. The dynamic hypothesis could explain the calm, nonconflicted emergence of previously repressed contents by assuming that they emerged as part of a compromise formation. In that case they would be opposed by defenses such as isolation. However, then the patient would not be able to link them to other contents and use his insight into them to advance his therapy.

Kris has reported observations that are in accord with the unconscious control hypothesis. He observed that in "the good analytic hour" important new material comes forth in a smooth and organized fashion as if "prepared" or "actually prepared"—but prepared outside of the patient's awareness (1956b). Kris suggested that this preparation takes place preconsciously and that the new material (which often includes ideas previously inaccessible to consciousness) is then brought forth under the ego's control.

Greenson (1967) observed that the analytic patient may be able to face particular repressed contents when it becomes safe for him to do so. For example, Greenson observed that Mrs. K became aware of strong homosexual feelings just after she became able, for the first time, to experience an orgasm during (heterosexual) intercourse. He concluded that her heterosexual success "gave her the courage" to face her homosexual feelings (p. 187). This example is analogous to crying at a happy ending.

Certain analytic authors, including Greenson and Rangell, have also observed that during analysis powerful regressions may take place and powerful transferences may be expressed when the patient feels safe enough to allow this to occur. Greenson, for example, noted that the analytic patient who "dares to regress" and to experience aspects of his neurosis in the transference, and who is then reassured by the analyst's response, becomes more willing to risk reviving further regressive transferences (1965, p. 172). Rangell observed that patients may develop powerful regressive transferences under their own control, and that they do so because the analytic attitude of the analyst has provided a "protective aegis" under which the patient can safely allow such regression (1968, pp. 22–23).

FOLLOW-UP STUDIES

Evidence suggesting unconscious control over transferences is also provided in the follow-up studies of Pfeffer (1959, 1961, 1963) and of Norman, Blacker, Oremland, and Barrett (1976). Both research groups discovered that the successfully analyzed patient, during a short series of follow-up research interviews with another analyst many years after termination, revives the major transferences in much the same sequence in which he manifested them in his analysis. The former analysand revives these transferences rapidly and spontaneously, and then overcomes them rapidly and without interpretive help. He recalls how the transferences were manifested during his analysis, and he also recovers the childhood memories pertaining to them. He carries out this entire process calmly.

We infer from these observations that the former analysand gained considerable control over his transferences during his analysis. He kept these transferences, and the memories pertaining to them, lightly repressed. When called upon to remember his analysis, he did so by first unconsciously reviving these transferences, and then analyzing them rapidly on his own, for the adaptive purpose of recalling his analysis in the follow-up interviews.

HOW THE RESEARCH BEARS ON THE TWO HYPOTHESES

Neither the clinical observations described in Part I nor the research presented in Part II rules out the possibility that some unconscious processes take place automatically in accordance with the pleasure principle. The clinical observations and the research, however, do support the thesis that much unconscious functioning is to some extent controlled unconsciously by the patient. The informal observations and the research also show that the analytic patient typically behaves in accordance with the expectations of the unconscious control hypothesis. Finally, the informal observations and the research would, if replicated, refute the automatic functioning hypothesis as formulated in Freud's early theory, for they show that not all, indeed not even most, unconscious behavior can be derived from the dynamic interplay (beyond the patient's control) of impersonal psychic forces.

THE EMPIRICAL STUDIES

We shall present in the next three chapters empirical studies that compare how well the unconscious control hypothesis and the dynamic hypothesis explain certain familiar psychoanalytic processes. In Chapter 12 we will compare how well the two hypotheses account for an analytic patient (Mrs. C) becoming conscious of previously unconscious contents that have not been interpreted. We shall compare predictions about this process derived from each of the hypotheses, and determine which predictions better fit our findings. In Chapter 13 we will compare how well the unconscious control hypothesis and the dynamic hypothesis account for Mrs. C overcoming her inhibitions and expressing warded-off strivings more directly in her behavior. In Chapter 14 we will examine whether the unconscious control hypothesis is compatible with our findings about how Mrs. C increased her awareness of, and began to gain some insight into, a particular domain of mental contents of conscious and unconscious concern to her.

12

THE EMERGENCE OF WARDED-OFF CONTENTS

SUZANNE GASSNER
HAROLD SAMPSON
SUZANNE BRUMER
JOSEPH WEISS

THE RESEARCH PROBLEM

In this chapter we shall report on research designed to throw light on the question: How, during psychoanalytic treatment, do repressed and uninterpreted mental contents typically become conscious? We investigated this question by comparing two different psychoanalytic hypotheses (see Chapter 11). The dynamic hypothesis, based on automatic functioning concepts, assumes that repressed mental contents typically become conscious as the result of dynamic shifts that take place beyond the patient's control.[1] The unconscious control hypothesis, based on higher mental functioning concepts, assumes that repressed contents typically come forth under the patient's unconscious control (Chapters 1, 2, and 11).

These two hypotheses may be compared empirically because, as we will show below, they lead to different predictions.

---

1. By a dynamic hypothesis, we mean a purely dynamic one, that is, one in which the ego does not exert control over the drives but interacts with them dynamically. The ego control hypothesis may contain dynamic elements. It may assume that the impulses and forces pushing to the surface have an impetus, but that these are ordinarily regulated by the ego.

Large portions of this chapter are adapted from S. Gassner, H. Sampson, J. Weiss, and S. Brumer, The emergence of warded-off contents. *Psychoanalysis and Contemporary Thought*, 1982, 5(1), 55–75. Copyright 1982 by International Universities Press. Adapted by permission of the publisher.

Portions of this chapter are also adapted from H. Sampson and J. Weiss, Testing hypotheses: The approach of the Mount Zion Psychotherapy Research Group. In L. S. Greenberg and W. M. Pinsof (Eds.), *The psychotherapeutic process: A research handbook*. Copyright 1986 by The Guilford Press. Adapted by permission of the publishers.

The authors wish to express their appreciation to Andy Propper for his help in analyzing the data.

PREDICTIONS BASED ON THE UNCONSCIOUS CONTROL HYPOTHESIS

The analytic patient's repressions, according to the theory of therapy set forth in Part I, are based on pathogenic beliefs (Chapters 1-4). The patient, because of the dangers foretold by these beliefs, maintains repressions against impulses, purposes, or goals that he believes would, if experienced, endanger him. In treatment the patient works unconsciously to change his pathogenic beliefs, both by testing them in relation to the analyst and by using the analyst's interpretations to understand and ultimately to disconfirm them. In an analysis that is progressing well the patient changes his pathogenic beliefs and so becomes less frightened of the dangers they foretell. He may, as a consequence, decide that he can safely experience certain previously repressed contents and so lifts the repressions opposing these contents and brings them forth.

According to the unconscious control hypothesis, which is part of the theory reviewed above, a patient may bring forth a particular repressed mental content when he unconsciously decides that he may safely experience it. His purpose in doing so is, in general, to master the content (increase his control over it). The unconscious control hypothesis was used in Chapter 1 to explain the observation that the patient may become conscious spontaneously of a previously repressed content, may remain calm as he discusses the content, may not come into conflict with it, may think about the content, and attempt to increase his understanding of it (e.g., the emergence of Mrs. G's beating fantasy).

We can derive from the unconscious control hypothesis certain expectations about the spontaneous emergence during a successful analytic treatment of previously warded-off mental contents:

1. The patient, even in the absence of interpretation, will frequently become aware of mental contents that he had previously warded off by defenses. This is because the patient, as he gradually changes his belief that certain repressed contents are dangerous, will decide that he may safely lift his defenses and make these contents conscious.

2. The patient experiences only a little anxiety about the content as it becomes conscious. This is because he will in general wait until, by unconsciously carrying out a piece of analytic work, he has weakened the pathogenic belief that gave rise to his anxiety about the content. After he has overcome or significantly reduced his anxiety about the content, he may make it conscious. If he does, he may be no more anxious while experiencing the previously repressed content than he is ordinarily. Indeed, since making the content conscious may be for him the culmination

of a good piece of analytic work, he may at that point experience a sense of satisfaction such as a person may feel when he has solved a puzzle. A patient may, on the other hand, feel considerable anxiety while experiencing the previously repressed content if he feels pressured—for example, by events, by the analyst, or by his own conscience—to experience it before he has unconsciously overcome his anxiety about it.

3. Because the patient typically makes a content conscious only after he has weakened the pathogenic belief from which his anxieties about it arose, he may not continue to defend against it after it has come forth. He is likely to experience the emerging content fully, think about its import, and use his insight about it to advance his therapy.

PREDICTIONS BASED ON THE DYNAMIC HYPOTHESIS

The dynamic hypothesis is based on automatic functioning concepts (Chapters 1 and 2). According to this hypothesis, repressions are regulated automatically beyond the patient's control by indications of pleasure and pain. Unconscious contents, unless interpreted, may remain repressed and are either unexpressed or expressed in symptoms. However, such contents may occasionally become conscious during analysis because of a shift in the dynamic balance between repressing and repressed forces in favor of the repressed.

An unconscious content that becomes conscious as a result of such a shift may, though rarely, become so powerful relative to the forces opposing it that it emerges in a scarcely disguised form. In this instance, the patient is likely to be intensely anxious when it emerges. Since the content is still dangerous to him, the patient is likely to remain in conflict with it after it has emerged and will attempt to rerepress it. More commonly, however, the repressed content will emerge in a well-disguised compromise formation. In this instance, the content is still defended against, however subtly, so the patient may not feel anxious about its emergence and may not come into intense conflict with it. However, since the content is still defended against, the patient cannot experience it fully, think about its significance for him, and use insight about it to advance his therapy.

The dynamic hypothesis, then, does not predict—and cannot readily account for—the combination of predictions derived from the unconscious control hypothesis. It can account for the analytic patient occasionally becoming aware, even without interpretation, of contents that he had previously warded off by defenses. It can also account for the patient not feeling anxious about the coming forth of previously warded-off contents. It cannot, however, account for his becoming aware of the contents without feeling anxious about them, experiencing them vividly, thinking about them, and using his insight into them to increase his understanding of his psychic life.

PLAN OF THE RESEARCH

Our research, which follows from the comparisons described above, re- quired us to take the following steps: first, to identify reliably, in the analytic sessions of a patient, a number of occasions when a previously warded-off, uninterpreted mental content became conscious; second, to examine how anxious the patient was while these contents were becom- ing conscious; third, to determine whether the patient thought about the contents, experienced them vividly, and used them to increase his control over his unconscious mental life.

THE ANALYTIC CASE

The studies by which we carried out these steps made use of the process notes and verbatim transcripts of the first 100 sessions of the analysis of Mrs. C, who was described in Chapter 10. These sessions lent themselves to our task of finding a number of occasions when previously warded-off mental contents had come forth without their having been interpreted. This is because the analyst made very few interpretations of any kind during this period of the analysis. He interpreted only a few previously repressed mental contents. Moreover, he made few resistance interpreta- tions except for occasional comments of a general nature such as "I notice you find it hard to begin today" or "What are you thinking about now?"

THE IDENTIFICATION OF PREVIOUSLY WARDED-OFF CONTENTS THAT HAD NOT BEEN INTERPRETED

The first task in testing our hypotheses was to identify a group of previously warded-off mental contents that came forth without having been interpreted. This task involved three steps: (1) identifying *new* con- tents—that is, contents which had not appeared previously—during a series of analytic sessions; (2) identifying within this pool of new con- tents those contents that previously had been warded off; and (3) determining which of these previously warded-off contents had never been interpreted.

IDENTIFYING PREVIOUSLY WARDED-OFF CONTENTS

In identifying previously warded-off contents, we used a method originally developed by Leonard Horowitz (who was at that time a member of our group) and other members of our research group (Horowitz, Sampson, Siegelman, Wolfson, & Weiss, 1975). The Horowitz *et al.* study demonstrated that experienced psychoanalytic clinicians working independently of each other could agree highly on which contents had been previously warded off. Moreover, the study demonstrated that the clinicians' judgments were based on complex clinical evaluations rather than on preconceptions of the kinds of mental contents that are likely to be warded off.

The present study (Gassner, Sampson, Weiss, & Brumer, 1982) used an improved version of the Horowitz *et al.* method. We began by identifying a group of new contents (e.g., new ideas, attitudes, affects, memories) that appeared for the first time during a particular series of sessions. This step was carried out by two judges, who examined the process notes of Mrs. C's analysis from sessions 41 to 100 inclusive and located in these all statements containing contents not contained in the process notes of sessions 1 to 40 inclusive. They identified approximately 500 statements containing new contents.

The 500 statements were then grouped according to a number of topics. These were the topics with which Mrs. C was preoccupied. They included, for example, Mrs. C's statements about her past and present relationships to her parents, siblings, husband, friends, and colleagues. They included too her statements about her feelings about submission and defiance, about rejection and acceptance, about her sense of responsibility, and about her sex life.

Our next step was to reduce the 500 statements to a more manageable 100. We did so by randomly selecting one-fifth of the statements in each topical group. We verified the accuracy of these statements, which were taken from the process notes, by checking each one against the corresponding statements in the verbatim transcripts.

We also verified that the 100 statements were new by showing that they were not similar to anything that appeared in the verbatim transcripts of the patient's first 10 treatment hours.

Seven of the 100 statements were prefaced by phrases that could cue judges that they contained previously warded-off contents. Examples of such phrases are: "Suddenly I realize that . . ."; "I had never let myself think or feel . . ."; "I can't believe that I'm saying that . . ."; "I never could allow myself to face . . . ." In order to avoid providing judges with such cues, we eliminated all such tell-tale phrases from the statements.

We now had a sample of 100 statements containing new, but not necessarily previously warded-off, mental contents. These new statements included contents that we assumed had been either conscious all along or were readily accessible to consciousness. We assumed that the statements also included contents that had been repressed or warded off by other defenses prior to the patient becoming aware of them and reporting them to the analyst. To identify this latter group of contents, we presented the sample of 100 statements to 19 judges, all of whom were trained in psychoanalytic therapy, and one-third of whom were practicing psychoanalysts. These judges were also provided with the process notes of the first 10 sessions of Mrs. C's analysis. The judges were asked first to read the process notes and make their own case formulations about Mrs. C from them, then to examine each of the 100 statements in the light of their formulations and decide whether the statement was warded off during the first 10 sessions. The judges were told that in carrying out this task they were not only to provide their own formulations but to define the state of "being warded off" by their own criteria. They were, in addition, urged to make full use of their clinical intuition. The judges were asked to rate each of the 100 statements on a 5-point scale, which indicated their degree of confidence that the statement contained a theme or content that was warded off during the first 10 sessions. A rating of "1" indicated a strong belief that the content had not been warded off; a rating of "5" indicated a strong belief that the content had been previously warded off.

In addition, the treating analyst (of the now completed case) was asked to perform the same task as the judges, namely, to rate each of the 100 statements so as to indicate how confident he was that the statement contained a content or theme that previously was warded off. However, the treating analyst was asked, in making his judgments, to use not just the first 10 sessions but all that he had learned about the patient in the entire analysis.

In order to decide from the judges' ratings which of the 100 new contents were warded off, we obtained the average rating of the 19 judges for each of the 100 statements, and the standard deviation for each. From these we calculated the mean for each statement, which we designated as the scale value for that statement.

The overall mean of the ratings for all of the statements was 2.89 and the standard deviation 0.74. Thirteen statements received a scale value of "4" or higher, 21 a scale value of "2" or less. We decided that for the purposes of the present study we would consider any content with a scale value of "4" or over to have been warded off.

Table 12-1 presents the 13 statements that received a scale value of "4" or over. It gives the scale value of each statement as determined by the judges and by the treating analyst. Table 12-1 makes clear that the judges' ratings and those of the treating analyst were in close agreement on 11 of the 13 warded-off items. Table 12-2 presents the 21 statements that received a scale value of "2" or less.

Table 12-1. Results for Items Rated Highly Warded Off

Statement	Mean of judges' ratings	Treating analyst's ratings
1. She recalls wanting to kill her brother.	4.56	5
2. She thought how she and Henry had had intercourse and she had wanted it and enjoyed it.	4.45	5
3. After she was very angry with me yesterday, she went home and felt very, very happy.	4.39	5
4. When she had to knock on her parents' bedroom door, she must have felt angry at being left out.	4.34	4
5. She had some kind of sexual attraction for her brother.	4.33	5
6. When she imagines her parents having intercourse, she thinks of her father being on the bottom because he just accepts it.	4.22	5
7. She looked at her bowel movements with the urge to see what she had done.	4.22	5
8. She knew how to work her parents, their guilt and their need to be absolutely fair.	4.22	2
9. It is as though her control while having intercourse is somehow disciplining Henry.	4.17	5
10. She feels some satisfaction seeing that she reacts just as her mother does.	4.17	5
11. The drawing she made turned out to be an elephant and when she went back and looked at it, the nose was a penis.	4.12	5
12. She couldn't have me raise a question without having to say that she had already thought of it.	4.07	2
13. She controls when Henry has an orgasm by whether she moves or not.	4.06	4

Table 12-2. Results for Items Rated Low Warded Off

Statement	Mean of judges' ratings
1. When she was in high school, she preferred the company of adults and wasn't comfortable being with kids her own age.	1.28
2. She has the worst eyesight, knock-knees, flat feet, teeth of anyone in her family.	1.33
3. She didn't want to have the kind of marriage her parents had.	1.44
4. Although she has many questions she would want to ask, the idea that they might look stupid just stops her and she can hardly think of any.	1.61
5. When she took up knitting, the results were disappointing.	1.67
6. Her mother told her that even though she didn't enjoy playing the piano, the day would come when she would appreciate it.	1.67
7. When her father yelled at her, she would just have to hide and wouldn't know what to do.	1.67
8. She got angry out of all proportion when a little boy acted up in her play group.	1.73
9. In college she was very confused about a career.	1.84
10. What she is mostly concerned about is the impression a gift will make on the other person and how that reflects on herself.	1.84
11. Because the patient is older, she feels she should be better than her co-worker.	1.84
12. With her grandmother she felt she could have a different kind of relationship where she could return something.	1.89
13. She felt that my voice indicated that I was irritated with her.	1.89
14. In the main she thinks she has no sense of humor.	1.89
15. She thought her father asked so much of her and gave so little.	1.95
16. Even if she is sick legitimately, she just has trouble making a decision not to go to work.	1.95
17. Her sense of insecurity makes her want to make her clients behave.	2.00
18. She feels guilty about wanting to see a light and romantic movie like *Gone with the Wind.*	2.00
19. She feels she is never on time and that I'll be very angry, will accept no excuse, and will have no forgiveness of her.	2.00
20. She thought that when I said "exactly," I was putting her down.	2.00
21. When the supervisor is too busy and can't talk to her, it is the way her mother was.	2.00

We calculated the split half reliability coefficient of ratings by correlating the mean values of one randomly selected group of nine judges' ratings with the mean value of the remaining group of ten judges' ratings. The reliability coefficient was .90. This finding demonstrates that raters were able to achieve a high consensus about whether an idea had been previously repressed.

WERE THE CONTENTS THAT THE JUDGES IDENTIFIED AS WARDED OFF OF CENTRAL IMPORTANCE TO THE PATIENT?

There is evidence from three sources—the patient, the treating analyst, and our research group—that the 13 statements rated highly warded off by the judges were not trivial but of central importance to the patient. Our evidence is this: The patient had prefaced seven of the 100 statements with comments that indicated that she was experiencing surprise at the contents of the statements or difficulty in facing the contents. These prefaces, which we have already described, were removed from the statements presented to the judges lest they cue the judges that the statement contained a previously warded-off content. Yet, according to the judges' ratings, the contents that *the patient* had cued as previously warded off (and which her cues indicated were of central importance) were indeed warded off. To demonstrate this we compared the mean ratings that the judges gave to the statements containing the seven cued contents with the mean ratings they gave to seven statements randomly selected from the remaining 93 statements. The mean for the cued statements was 3.96, and the mean for the random statements, 2.86. This difference in scale values is statistically significant ($p < .05$).

Evidence that the treating analyst agreed with the judges is presented in Table 12-1, which shows that the treating analyst, drawing on his knowledge of the entire analysis, rated 11 of the 13 statements as previously warded off. Moreover, the treating analyst considered several of the statements to which our judges gave the highest ratings as especially important to the patient and revealing of her difficulties. Indeed, he was so impressed with their centrality that he asked us to disguise these contents for the purposes of this publication.

The evidence that our research group considered the same 13 statements as warded off is also impressive. Our group, working entirely independently of the 19 judges, had made its own case formulation. Moreover, we predicted, on the basis of our formulation, the kinds of impulses, affects, goals, memories, and ideas the patient would have to become conscious of in order for the analysis to be successful. The contents the judges selected were of the kind predicted by our group (see Chapter 10).

DID THE CONTENTS JUDGED WARDED OFF EMERGE WITHOUT BENEFIT OF INTERPRETATION?

We used a simple, straightforward method to investigate whether the contents judged warded off emerged without benefit of interpretation.

Before describing this method, let us present an overall picture of the analyst's activity during these 100 sessions. During this phase of the treatment, the analyst made 846 interventions.[2] Two members of our research group[3] studied these interventions to identify all instances in which suggestions, clarifications, or interpretations were made. They found that 78% of the interventions were intended as simple clarifications or questions such as, "When did that happen?"

We looked at each of the analyst's interventions to determine whether anything he had said prior to the emergence of the contents judged previously warded off was related *in any way* to these contents. One judge read through all 846 statements to identify any analytic interventions that might pertain to the 13 statements judged previously warded off. This judge was instructed to identify interventions even if they were only vaguely related to the contents judged warded off. Although we had anticipated using additional judges for this task, it turned out that the findings were so clear-cut that additional judges were unnecessary. The judge was able to find only one analytic interpretation that related to a content judged previously warded off. The one interpretation occurred 14 sessions prior to the patient's stating that whenever the analyst raised a question she felt compelled to say that she had already thought of it. The analyst had said: "If I say anything you did not already know or did know but didn't think of, you feel it reveals some inferiority on your part."

Thus it was found that 12 of the 13 statements had emerged without any previous interpretation pertaining directly or indirectly to the ideas expressed. Perhaps the reason for this is that, in this early part of the treatment, the analyst's interpretations did not focus on the contents themselves but, in a general way, on the patient's reluctance to talk. For example, the analyst would say, "I notice you find it hard to begin."

2. Two members of our research group, Carol Drucker and Marla Isaacs, catalogued all the interventions the analyst made during the first 100 hours.

3. Saul Rosenberg and Lynn Campbell.

HOW ANXIOUS DID THE PATIENT FEEL WHEN
THE PREVIOUSLY WARDED-OFF CONTENTS
BECAME CONSCIOUS?

Having located 12 contents that emerged without interpretation, we next attempted to determine how the patient felt about them as they were emerging. Was she anxious or calm? We used three techniques to assess the patient's anxiety at any given moment in the treatment: the Speech Disturbance Ratio (Mahl, 1956), the Gottschalk–Gleser Content Analysis Scale (Gottschalk & Gleser, 1969), and clinical ratings.

Mahl's Speech Disturbance Ratio investigates momentary anxiety in patients by quantifying aspects of how they speak. Disturbances in speech such as sentence changes, stutters, slips of the tongue, intruding incoherent sounds, repetitions, omissions, and sentence incompletions are identified. A speech disturbance ratio can be obtained for any segment of speech by compiling the ratio of speech disturbances to the total number of words spoken. Numerous studies have been conducted using the Mahl measure to assess anxiety and its correlates in psychiatric patients (Mahl, 1956, 1959a, 1959b, 1961). It has been found to be an objective approach to the quantification of anxiety, and a reliably discriminating measure.

The Gottschalk–Gleser Content Analysis Scale is designed to assess immediate anxiety by measuring manifest anxiety-related verbal content. Phrases that focus on any of the following six contents are viewed as evidence of the presence of anxiety in the speaker: mutilation, death, shame, guilt, separation, and diffuse or nonspecific anxiety. Since the six sources of anxiety are considered of equal importance, their manifestations are added together to obtain a measure of the magnitude of a person's anxiety.

Any direct expression of the six types of anxiety is considered evidence that an internal state of anxiety has been activated. In addition, defensive and adaptive manifestations of anxiety are inferred when the speaker (1) imputes anxiety or anxiety-motivated behavior to other people, to animals, or to inanimate objects; (2) repudiates or denies the affect of anxiety; or (3) reports the affect in an attenuated form. There have been numerous studies demonstrating the reliability and the predictive validity for this measure, and there is some evidence for its construct validity (Gottschalk & Gleser, 1969; Gottschalk, 1974a, 1974b).

The third method we used to determine the patient's anxiety involved clinical judgments of anxiety. Judges were given the following instructions:

You will be listening to and reading the typescripts of sequences of patient talk on a variety of themes. I would like you to rate each episode along the following 5-point scale of anxiety (with "1" designated as "relaxed, not anxious"; "5" designated as "very anxious"). This is a rating of manifest anxiety, that is, anxiety which either the patient is experiencing or potentially would experience if asked whether she were anxious. As you listen, consider the patient's general mood during the episode; try to get a feel for her emotional state at the time she is saying these words. Content may or may not be important. Rely on your clinical impressions, using whatever cues make sense to you. Try to use the entire scale, with "3" as the center point representing the average anxiety level for the patient. In order to obtain a sense of what the patient sounds like, listen to the first five episodes without rating them, and then start rating with episode six.

Interrater reliability was high for each of the three anxiety measures. A .91 reliability coefficient was obtained by the two judges who applied Mahl's Speech Disturbance measure to 103 episodes (from verbatim transcripts) in which the 12 warded-off statements and 91 randomly selected statements appeared.[4] Four judges applied the Gottschalk–Gleser Scale to the same 103 episodes, with an interrater reliability coefficient of .80. An intraclass correlation coefficient of .74 was obtained for the average intercorrelation between pairs of six raters who made clinical judgments about the amount of anxiety the patient was expressing in episodes containing the 12 warded-off contents and episodes containing the 20 statements the judges did not believe were strongly warded off. Graduate students served as judges for the Mahl and Gottschalk–Gleser ratings. The clinical ratings of anxiety were made by clinicians who had 2–10 years of clinical experience. These clinical ratings were made by judges listening to audiotape recordings of the episodes while reading the transcripts.

For all three methods used, it was found that there was *no* evidence that the patient was more anxious when previously warded-off contents were emerging than at other times during the analysis (see Tables 12-3 and 12-4). Indeed, in the data produced by the Mahl measure, randomly selected statements were accompanied by considerably *more* anxiety than were previously warded-off statements. This difference was statistically significant ($p < .025$).

---

4. One hundred statements were selected by a random stratified procedure from the first 100 hours of the analysis. Nine of these were found to be too brief to score on the Gottschalk–Gleser Scale. The remaining 91 statements constituted the sample of random items that was used as a comparison group.

Table 12-3. Means and Standard Deviations of Anxiety Ratings on Episodes Containing Statements Judged Highly Warded Off (JHWO) and Randomly Selected Statements

	JHWO statements (N = 12)	Random statements (N = 91)	t
Mahl Speech Disturbance Ratio	.247 (SD = .102)	.319 (SD = .159)	2.25*
Gottschalk–Gleser Content Analysis Scale	2.58 (SD = 0.318)	2.48 (SD = 0.663)	N.S.

*$\alpha < .025$.

EXPERIENCING THE EMERGING CONTENT

In our final study in this research we tested the prediction, based on the unconscious control hypothesis, that the patient is likely to experience the emerging content fully, think about its import, and use it to advance his therapy. This prediction is in contrast to that of the dynamic hypothesis, which assumes, if the patient is calm, that because he is continuing (however subtly) to defend against the content, will not experience the content fully, will not think about its import, and will not use it to advance his therapy.

In order to study these contrasting predictions, we applied the Experiencing Scale (described below) to the 12 statements containing previously warded-off contents. To obtain a control, we also applied it to 91 randomly selected statements.

Table 12-4. Means and Standard Deviations of Clinical Judges' Ratings of Anxiety during Episodes Containing Statements Judged Highly Warded Off (JHWO) and Low Warded Off (JLWO)

	JHWO statements (N = 12)	JLWO statements (N = 20)
$\bar{X}$	2.620	2.580
SD	0.624	0.448
t	N.S.	N.S.

The Experiencing Scale is used to assess the degree to which a patient focuses on his changing feelings as they occur during psychotherapy, the degree to which he reflects on these feelings, and the degree to which he uses such reflections to work at solving his problems. The scale is "sensitive to shifts in patient involvement: this makes it useful for microscopic process studies" (Klein, Mathieu, Gendlin, & Kiesler, 1970, p. 1). The Experiencing Scale, which has been used widely for many years, is considered to be an especially good measure for the study of how patients progress in psychotherapy.

The Experiencing Scale yields two kinds of scores. One is the modal score, which measures the overall experiencing level of a patient during a particular segment of therapy. The other is the peak score, which measures the highest level of a patient's experiencing during this segment.

We calculated the modal and the peak scores both for segments in which previously warded-off contents emerged and for segments containing the randomly selected statements. This work was carried out by four trained judges, all graduate students. Their interrater reliability was .75.

Table 12-5 shows that the patient's experiencing during the analytic segments in which previously warded-off contents emerged was considerably higher than in randomly selected segments. When the modal measure was used, the difference was significant at the .05 level. When the peak measure was used the difference approached significance at the .10 level. This means that the patient, according to our findings, was more involved with reflecting on the feelings she associated with the previously warded-off contents than with those associated with randomly selected contents. She evidently did not ward off the emerging contents with defenses. Indeed, the opposite seemed to be the case. As previously

Table 12-5. Means and Standard Deviations of Experiencing Scores on Episodes Containing Statements Judged Highly Warded Off (JHWO) and Randomly Selected Statements

	JHWO statements ($N = 12$)	Random statements ($N = 91$)	t
Modal Experiencing Scale score	3.400 (SD = 0.632)	3.000 (SD = 0.791)	1.7*
Peak Experiencing Scale score	3.960 (SD = 0.554)	3.610 (SD = 0.749)	1.61**

*$\alpha < .05$.

**$\alpha < .10$.

warded-off contents were becoming conscious, the patient was calmly and without anxiety focusing on them and thinking about them.

A high level of experiencing has been found by a number of investigators to be strongly connected with progress in therapy. The patient's powerful but nonanxious involvement with the emerging warded-off contents and her lack of defensiveness about them is compatible with the idea that she was using her reflections on them to advance her therapy.

DISCUSSION

Our research findings may be summarized as follows: During the first 100 sessions of the analysis, Mrs. C became conscious of a number of previously repressed mental contents without benefit of interpretation. She became conscious of these contents without experiencing any more anxiety about them than about randomly selected new contents. Indeed, according to one measure, she experienced significantly less anxiety. As these previously repressed contents became conscious, Mrs. C experienced them more vividly than she experienced randomly selected contents. She was especially interested in and reflective about them.

These findings are explained simply and directly by the unconscious control hypothesis. According to this hypothesis, a number of previously warded-off contents that had not been interpreted became conscious because the patient herself wished unconsciously to make them conscious. She possessed the capacity to bring them forth and did bring them forth when she unconsciously decided that she could safely experience them. The contents emerged without arousing anxiety because Mrs. C kept them warded off until she unconsciously had overcome her anxieties about them, and only then did she make them conscious. She was able to experience the contents fully, think about them, and use them therapeutically because they no longer endangered her. She had no need, therefore, to defend against them.

The dynamic hypothesis is unable to account convincingly for our combination of findings. It could explain, on the basis of shifts in dynamic equilibria, the coming-to-consciousness of a number of previously warded-off contents. It could explain the patient's lack of anxiety about the emergence of previously warded-off contents by assuming that they continued to be defended against (i.e., they were part of compromise formations). However, it could not explain the patient's experiencing these contents vividly and fully, reflecting upon them, and working with them after their emergence to advance the analysis.

A FINAL POINT

Our observation—that most of the previously warded-off contents which Mrs. C brought forth during these sessions had not been interpreted—is of great interest to psychoanalysts and other students of human behavior. Yet, it is an observation that the psychoanalyst is unlikely to make in the course of his daily work. The analyst ordinarily cannot remember in sufficient detail what was repressed at the beginning of treatment to know whether a particular content was repressed. Moreover, if the analyst happens to understand the analytic process in terms of a purely dynamic hypothesis, he may assume that a content that comes into the patient's focus of attention unobtrusively and without benefit of interpretation was not previously repressed. That is, he may reason from his theory and so assume that an uninterpreted content that comes forth without benefit of interpretation and without arousing anxiety was from the beginning available to consciousness.

The fact that the practicing analyst is not normally in a position to make certain important observations highlights the importance, for the advancement of theory, of formal research.

13

EXPRESSING WARDED-OFF CONTENTS IN BEHAVIOR

JOHN T. CURTIS
PAUL RANSOHOFF
FRANCES SAMPSON
SUZANNE BRUMER
ABBOT A. BRONSTEIN

THE RESEARCH PROBLEM

In this chapter we will compare how well the unconscious control hypothesis and the dynamic hypothesis account for an analytic patient overcoming certain inhibitions and thus expressing warded-off tendencies more directly and openly in behavior.

THE UNCONSCIOUS CONTROL HYPOTHESIS

According to the unconscious control hypothesis, as the patient changes certain pathogenic beliefs and as the anxieties that stem from them are overcome, he will feel less endangered by a particular content. Feeling less threatened, the patient may express that content more prominently in behavior. Because the patient is unconsciously controlling the emergence of the previously warded-off content, it may be expressed more confidently, with a greater sense of control, and persistently over a period of analytic sessions. Moreover, because the patient no longer actively defends against the previously warded-off content, he may think about it and gain insight into its significance.

As noted in the previous chapter, there are certain exceptions to these expectations. For instance, if the patient feels pressured by the analyst, external events, or his conscience to openly express the content before he has overcome his anxiety about it, then the expression of the content may be accompanied by considerable anxiety. In general, however, the patient unconsciously will inhibit or repress the expression of the content in behavior until he feels less endangered by it.

THE DYNAMIC HYPOTHESIS

In contrast, the dynamic hypothesis, based on automatic functioning concepts, attributes changes in the expression of inhibited or warded-off tendencies in the analytic patient's behavior to shifts in the dynamic balance between the patient's impulses and defenses. According to the dynamic hypothesis contained in Freud's early theorizing, the analytic situation leads to a mobilization of conflict. The frustration of the patient's unconscious instinctual wishes in the transference and the undermining of his defenses produce this mobilization of conflict. Both the patient's repressed strivings and the defenses against them are intensified.

According to this hypothesis, the patient may express warded-off strivings more directly and openly because they have become more intense. As these strivings find open expression, the patient is likely to be in conflict with them, feel that they are alien and out of control, and experience heightened anxiety. Sometimes, because of subtle shifts in the dynamic equilibrium between the repressed and repressing forces, the warded-off contents may be expressed only gradually and in the form of successfully disguised compromise formations. In this circumstance, the patient may experience little overt anxiety over or conflict with the contents being expressed in behavior. However, whether or not the contents are expressed with anxiety and conflict, the patient is unlikely to feel an increased sense of control over the expression of these contents. Moreover, the patient is unlikely to express these strivings calmly and persistently, to think about them, or to gain insights into them.

PLAN OF THE STUDY

The first step we took was to find a situation in which an analytic patient, over time, expressed more directly and openly in behavior certain strivings that had been inhibited or warded off previously. The second step was to investigate whether this change in behavior took place in ways more compatible with the unconscious control hypothesis or the dynamic hypothesis.

The patient we studied was Mrs. C. When she began analysis, Mrs. C suffered from severe inhibitions in her ability to be assertive—for example, to disagree directly and openly with others, to express her own opinions and hold to them, and to criticize or blame others. She was also severely inhibited in her capacity to be close to others—for example, to be cooperative, affectionate, and sexual (see Chapter 10).

In our formulation of Mrs. C's unconscious plan for treatment (Chapter 10), we inferred that she would work persistently to overcome these inhibitions and repressions and to be both more assertive–aggressive and more friendly–affectionate–sexual. In the first study described below, we investigated whether during the first 100 sessions of her analysis Mrs. C actually overcame these inhibitions and expressed both types of behaviors more directly. The second study tested whether the changes that had been observed represented a mobilization of conflict or took place under the patient's unconscious control.

THE FIRST STUDY: CHANGES IN TWO TYPES OF BEHAVIOR

The first study, carried out by Horowitz, Sampson, Siegelman, Weiss, and Goodfriend (1978), used the process notes of the first 100 hours of Mrs. C's psychoanalysis to examine changes in two types of behavior. The first type of behavior (termed "Distancing" or "Type D" by Horowitz *et al.*) was assertive or aggressive; it included criticizing, disagreeing with, blaming, or opposing another person. The second type of behavior (termed "Closeness" or Type C" by Horowitz *et al.*) was affectionate, friendly, or sexual behavior; it included such behaviors as complimenting someone, expressing affection/sexual feelings or behaving sexually toward someone, and expressing compassion toward someone.

METHODS OF PROCEDURE

The Process Notes

The analyst took detailed notes during each session. As the patient was talking, the analyst was writing. He took special care to be comprehensive and accurate because he intended to use the notes in his own research. The analyst was unfamiliar with the ideas of our research group, and indeed had completed the analysis before the present study was undertaken.

Item Selection

Three clinicians independently read the process notes of the first 100 hours in unsystematic order (to avoid bias), looking for all passages in the notes that described Type D behaviors. Such behaviors could have taken place in the present or in the past, and could have been expressed toward the therapist or anyone else. Then the three clinicians together reviewed all the passages that they had identified and retained the ones that they all agreed were instances of Type D behavior. An identical procedure—except that it was carried out by only two clinicians—was used to identify instances of Type C behavior.

A total of 190 passages of Type D behavior were identified, including instances of directly observable behaviors (e.g., criticizing the analyst) and self-reports of such behaviors. A total of 106 passages of Type C behaviors were identified, including both directly observable behaviors and self-reports of such behaviors.

Rating Scales

The investigators developed a 4-point rating scale to assess the directness of expression of the Type D and C behaviors identified in the preceding step. If the behavior was only implied or if it was expressed tentatively, the scale value was "1" (e.g., "She was also troubled with not getting reactions from me, no interaction. She was afraid she needed approval."). As the behavior became more explicit and direct, the scale value increased. A behavior that was expressed but was then immediately undone was rated "2." A rating of "3" was given when the behavior was overtly expressed by telling a third party about it (e.g., criticizing one person to another). If the behavior was expressed directly to the first person, it was rated "4" (e.g., "Then she said she just realized that actually she had intercourse Sunday morning."). If the behavior occurred in the present (i.e., since the start of therapy) rather than in the past (before starting therapy), the rating was increased by 0.5. Consequently, the range of possible scores for a given C or D behavior was 1.0 to 4.5. Explicit scoring rules were developed for rating the D and C passages, and the judges followed these rules in rating each behavior.

Rating D and C Segments on the Scales

The Type D passages were divided into two subsets for rating. Two groups of four clinical psychologists who were naive to the case served as raters. Each group rated a different subset of the D items. The passages were presented to the judges independently and in random order. A similar procedure was used for rating the Type C passages, except that there was only one set of C passages to rate.

(See Appendices 1 and 2 for further details about the rating scales.)

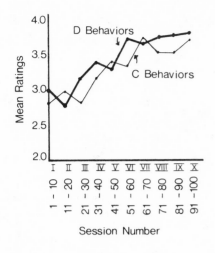

Figure 13-1. Mean rating of passages in each block of hours. From L. M. Horowitz, H. Sampson, E. Y. Siegelman, J. Weiss, and S. Goodfriend, Cohesive and dispersal behaviors: Two classes of concomitant change in psychotherapy. *Journal of Consulting and Clinical Psychology,* 1978, *46*(3), 556–564. Copyright 1978 by the American Psychological Association. Reprinted by permission of the publisher.

RESULTS[1]

Type D Behaviors

The reliability of the judges' ratings was computed for each set of judges through an analysis of variance. The reliability was .89 for one set, .90 for the other set. The 100 sessions were then grouped into 10-session blocks denoted I, II, . . . , X. The number of passages within each block were I = 31; II = 13; III = 18; IV = 9; V = 35; VI = 13; VII = 13; VIII = 10; IX = 29; and X = 19. The ratings of passages within each block were averaged, and the means ranged from 2.62 to 3.81. These means are reported in Figure 13-1.

To examine changes in Type D behaviors more closely, all passages rated alike were examined as a group. Because of the small frequencies in some categories, passages rated 2.0 and 2.5 were combined, as were passages rated 4.0 and 4.5. Also, to obtain more stable frequencies, the sessions were grouped into 20-session blocks.

The relative frequency for each rating was computed for each block (Figure 13-2). The top two graphs show a steady decline for passages rated 1.0–2.5. Figure 13-2 also shows a decline in 3.0's (criticizing someone for a past event) but an increase in 3.5's (criticizing someone for a

1. This section is taken in its entirety from L. M. Horowitz, H. Sampson, E. Y. Siegelman, J. Weiss, and S. Goodfriend, Cohesive and dispersal behaviors: Two classes of concomitant change in psychotherapy. *Journal of Consulting and Clinical Psychology,* 1978, *46*(3), 556–564. Copyright 1978 by the American Psychological Association. Reprinted by permission of the publisher.

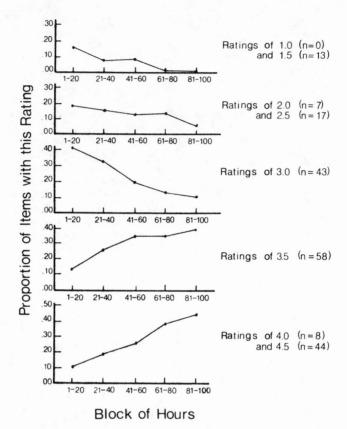

Block of Hours

Figure 13-2. Relative frequency of passages in each rating category for successive blocks of hours (Type D). From L. M. Horowitz, H. Sampson, E. Y. Siegelman, J. Weiss, and S. Goodfriend, Cohesive and dispersal behaviors: Two classes of concomitant change in psychotherapy. *Journal of Consulting and Clinical Psychology,* 1978, *46*(3), 556–564. Copyright 1978 by the American Psychological Association. Reprinted by permission of the publisher.

current event). Direct confrontations (4.0 and 4.5) also became more frequent throughout the treatment. The graphs reflect major changes that occurred in the patient's behavior during the treatment.

To compare the frequencies of past and present events, the relative frequencies of 3.0's and 3.5's were compared. There were 101 passages with these ratings. For each block of 20 sessions, the relative frequency of 3.5's (present tense) was computed. For successive 20-session blocks, the values were 6/24 (i.e., 6 cases were reported in the present tense, 18 were reported in the past tense) = .25; 8/16 = .50; 17/26 = .65; 8/11 = .73; and

19/24 = .79. Thus, the patient increasingly came to criticize others for events in her current life. It is assumed that events from the past were less threatening for her and provided a convenient starting point for the therapy, but as the sessions progressed, she shifted her focus to her current life. Thus, *part* of the increment in Figure 13-1 is due to the patient's shift to present tense events, and *part* is due to the decline in lower ratings (primarily 1.5 and 2.5).

Type C Behaviors

The reliability of the 106 Type C ratings was also assessed by an analysis of variance; the reliability of the four judges' means was .83. The 100 sessions were grouped into 10-session blocks, with the following frequencies within each block: I = 11; II = 9; III = 15; IV = 10; V = 9; VI = 12; VII = 14; VIII = 9; IX = 5, X = 12. The ratings of the passages within each block were then averaged, and the resulting means ranged from 2.67 to 3.75. Figure 13-1 shows the expression of the Type C behaviors across successive blocks of sessions.

To examine the change in Type C behaviors more closely, all passages rated alike were examined as a group. Since the frequencies were smaller than those concerning Type D behaviors, all of the ratings from 1.0 to 3.0 were pooled. (These were the categories that had shown declining relative frequencies in Type D behaviors.) Likewise, all of the ratings from 3.5 to 4.5 were pooled. (These were the categories that had shown increasing relative frequencies in Type D behaviors.) Relative frequencies of occurrence were computed for each block of 20 sessions, as shown in Figure 13-3. One graph shows a progressive decline in the relative frequencies of the lower ratings, and the other graph shows a progressive increase in the relative frequencies of the higher ratings. The two graphs thus resemble those obtained for the Type D behaviors. Events in the past tense were also examined, but their frequencies were too small (only 23 cases) to permit any inference.

Thus, two types of changes clearly occurred, but it still needed to be demonstrated that a change occurred in the patient's presenting complaint, sexual frigidity. Therefore, every reference by the patient to her sexual behavior was noted throughout the 100 hours. There were 18 such references (comprising a subset of the 106 Type C passages), all occurring between hours 28 and 100. Each passage contained the word *intercourse* except one, which contained the phrase *sexual interest*. Here are some examples: From hour 33 (rated 2.5): "Sometimes when she is trying to

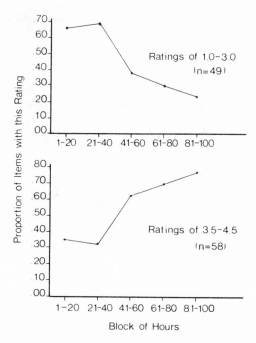

Figure 13-3. Relative frequency of passages in different rating categories for successive blocks of hours (Type C). From L. M. Horowitz, H. Sampson, E. Y. Siegelman, J. Weiss, and S. Goodfriend, Cohesive and dispersal behaviors: Two classes of concomitant change in psychotherapy. *Journal of Consulting and Clinical Psychology,* 1978, *46*(3), 556–564. Copyright 1978 by the American Psychological Association. Reprinted by permission of the publisher.

make herself have intercourse with Henry, she feels as though she wants to hurt him. She just doesn't understand it. She'll go from feeling very warm to feeling nothing toward him suddenly." From hour 67 (rated 4.5): "This weekend she and Henry had intercourse, and she was thinking how different it can be when she's thinking about him and feeling close to him and not all wrapped up in herself."

Seven passages occurred in the first 50 sessions, and 11 occurred in the last 50 sessions. The C rating assigned to each passage was noted. For those in the early block, 6 had ratings of 1.5 to 2.5, and 1 (in hour 43) had a rating of 3.5 to 4.5. Of the 11 passages in the later block, 4 had ratings of 1.5 to 2.5, and 7 had ratings of 3.5 to 4.5. The difference in the ratings (from the first 50 hours to the last 50) was significant (Fisher probability $< .05$), indicating that Mrs. C became more direct in her expressions of sexual behavior over the course of the first 100 sessions.

CHECKING FINDINGS IN A RANDOM SAMPLE
OF TRANSCRIPTS

Curtis and Ransohoff checked the accuracy of findings obtained in the process notes study above by comparing them to findings obtained for a random sample of verbatim transcripts taken from the same 100 hours. The transcripts were divided into ten 10-session blocks. Two therapy sessions were randomly selected for study from each of the 10-session blocks, for a total of 20 sessions. The methods used to select passages containing Type C and D behaviors and to rate these items were analogous to those used in the Horowitz *et al.* study above.

Results

A total of 133 D segments and 85 C segments were identified in the sample of verbatim transcripts. Four experienced clinician judges independently rated all the D segments, and a separate group of four experienced clinician judges independently rated all of the C segments. The intrarater reliability for ratings of the D scale, computed using the interclass correlation coefficient (Tinsley & Weiss, 1975), was .66. The analogous reliability coefficient for the 85 C segments was .68.

As the number of both C and D items in each 10-hour block (i.e., in the two random sessions drawn from each 10-session block) varied considerably, ratings were analyzed in terms of 20-session blocks (i.e., sessions 1–20; 21–40; etc.). The judges' ratings for C and D items within each 20-hour block were averaged, providing a mean D item score and a mean C item score for each of the five blocks (see Table 13-1). Figure 13-4 illustrates the increase in level of directness with which both C and D behaviors were expressed across the first 100 hours of therapy. The correlation between the level of directness of the D items and time (i.e., block of hours) was .87 ($p < .05$); for C items it was .79 ($p < .10$).

Although the correlation for C items was not statistically significant, the results from the random sample of transcripts were consistent with findings in the process notes study. Additional support for the findings of the Horowitz *et al.* study were obtained by comparing the mean scores for D and C behaviors in comparable 20-hour blocks. The correlations between the scores from the transcript study and the process notes study were .86 for D behaviors ($p < .05$) and .90 for C behaviors ($p < .05$). These correlations further demonstrate the similarities between the findings from verbatim transcripts and from process notes.

Table 13-1. Mean Directness Ratings for Type D and C Behaviors in 20-Hour Blocks

	Mean directness ratings[b]			
	Transcripts		Process notes[c]	
Block of sessions[a]	D segments ($N = 133$)	C segments ($N = 85$)	D segments ($N = 190$)	C segments ($N = 106$)
I (1–20)	2.65 (35)	2.46 (23)	2.76 (44)	2.77 (20)
II (21–40)	2.99 (28)	2.55 (23)	3.09 (27)	2.84 (25)
III (41–60)	3.34 (21)	2.73 (15)	3.37 (48)	3.33 (21)
IV (61–80)	3.12 (24)	2.84 (13)	3.69 (23)	3.65 (23)
V (81–100)	3.44 (25)	2.69 (11)	3.78 (48)	3.65 (17)

[a]Numbers in parentheses are the sessions included within each block.

[b]Numbers in parentheses are the numbers of Type C or D segments identified in each block.

[c]From raw data of Horowitz *et al.* (1978).

Conclusion

The Curtis–Ransohoff study of verbatim transcripts supports the finding from the Horowitz *et al.* process notes study: There was a progressive increase in the directness of expression of both assertive–aggressive behaviors and friendly–affectionate–sexual behaviors by Mrs. C during the first 100 sessions of her analysis.

THE SECOND STUDY: UNCONSCIOUS CONTROL OR MOBILIZATION OF CONFLICT

Our next task was to determine whether Mrs. C was expressing previously warded-off contents more directly and openly under her own control or because of a mobilization of conflict. We used various kinds of evidence to provide information about this question: clinical judgments, formal measures of anxiety, a rating of freedom versus beleaguerment, and a measure of the patient's drivenness versus sense of control.

The studies designed to answer this question were carried out by Frances Sampson, Abbot Bronstein, and Suzanne Brumer, under the direction of Elizabeth Mayer.

CLINICAL JUDGMENTS

Independent Psychoanalytic Clinicians

Two training analysts who were not members of the research group, and who were unfamiliar with the case of Mrs. C, studied the process notes of the first 100 sessions of her analysis. Their task was simply to formulate their own agreed-upon impression of the most important emerging theme in hours 41–100. They were given no further orientation as to how to define their task or what to attend to. Indeed, the task we assigned them was not intended for the present purpose, although their response is pertinent to it. They summarized the most important emerging theme as follows:

The patient is now able to experience intermittently and enjoy relaxation of control in various areas. This is demonstrated, for example, in a new if limited capacity to respond sexually; free-associate and reveal symptoms and preoccupations; think and work more spontaneously and productively; tolerate and express

Figure 13-4. Level of directness of Type C and D behaviors.

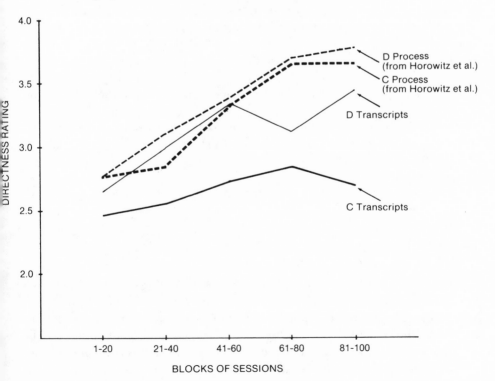

strong affects—especially anger—more readily; exercise a more modulated discipline over colleagues in her charge.

It is evident that these experienced psychoanalysts saw Mrs. C as becoming increasingly relaxed, less anxious, and freer over the course of hours 41–100. This means that as the patient was expressing assertive and friendly–affectionate behaviors more openly and directly, she was also, as perceived by these independent judges, becoming more relaxed, spontaneous, and comfortable with herself.

The Research Group

A number of members of the research group informally studied the process notes of the first 100 sessions of Mrs. C's psychoanalysis more than a year before the present study was conceptualized. No attempt was made to formalize the clinical impressions of these members of the research group, but brief notations were made about their impressions of these hours. These notations suggest that the group formed an impression very similar to that of the two independent training analysts cited above: Mrs. C was becoming more free, spontaneous, and relaxed. This is indicated by such notations as the following:

Hour 38: "Mrs. C acknowledges feeling freer in the sessions."
Hour 41: "Mrs. C feels freer to talk."
Hour 49: "We see much more relaxation in the analysis . . . working on relaxing control."
Hour 53: "Much freer, less fear of intercourse, less formal, more intimate . . . more relaxation in analysis and at the agency."
Hour 75: "Enjoys self more."

There were no notations indicating increased anxiety, tension, or constriction.

Comment

There is a striking similarity in the clinical impressions of the two training analysts and of the research group members. Both sets of observations emphasize the patient's progressive relaxation and freedom. Thus, the patient's behavior, according to these judgments, was fully in accord with expectations derived from the unconscious control hypothesis. The patient, as she began to express previously warded-off contents more directly in her behavior, was becoming more relaxed rather than more anxious, more confident, less driven. There was no evidence of a mobilization of conflict.

No measures presently exist that can replicate the complex weighing and integration of information provided by sophisticated clinical judgment. Moreover, these clinical impressions are based on the reading of all of the hours in sequence, rather than on reading selected excerpts. These spontaneous clinical impressions provide a broader and more complex assessment of the patient's mental state and behavior than the formal measures we applied subsequently. Nonetheless, formal measures may avoid potential biases and are based on judgments that can be made reliably by independent judges.

FORMAL MEASURES OF ANXIETY

We used two standardized measures of anxiety to address the question of whether Mrs. C became more anxious as she expressed warded-off contents more directly in her behavior. We would expect her to have become increasingly anxious if there was a mobilization of conflict. We would not anticipate an increase of anxiety over the first 100 sessions if she was expressing warded-off contents under her own unconscious control.

The two measures we used were the Gottschalk–Gleser Content Analysis Scale and the Mahl Speech Disturbance Ratio (see Chapter 12). The Gottschalk–Gleser Scale was applied to transcript episodes selected from the same 20 hours used by Curtis and Ransohoff in their study of changes in Type D and C behaviors. For the current study, the transcripts of the 20 hours were divided into segments of 10–20 lines of patient speech uninterrupted by the analyst. Five of these segments were then randomly selected from each of the 20 hours for a total of 100 segments.

Four judges independently rated the 100 segments on the Gottschalk–Gleser Scale. Good interrater reliability (intraclass correlations using the means of the four judges' ratings) were obtained ($r = .80$, $p < .01$). An average rating for the measure was then calculated for each hour, and these averages were correlated with hour number to yield a trend over time. Essentially there was no correlation between changes in the Gottschalk–Gleser ratings and time ($r = .04$, N.S.).

The Mahl Speech Disturbance measure was applied to the same 100 segments selected for the Gottschalk–Gleser Scale. Two judges independently rated each segment on this scale, and excellent interrater reliability (Pearson r) was obtained ($r = .92$, $p < .01$). Averages for the Mahl measure ratings within each hour were computed and then correlated with hour number to yield a trend over time. Again, there was essentially no correlation of this measure with time ($r = -.255$, N.S.).

Comment

We found no evidence on the two measures used that Mrs. C's anxiety increased over the first 100 sessions. Thus, our findings do not support the expectation, based on the dynamic hypothesis, that Mrs. C would experience intensified conflict as she expressed warded-off impulses more directly in her behavior.

A MEASURE OF FREEDOM VERSUS BELEAGUERMENT

We sought to measure the psychic state of freedom, relaxation, and comfort versus that of anxiety, drivenness, and beleaguerment. No standardized instrument available entirely captured this broad dimension. Therefore, we decided to develop our own scale. The following definitions were employed:

The patient would be considered to be feeling "free" or "relaxed" if displaying any or all of the following behaviors:

The patient is able to associate freely and easily be playful, and experience a wide range of feelings without feeling driven. She is able to play with ideas and explore connections between thoughts in an uninhibited, spontaneous kind of way. She feels generally on top of things. She may be feeling bad (depressed, anxious, etc.); but if so, she is able freely to experience and explore these feelings. She is creative, confident, optimistic, flexible, or especially bold and relaxed in tackling tasks. She seems generally comfortable with the way she is.

Similarly, any or all of the following behaviors would be considered to reflect feeling "beleaguered":

The patient is constricted and narrow in her associations; she is driven to think, feel, or behave in certain ways. She seems compelled by things beyond her control. She is tense, rigid, tight, grim. She may feel weak, ineffectual, or inadequate. She seems halting, timid, or bothered by the train of her thoughts and makes connections with difficulty. She is stuck and without vitality or hope. She seems generally uncomfortable with the way she is. She is anxious and driven.

A 5-point rating scale was developed by Mayer, Sampson, Bronstein, and Brumer to rate brief transcript episodes. At the low end of the scale

(1), the "patient seems uncomfortable, beleaguered, driven, defensive, constricted, tense, tight." At midrange (3) the "patient seems just about as constricted and tense as she is free and relaxed." At the high end of the scale (5), the "patient seems free, unconstricted, spontaneous, relaxed (relatively more so than in 4)." Cues used to infer freedom and relaxation (the high end of the scale) include:

a. The patient is able to associate freely, easily, and flexibly.
b. The patient is able to be playful with ideas and explore connections between thoughts in an uninhibited, spontaneous manner.
c. The patient is able to experience and explore her feelings fully and undefensively.

Cues for inferring anxiety, beleaguerment, and drivenness (the low end of the scale) include:

a. The patient is defensive, constricted, or narrow in her associations.
b. The patient feels compelled by things beyond her control.
c. The patient feels anxious, tense, rigid, tight, or grim.
d. The patient seems halting, timid, or bothered by her train of thoughts, and her associations come with difficulty.
e. The patient seems stuck, without vitality or hope.

(See Appendix 3 for a fuller description of the scale.)

Four judges independently applied the Freedom versus Beleaguerment Scale to the same 100 brief transcript episodes employed with the Mahl and Gottschalk-Gleser scales. Good interrater reliabilities were obtained; the intraclass correlation was .73 ($p < .01$). The judges' ratings for each item were averaged, and a mean rating of the items for each hour was then calculated. These means for each hour were then correlated with the hour number to test for changes in Mrs. C's feelings of anxiety and drivenness over the course of the analysis. The correlation obtained was $-.43$ ($p > .10$). The relationship is in the direction of *increased* beleaguerment over time, but it is not statistically significant, and there was considerable fluctuation in Mrs. C's feelings of freedom and beleaguerment over the first 100 hours of her psychoanalysis.

Comment

This finding, although in the direction predicted by the dynamic hypothesis, does not enable us to reject the null hypothesis that no changes occurred in the patient's feelings of anxiety and control while she was expressing previously warded-off contents. We shall comment on the discrepancy between this measure and certain other measures in the Discussion, later in the chapter.

A MEASURE OF DRIVENNESS VERSUS CONTROL

The scale developed by Horowitz *et al.* (1978) reported earlier in this chapter provides a direct measure of the degree of control a patient experiences over behavior. It thus provides a way of discriminating between behavior that is experienced by the patient as under his control, and behavior experienced by the patient as driven, forced, and inflexible. Horowitz called this measure the Drivenness Scale.

This scale (see Appendix 4) includes two kinds of complaint statements. One kind of complaint statement is of having to act in a certain way although one does not wish to do so—for example, a complaint by Mrs. C that she feels she *has to* fight with her husband. The other kind of complaint statement is of being unable to act in a certain way although one would like to—for example, a complaint by Mrs. C that she *cannot* praise her colleague at work. Both kinds of complaints convey a sense of behaving in a driven, inflexible, compelled way. The scale simply measures the frequency with which such complaints appear over specified intervals of time or in relation to specified kinds of behavior (such as Type D and Type C behaviors).

Horowitz *et al.* applied the Drivenness Scale to the process notes of the first 100 hours of Mrs. C's psychoanalysis. A total of 351 pertinent complaint statements were identified. All of the complaints referred to the present; that is, statements of a past limitation that had been overcome were not counted.

Horowitz *et al.* identified changes in drivenness over time. The first 100 sessions were broken into 20-hour blocks, and the number of Drivenness statements within each block was calculated. The number of these statements occurring within consecutive blocks of sessions dropped significantly over the first 100 sessions. The percentage of the total number of Drivenness statements for the five blocks were: I = 26%; II = 24%; III = 17%; IV = 19%, and V = 15% ($\chi^2 = 15.48$, $p < .01$). Further, when the total number of Drivenness statements per hour was correlated with time (hour number), there was a statistically significant decline in the number of such statements over the course of the 100 sessions ($r = -.28$, $p < .01$).

We tested whether these findings would hold in a random sample of verbatim transcripts. F. Sampson replicated the study on verbatim transcripts using the same 20 hours employed by Curtis and Ransohoff in testing the D and C measures. The product–moment correlation coefficient of the number of Drivenness items in *each* of the 20 transcript hours with the number of such items in the corresponding process note for each of these hours was .73 ($p < .001$). The number of Drivenness statements per transcript hour correlated with time (hour number) was −.63 ($p < .001$), indicating a marked decrease in Mrs. C's expressions of Drivenness across the first 100 sessions of her analysis. Thus, the transcript study supports the findings from the process notes study: Mrs. C, according to the Drivenness Scale, progressively experienced herself as less driven and more flexible and free in her behavior over the course of the first 100 sessions.

DISCUSSION

The studies reported in this chapter indicate that Mrs. C, over the course of the first 100 hours, became progressively more direct in expressing previously warded-off contents: She became more direct and open in expressions of self-assertion and aggression; and she became more direct and open in expressions of friendliness, affection, and sexuality. At the same time that these changes in behavior were occurring, the patient, according to two independent clinical studies, became less anxious and more relaxed, free, and spontaneous. She also enjoyed herself more, felt more comfortable with herself, and was confident enough to relax controls somewhat in various areas. These clinical impressions were supported when the Drivenness Scale was applied to the first 100 sessions. According to this scale, Mrs. C steadily and progressively experienced her behavior as under her control and as less driven and involuntary.

However, another formal measure (the Freedom versus Beleaguerment Scale) did not detect any significant change in Mrs. C's feelings of freedom or beleaguerment during these same 100 hours. Similarly, two other standardized measures of anxiety (Mahl and Gottschalk–Gleser scales), when applied to brief episodes of patient speech, failed to detect any significant increase or decrease in anxiety over the same period. According to these three measures, Mrs. C was working within a relatively constant range of anxiety over the first 100 hours. We cannot be sure how to account for this discrepancy, but we venture a possible explanation: The anxiety measures and the Freedom versus Beleaguerment Scale measure momentary states. They fluctuate markedly from moment to moment. The average of a sample of these momentary states may not provide an adequate index of the patient's overall sense of calmness, relaxation, and control. Moreover, each of these measures was applied to brief speech episodes taken from a random sample of 20 sessions. This limited sampling of hours over time may not have provided an adequate basis for detecting change (increase or decrease) in the patient's underlying sense of freedom, calm, and relaxation over the 100 sessions. In contrast, the clinical studies were based on consecutive reading of all of the sessions, and the Drivenness Scale was based on all pertinent items in all sessions.

IMPLICATION OF FINDINGS IN RELATION TO OUR RESEARCH QUESTION

Our key research question in this chapter is whether Mrs. C's expression of warded-off contents was taking place under her unconscious control or beyond her control as a product of the dynamic interaction of her impulses and defenses. To test this question, we studied whether Mrs. C's anxiety and drivenness increased over time in conjunction with the more direct expression of these tendencies. In light of the fact that over the first 100 hours of her psychoanalysis Mrs. C was developing new insights and expressing certain thoughts and behaviors more freely and directly, the clinical impressions that she appeared less anxious and driven, in combination with the results from the Drivenness Scale, support the hypothesis that the expression of warded-off contents was taking place under her unconscious control. Similarly, findings of no significant change on the other three formal measures (the Gottschalk–Gleser, Mahl, and Freedom versus Beleaguerment scales) are consistent with this hypothesis. However, these latter findings of no change may be questioned because they involve acceptance of the null hypothesis and thus do not provide statistical support for the unconscious control hypothesis. Also, the findings from the Freedom versus Beleaguerment Scale, though not statistically significant, were in the direction of Mrs. C appearing less free and more beleaguered. Nonetheless, the clinical findings and the results from the four clinical scales can be regarded as converging lines of evidence for the proposition that the changes noted in Mrs. C's thoughts and actions during the first 100 hours of her analysis occurred under the control of her ego and as a consequence of her deliberately bringing them forth.

The overall pattern of findings does not support the dynamic hypothesis that Mrs. C was expressing warded-off impulses more overtly in her behavior because of a mobilization of conflict. Mrs. C showed no increased anxiety or conflict. There was a decrease rather than an increase in the drivenness of her behavior. She became more confident of herself, had more sense of control, and, according to clinical judgments, also had more freedom to relax her controls and behave spontaneously. Nor was there evidence of a gradual shift in the dynamic balance of impulses and defenses leading to a gradual and more disguised expression of impulses. In a gradual and well-disguised shift toward greater impulse expression, the patient might not manifest an increase in anxiety, for the impulse expression would be disguised in a compromise formation. The patient would not, however, be expected to feel an increased sense of comfort and control over her behavior, nor an ability to relax controls and to be spontaneous.

Thus, the network of findings reported in this chapter and Chapters 12 and 14 support the hypothesis that Mrs. C's expression of warded-off contents took place under her unconscious control, not as a consequence of a dynamic interaction of impulses and defenses.

14

THE ACQUISITION OF INSIGHT

CYNTHIA SHILKRET
MARLA ISAACS
CAROL DRUCKER
JOHN T. CURTIS

THE RESEARCH PROBLEM

In this chapter we shall report research investigating whether the unconscious control hypothesis is compatible with findings about how Mrs. C increased her awareness of a particular domain of conscious, preconscious, and unconscious concern to her. The domain is that of her irrational feelings of responsibility and guilt toward others and the pathogenic beliefs about her power to harm others, which provoke these feelings.

Our case formulation for Mrs. C, presented in Chapter 10, identified the domain described above as of central importance for her psychopathology. We inferred that Mrs. C's symptoms and inhibitions were based to a considerable extent on largely unconscious fears of her power to harm others and that these fears stemmed from pathogenic beliefs developed in childhood about her parents' and siblings' vulnerabilities. She believed they would be severely damaged if she held different ideas or values than they; if she led a life that was less burdened and joyless than she perceived theirs to be; if she was strong, assertive, able to think for herself, self-confident, and decisive; or if she was able to be close to others, to be sexual, and to enjoy sexual intercourse with her husband.

Because this domain was central to our case formulation, we decided to study it systematically. The first study, carried out by Cynthia Shilkret, investigated these questions: Did Mrs. C work steadily and persistently on her thoughts and feelings in this domain during the first 100 sessions of her analysis? If so, did she make progress in becoming more aware of, and in beginning to gain some insights about, her thoughts and feelings in this domain? The second study, carried out by Carol Drucker and

Marla Isaacs, investigated this question: If Mrs. C did focus on this domain and made progress in becoming more aware of and insightful about it, was this because the analyst was guiding her in this direction by focusing her attention on these issues and conveying insights to her? Or did Mrs. C focus on this domain and begin to acquire increased awareness and insight largely on her own?

The theory of therapy presented in Part I assumes that Mrs. C would have powerful unconscious motivations to understand and eventually to change her pathogenic beliefs. Moreover, according to this theory, as Mrs. C made some progress in changing her pathogenic beliefs, she would be less endangered by feelings of anxiety, guilt, and responsibility stemming from these beliefs. She would be able to unconsciously lift her defenses against these contents and become more aware of feelings of guilt and responsibility. She might also be able to begin to gain insight into her problems with these feelings, as well as into the pathogenic beliefs themselves. Although pertinent interpretations would be helpful to her in making this progress, she might be able to do so on her own even without much interpretive help from the analyst.

In contrast, a purely dynamic hypothesis could not account convincingly for Mrs. C's lifting her defenses without interpretation and developing insight into unconscious conflicts without interpretive help.

THE FIRST STUDY

The purpose of the first study was to determine if Mrs. C did work persistently during the first 100 sessions of her psychoanalysis in the domain of her feelings of responsibility, guilt, and irrational feelings of power to hurt others and, if so, whether she made progress in acquiring insights into this domain.

METHOD

Our method of answering these questions involved three steps. The first step was to select all patient statements during the first 100 sessions that pertained unambiguously to her irrational feelings of responsibility, guilt, and power to hurt others. The second step was to describe different levels of Mrs. C's insight into her irrational ideas. The third step was to have the selected ideas rated by independent judges in order to determine whether Mrs. C did achieve higher levels of awareness and insight over the course of the 100 hours.

Item Selection

Seven clinicians carefully read the process notes of the first 100 hours of Mrs. C's psychoanalysis and extracted all statements by the patient that pertained to her preoccupations with feelings of responsibility, guilt, power to harm others, and so forth. These clinicians were guided in this task by a list of instructions (see Appendix 5) that described the kinds of items pertinent to the domain. For purposes of this scale, only statements demonstrating conscious awareness of, preoccupation with, or understanding of the problem area were relevant; that is, the clinicians were asked to select statements pertaining to what the patient was *aware of* or *understood*, rather than *behavioral manifestations* of the problem area.

For this initial selection of items, the intent was to be overinclusive in obtaining a preliminary item pool. Shilkret and four colleagues reviewed together each item from the preliminary pool. On the basis of discussion and consensus, they eliminated from further consideration all items judged ambiguous or not relevant to the domain. After these items were dropped from the preliminary pool, a total of 144 items remained.

Scale Development

Shilkret then studied the 144 items to determine if they contained differing levels of awareness of and insight into the problem area.[1] She defined five distinguishable levels of awareness by the patient into her irrational fear of hurting others[2]:

At *Level 1*, the patient is virtually unaware of her irrational sense of power to harm others. She is aware instead of feeling weak, helpless, impotent, or unable to exert control in her relations with others. She cannot do things she wants to do in these relationships, or she feels compelled to do things she does not want to do; that is, she feels either inhibited or compulsive in relation to others. For example, "She wanted to behave differently, but she found herself doing the same old things."

At *Level 2*, the patient is aware of typically vague and unfocused feelings of responsibility or guilt. She is not aware of why she has these feelings. For example, "She feels responsible when other people criticize someone close to her."

1. Shilkret was not entirely blind to when these items appeared during the 100 sessions, for she had led the team selecting the original item pool.

2. Robert Shilkret and Georgine Marrott also took part in this phase of the research and worked with Cynthia Shilkret to prepare the scale in its final form.

At *Level 3*, the patient is not only aware of feelings of responsibility or guilt, but links these feelings to the idea that she can harm others by her thoughts or actions or failure to act. She is not aware explicitly that her fear of harming others may at times be irrational, nor is she aware that having control in a relationship is something she may want or enjoy. She is aware of feeling uncomfortable if she feels she has any control in a relationship, for she may harm others by that control. For instance, "She thinks it is terrible that she can make people do what she wants them to." "She can hurt people if she isn't careful."

At *Level 4*, the patient is aware of comfort, and even at times of enjoyment, about feeling that she has power and control over others. We may infer that, at Level 4, the patient knows implicitly that she is not in danger of harming others by having power and control over them. She is not, however, explicitly aware that her fears of having power and control are, in many regards, irrational. For example, "She can make people obey her." "She really enjoys making people obey her."

At *Level 5*, the patient is beginning to be explicitly aware that her concerns over her power to harm others are at times irrational. She makes an explicit distinction between thoughts and actions (e.g., "She realizes it's not what she did that bothers her, but rather what she was thinking."); or she realistically explores and assesses the extent of her ability to control others ("She's trying to figure out just how much control she has over others.") and whether or not that control is harmful; or she begins to examine the genetic origins of her irrational sense of harmful power in present relationships.

(Shilkret's scale is presented in Appendix 6.)

The five levels of this scale may be combined into a single sentence (formulated by Estelle Weiss). In this sentence each level is related to the next higher level by an explanatory term or phrase: (1) I have felt helpless in my relationships with others *in order to avoid* (2) feeling responsible and guilty toward them *because* (3) if I have any control or power in relation to them I will hurt them by my thoughts and actions; *however*, (4) I need not feel anxious and guilty if I have power in relation to them, *because* (5) my fear of hurting them is irrational.

Ratings

Following development of the scale, three new judges were trained in its application. They were then given the 144 statements and asked to rate each for the scale level it most closely represented. The statements were typed on individual cards and presented to the judges in random order.

Interrater reliabilities (Pearson r) were .54, .60, and .68 (all $p < .001$). Two or more of the judges agreed on the absolute rating of 131 of the 144 original items. The 13 items upon which no two judges agreed were deemed ambiguous (generally because of being too brief or so out of context that they were difficult to rate), and these items were eliminated from further consideration. The remaining 131 statements were given the rating that two or more judges agreed upon. All five levels were represented in the ratings, though very few statements within the first 100 sessions were rated at Level 5.

RESULTS

The 131 statements were grouped into 10-hour blocks (I: hours 1–10; II: hours 11–20; . . . ; X: hours 91–100) and mean ratings of the statements within each block were calculated (see Table 14-1).

Table 14-1. Mean Ratings of Patient's Awareness into
Irrational Fears

Block of sessions[a]	Stage of awareness[b]				
	I	II	III	IV	V
I	11	2	4	0	0
(1–10)	(65)	(12)	(24)	—	—
II	2	5	7	2	0
(11–20)	(12)	(31)	(44)	(12)	—
III	3	12	2	0	0
(21–30)	(18)	(70)	(12)	—	—
IV	3	6	4	1	0
(31–40)	(21)	(42)	(29)	(7)	—
V	5	4	4	1	0
(41–50)	(36)	(29)	(29)	(7)	—
VI	2	6	3	0	0
(51–60)	(18)	(55)	(27)	—	—
VII	2	3	4	5	1
(61–70)	(13)	(20)	(26)	(33)	(7)
VIII	1	1	3	0	0
(71–80)	(20)	(20)	(60)	—	—
IX	3	3	5	3	1
(81–90)	(20)	(20)	(33)	(20)	(7)
X	1	2	2	2	0
(91–100)	(14)	(28)	(28)	(28)	—

[a]Numbers in parentheses are sessions included in each block.

[b]Numbers in parentheses are row percentages.

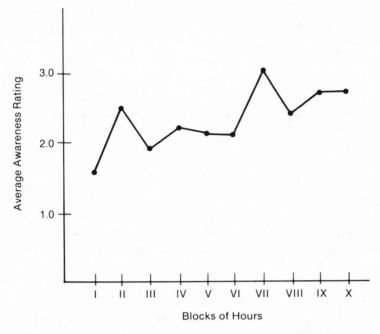

Figure 14-1. Average awareness rating across 10-hour blocks.

As illustrated in Figure 14-1, the average rating of statements within the 10-hour blocks gradually increased over time. Indeed, a correlation (Pearson r) of .72 ($p < .01$) was obtained between the mean ratings and time. This finding indicates that during the first 100 sessions of her psychoanalysis, Mrs. C became increasingly aware of and insightful about her problems in the domain we are considering.

Table 14-1 shows that from the beginning of her analysis Mrs. C shifted among the first three levels of insight, most likely because she was somewhat aware of issues of responsibility and guilt even before she entered treatment. Nonetheless, the majority of Mrs. C's statements in the first 10 hours were at Level 1, which means that at the beginning of her analysis she was primarily aware of feelings of weakness and helplessness. Vague awareness of responsibility and guilt (Level 2) and then more focused awareness of these feelings (Level 3) increased in subsequent blocks of hours, indicating that she became increasingly conscious of feelings of guilt and responsibility as the analysis continued. She became aware of being comfortable with feelings of control and power (Level 4) and began to assess overtly her fears of harming others (Level 5) essentially from block VII onwards.

Thus, both the mean values over time and the distribution of the item ratings across the first 100 hours of her psychoanalysis support the idea that Mrs. C gained awareness of feelings of responsibility and guilt and of fears of harming others. She also began to develop some insight into the irrationality of these fears. We will discuss these findings more fully in the Results.

THE SECOND STUDY

The second study is concerned with whether the insights Mrs. C acquired were conveyed to her by the analyst's interpretations or whether she developed increased awareness and insight largely on her own.

METHOD

The method for this study is similar to that of the first study. Initially, all the analyst's interpretations pertaining to the patient's irrational feelings of responsibility, guilt, and power were identified. Then these statements were rated on a scale composed of stages or levels that parallel those used to rate Mrs. C's statements. Finally, the temporal relationship between the analyst's and patient's statements at different stages or levels were examined.

Item Selection

All of the analyst's statements during the first 100 hours were selected from the verbatim transcripts of these hours. The analyst made 152 interpretations.[3] These 152 interpretations were reviewed independently by two judges who were instructed to select all statements pertaining to the domain we had used in selecting the patient's items. In fact, they used the patient scale to identify analyst remarks pertinent to the domain. Only 21 interventions were so identified.

Before submitting the 21 items to a second set of judges for rating, Drucker and Isaacs independently rated these interventions on the scale below. Since they rated none of the analyst's interventions as being at

---

3. These data are based on a study carried out by Saul Rosenberg and Lynn Campbell of our research group. They had all the analyst's interventions classified reliably by independent judges.

Level 5, the authors constructed three Level 5 "dummy" interventions to assure that all of the levels of the scale would be represented in the items rated by judges. This brought the total number of items to be rated to 24.

The Scale

The scale for rating the analyst's interventions was constructed to parallel the 5-point scale used in the first study to rate the patient's statements (see Appendix 6). A brief summary of this scale is presented below:

At *Level 1*, the analyst notes that the patient feels weak, helpless, impotent, or unable to exert control in situations involving other people.

At *Level 2*, the analyst comments that the patient feels responsible for other people, or guilty. He does not interpret a reason for her feeling this way.

At *Level 3*, the analyst interprets that the patient is afraid that she can harm people or that she is feeling uncomfortable because she feels in control in a relationship.

At *Level 4*, the analyst comments on the patient's idea that she is controlling others. He may or may not note that she is no longer frightened, guilty, or bothered by this control.

At *Level 5*, the analyst points out the realistic limitations of the patient's ability to influence and control others or alludes to the genetic origins of the patient's concerns about her feelings of responsibility and power or points to the distinction between thought and action.

Ratings

Three judges were trained in the use of the intervention scale. They were then given the 24 statements described above and asked to rate each item for the scale level it most closely represented. The statements had been typed on individual cards and were presented to the judges in random order.

Interrater reliabilities (Pearson r) between the three judges for the 24 items were .72, .84, and .92 (all $p < .01$). Each item was given the mean score of the three judges. None of the therapist's statements (excluding the three "dummy" items) was rated Level 5. The distributions of ratings among the 21 analyst statements is summarized in Table 14-2 below.

RESULTS

A comparison was made between the hours in which the analyst first made a comment at a given level and the hour in which the patient first

Table 14-2. Ratings of Analyst Interpretations

Level	N	Percentage of total
1	5	24
2	4	19
3	8	38
4	4	19
5	0	0
Totals	21	100

made a statement at the equivalent level. Table 14-3 summarizes these observations. These findings demonstrate that Mrs. C made progress toward each new level of insight into her irrational feelings of responsibility and guilt in advance of the analyst's making an intervention at that level. Indeed, it should be emphasized that the analyst rarely commented on the domain under consideration. Referring back to Figure 14-1, it will be noted that the vast majority of statements made by Mrs. C during the first 60 hours of her analysis (blocks I–VI) were rated as being at Levels 1, 2, and 3. In fact, relatively early in the treatment (within the first 20 hours), both Mrs. C and the analyst made statements rated as being at Levels 1–3. Thus it appears that during this period of the analysis both Mrs. C's and the analyst's statements concerning her feelings of power and responsibility focused predominantly on her feelings of helplessness and then guilt. Mrs. C did make a few rare and isolated statements rated as level 4 during this period, but the analyst failed to make interventions at a corresponding level. However, during block VII, an interesting development occurred. Following three Level 4 statements by Mrs. C in hour 62, the analyst, in the same hour, made his first Level 4 intervention. Subsequently, in the same block of hours, Mrs. C made additional Level 4 statements as well as her first Level 5 statement; and in the following blocks of hours she made a greater proportion of Level 4 and 5 statements than were made in the earlier hours of the treatment.

In some respects, Level 4 patient statements and analyst interventions may be regarded as qualitatively different from lower-level statements and interventions, for at this level there first appears explicitly the notion that the patient's feelings of responsibility and guilt (the *awareness* of which is emphasized in Levels 1–3) may be irrational in some instances. It can be speculated that Mrs. C, who had first made a Level 4 comment more than 50 hours before the analyst, was assisted by his later intervention and thus was able subsequently to focus more explicitly and intensely on her irrational feelings of guilt and responsibility. However much she was assisted in so doing by the analyst's Level 4 intervention, it still must be emphasized that Mrs. C consistently made higher-level statements well in advance of the analyst (e.g., the analyst made no Level 5 interventions within the first 100 sessions). Consequently, the analyst's interventions may be seen as helpful and facilitative but, in this case, not entirely necessary to the patient's progressive work toward the preliminary acquisition of insight into her irrational feelings of power, responsibility, and guilt.

DISCUSSION

The findings show that throughout the first 100 sessions of her psychoanalysis, Mrs. C did focus steadily and persistently on the related issues of responsibility, guilt, and power to harm others. Moreover, the findings indicate that Mrs. C worked progressively in this domain during the first 100 hours of her treatment. She became increasingly aware of feelings of responsibility and guilt and of discomfort about having control over others. She developed a greater awareness of her fear of hurting others if she had power or control in a relationship with them. She became more comfortable with feelings of power and control, and she acquired the beginnings of insight into the irrationality of some of her fears of harming others by her strength, power, and control.

Mrs. C made the aforementioned gains largely without interpretative help from the analyst. In fact, after the analysis was completed, we had an opportunity to discuss the case with the treating analyst, and we learned

Table 14-3. Hours in Which Patient and Analyst First Made Comments at Given Levels of Awareness

Level	Patient statement	Analyst statement
1	Hour 2	Hour 3
2	Hour 5	Hour 18
3	Hour 2	Hour 12
4	Hour 11	Hour 62
5	Hour 66	(None in hours 1–100)

that his case formulation included no references to this domain and that he had scarcely any interest in it. As we have seen, the analyst made few interventions in this area. The interpretations he did make always followed the patient's current or earlier level of insight. He never interpreted in this domain at a more advanced level than the patient had reached.

Nonetheless, we inferred that the analyst's comments concerning the patient's concerns about power, guilt, and responsibility *did* facilitate the patient's progress *in the direction she was already moving.* For instance, in hour 62, when the patient was already working at an advanced level and the analyst made his first intervention at the same level, Mrs. C responded with a flurry of further work at that level. The analyst's intervention did not serve as a suggestion to direct the patient toward the analyst's theories (the analyst, as noted, did not include this domain in his own case formulation). Rather, it served as an interpretation congruent with the patient's own goals and plans and therefore likely to facilitate her progress. In later chapters, we will report studies suggesting that the analyst's interpretations are facilitative when they are in accord with the patient's own goals.

Findings similar to those described here have been reported by Sampson *et al.* (1972). They found that an analytic patient made considerable progress toward understanding his defense of "undoing" before the analyst's first interpretation pertaining to this defense. However, the analyst's first interpretation of undoing was slightly ahead of the patient's own level of insight. The patient responded with an immediate flurry of insights at the new level and then developed and extended these insights rapidly in the following sessions.

The present findings lend support to the theory of therapy presented in Part I. They are compatible with the idea that patients have unconscious goals and plans and may work successfully toward these goals even without direction or interpretive help from the analyst. The findings further suggest that the analyst's interpretations will help the patient move toward his goals if the interpretations are congruent with those goals.

The present studies also lend support to the view developed in the preceding two chapters that the patient may control repressions, may lift them when it is safe to do so, and may bring forth and use for therapeutic purposes previously warded-off contents and themes. Mrs. C deepened her awareness of feelings of guilt and responsibility, and her understanding of the pathogenic beliefs from which these feelings stemmed, largely without interpretive help. It would be difficult to account for these observations by a purely automatic functioning hypothesis.

Finally, the present study demonstrates that the analytic patient is not a *tabula rasa* who produces material primarily in response to the analyst's suggestions and reinforcements (Grünbaum, 1979). Our findings suggest that Mrs. C was pursuing her own path in exploring certain issues, and that she did so in spite of the analyst's lack of interest in this domain and limited awareness of her preoccupation with it.

D: THE PATIENT'S WORK

15

INTRODUCTION TO EMPIRICAL STUDIES OF THE PLAN CONCEPT

HAROLD SAMPSON

REVIEW OF THE CONCEPT

We will in this section take up evidence for the concept developed in Chapters 5 and 6 that the analytic patient's behavior is guided by certain unconscious plans, which the patient unconsciously devises for working with the analyst to overcome his problems. I shall refer to this concept, and the network of ideas it contains, as the *plan concept*.

In this chapter I shall review the plan concept, comment on its scientific status, remind the reader of clinical observations from Part I that provide informal support for it, and introduce the series of research studies we undertook to test its fruitfulness and explanatory power.

The plan concept assumes that the patient's psychopathology stems largely from unconscious pathogenic beliefs. In obedience to such beliefs the patient may decide to repress impulses, affects, behaviors, or goals that put him in a situation of danger. He is burdened by his pathogenic beliefs and so has a strong unconscious wish to change them and to overcome the problems to which they give rise.

The patient works, unconsciously as well as consciously, to overcome his problems. He is guided in his work by certain goals and plans. Weiss has referred to these as *ego* goals and plans to distinguish them from impulses of the id or pressures of the superego.

The patient's plans are not like blueprints. Indeed, they may merely point him in a particular direction. They reflect the patient's decisions about what dangers he will work to overcome at a given time, and what dangers he will defer working to overcome until later. For example, Mrs. G (Chapter 1) was guided early in her analysis by the goal of assuring herself that she could not be dominated by the analyst. The attainment of this goal was for this patient a precondition to tackling other analytic tasks.

A patient may work in accord with his particular plans to change his pathogenic beliefs, by testing them in his relation to the analyst in the hope of disconfirming them, and by using the analyst's comments and interpretations to acquire insight into them.

NATURE OF THE EVIDENCE: GENERAL CONSIDERATIONS

The plan concept both explains the patient's behavior in terms of his use of higher mental functions, and takes account of his goals. As Weiss has argued (Chapter 2), attempts to explain behavior by the plan concept are neither more nor less acceptable on philosophical grounds than are attempts to explain it in terms of the dynamic interactions of psychic forces. A rational choice between the two kinds of concepts should be based on empirical grounds.

Both higher mental functioning concepts and dynamic interaction concepts are constructions derived by inference from behavior; that is, both are inferred from a person's thoughts, fantasies, affects, and actions. Both kinds of concepts assume that behavior is lawful, and both can lead to potentially testable propositions about nature. Thus, neither kind of explanatory concept can be dismissed on philosophical grounds alone. Each must stand or fall on its demonstrable capacity to explain and to predict relationships in nature.

The plan concept is a hypothetical construct (MacCorquodale & Meehl, 1948) invoked to explain a wide range of observations. The explanatory power of the construct cannot be judged adequately by single pieces of evidence considered in isolation; such judgment requires a broad assessment of converging lines of evidence.

We shall take up various kinds of evidence that bear on this concept. In deciding what is evidence for the concept, we ask: If the analytic patient's behavior during treatment is guided by (largely unconscious) goals and plans, how may we expect him to behave? What do we predict he will do in specified situations?

I shall introduce briefly certain answers to these questions now, and then expand on them below.

1. We may expect, if the patient is guided by a plan, that his behavior during any period of his analysis is likely to show *goal-directedness*; that is, the patient will move, or more precisely he will *attempt* to move, in a particular direction, toward a particular goal or interrelated set of goals. He may of course be unable to attain these goals, even as a person pursuing a conscious goal—for example, admission to college—may be unable, for various inner and outer reasons, to attain his goal.

2. We may expect, further, that the patient may modify to some extent the means he uses to pursue his goal if his initial means prove unsuccessful. That is, the patient may show *flexibility* in moving toward a particular goal. Once again, we may consider the analogy to conscious plans. For example, a person who planned to walk downtown to shop may change his mind when it begins to rain. He may decide to shop locally, or to drive downtown, or to defer his shopping until another day.

3. If the patient's behavior during a particular period of his analysis is guided by goals and plans to change certain pathogenic beliefs, he is likely to test these beliefs, and the dangers they foretell, in his relationship to the analyst. If the analyst's responses to the tests are experienced by the patient as disconfirming the pathogenic beliefs, the patient is likely to become less anxious, more relaxed, more confident in the analyst, and bolder in tackling his problems. If, in contrast, the analyst's responses tend to support the pathogenic beliefs the patient is testing, the patient may temporarily become more anxious, more tense, less confident in the analyst, and less bold in tackling his problems.

4. If the patient's behavior during a particular period of his analysis is guided by specific goals and plans, he is likely to *respond differently* to the analyst's comments and interpretations depending on whether what the analyst says can be used to support the patient in moving toward his goals or impedes him from doing so. This expectation provides a basis for classifying the analyst's comments and interpretations during a period of treatment as facilitative or hindering, and then observing whether the patient's responses correspond to that prediction.

I shall turn now to a brief review of clinical observations, mostly from Part I, which will illustrate each of these types of evidence and provide *informal* support for the explanatory power of the plan concept. I will show, in addition, how these observations provide a paradigm for our research studies of the plan concept.

DIRECTEDNESS: THE PATIENT WORKS TOWARD PARTICULAR GOALS

According to the plan concept, the analytic patient may be expected, in each stage of his analysis, to work in a particular direction, that is, toward overcoming a particular danger or group of dangers and so attaining certain goals. Therefore, evidence that the patient is working persistently toward overcoming certain dangers and reaching certain goals would support the plan concept. Of course, the attainment of a goal, or even persistent movement toward a goal, does not demonstrate that the patient necessarily *planned* to attain the goal or moved purposively toward it. Among possible alternative explanations, two are particularly plausible. The first is that the patient's directedness is foisted upon him by the analyst; the second is that the patient's directedness is determined by the dynamic interactions of persisting impulses and defenses. Let us consider each of these alternatives.

The analytic patient may move persistently toward certain goals and overcoming certain dangers because of direct or indirect suggestions or pressures from the analyst. Fisher and Greenberg (1977), in a review of numerous empirical studies, concluded that all psychotherapists reinforce certain types of patient communication. Grünbaum (1979) has argued that the analyst may persuade the patient that he harbors particular unconscious fears, or may induce the patient to produce particular "insights" or "memories." That is, the patient may move toward particular goals or even focus on particular dangers because the analyst is pushing him, overtly or covertly, in this direction. Therefore, in assessing whether or not a patient's goal-directedness lends support to the idea that the patient is working in accord with his own plan, it is important to determine whether or not that directedness can be attributed to the analyst rather than the patient.

The patient's goal-directedness might, according to the automatic functioning hypothesis, also be due to a blind play of forces—impulses and defenses, transferences and resistances—outside of the patient's control, rather than to the patient's pursuit of certain goals. Consider, for example, an obsessive–compulsive man who in his treatment shifts repeatedly between defiant and submissive behavior. An investigator might perceive him as "working" persistently on problems of defiance and submission during a period of his analysis. However, according to the automatic functioning hypothesis, his behavior may be the expression of a persisting conflict that has been intensified by the treatment and that is outside the patient's control. Thus, in assessing whether a patient's goal-directedness lends support to the idea that the patient is working in accord with his own plan, it is important to determine whether or not his directedness is explicable by the dynamic interactions of his impulses and defenses.

SUMMARY OF OBSERVATIONS FROM THE CASE OF MRS. G

I should now like to review observations from the case of Mrs. G (Chapters 1 and 5), which provide informal evidence that an analytic patient may work persistently during a period of analysis toward particular therapeutic goals, and that he may do so under his own control, independently of the analyst's implicit or explicit suggestions. In the case of Mrs. G, the analyst made no inferences about either the patient's unconscious work or her unconscious goals until after the termination of the case, when he made a study of part of her analysis.

Mrs. G became conscious, after 20 months of treatment, of a previously repressed sexual fantasy of being beaten by the analyst. This important new material came to consciousness without interpretation, calmly, and, from the viewpoint of the analyst, unexpectedly. How could this event be understood? In an attempt to answer this question, Weiss studied closely the process notes for the preceding 10 months of the analysis. I shall summarize his conclusions:

At the beginning of the 10-month period preceding the emergence of her beating fantasy, Mrs. G unconsciously feared a powerful urge to submit to the analyst. She feared that if she did submit to him, she would be trapped in a masochistic relationship with him from which she would be unable to extricate herself. She feared that once she submitted to him she would be unable comfortably to stop submitting to him, for she assumed that if she defied him she would hurt him as she believed she had hurt her parents (especially her father) when she defied them.

Mrs. G's initial goal during this period (as inferred by Weiss from his study of the process notes) was to overcome her fear of hurting the analyst, and thereby to acquire the capacity to disagree with him and to make decisions without undue regard for his opinions. She hoped that once she had attained this goal, she would be able safely to experience and analyze her powerful masochistic urge to submit to him.

Mrs. G worked to attain this goal by testing the analyst in various ways over the 10-month period. As a consequence of this work (described in detail in Chapter 1), Mrs. G became progressively less anxious and guilty about her assertiveness. She became more able to disagree comfortably with the analyst, to make her own decisions, and to express her own opinions. She made considerable progress, both in her sessions and in her everyday behavior. She became freer, more able to be close to people, less anxious about both her assertiveness and about her cooperativeness and submissiveness. She acquired greater control over her behavior as well as significant insights into her relationship with her parents and with the analyst. Her progress in analysis is epitomized by the ease with which at the end of the period studied she spontaneously disclosed to the analyst a previously repressed sexual fantasy of being beaten by him, and then proceeded to explore the meanings and the genetic origins of the fantasy.

Weiss's conclusions, based on a thorough study of the process notes of a 10-month period of Mrs. G's analysis, account well for the observable changes in the patient's behavior. In addition, they strongly suggest that Mrs. G was working in a particular direction (toward a particular goal or family of goals, and toward the overcoming of a particular danger) during this period of her analysis.

This patient's goal-directedness cannot be attributed convincingly to compliance on her part with overt or covert suggestions or interpretations by the analyst. The patient initiated this direction of work. The analyst made only a few interpretations during the period of analysis with which we are concerned: He told Mrs. G on four occasions that she seemed reluctant to disagree with him for fear of hurting him. The patient, after each such interpretation, was relieved and produced confirmatory material, including, in some of these instances, new memories of fear of hurting her parents by disagreeing with them. She also responded to such interpretations by increased freedom during subsequent sessions in disagreeing with him. We may conclude that Mrs. G moved rapidly and productively toward increasing assertiveness and spontaneous insight into the origins of her conflict about assertiveness, following the analyst's occasional interpretations of her fear of hurting him by disagreeing with him. However, the analyst's interpretations followed rather than preceded the patient's own movement toward increased assertiveness. We infer that Mrs. G responded productively to such interpretations because they directly disconfirmed a pathogenic belief (that disagreeing with the analyst would hurt him), reduced the danger of disagreeing with the analyst, and thereby helped her to move in the direction in which she herself was attempting to move.

The idea that the analyst's interpretations helped the patient to move in the direction she herself wished to move is supported by another observation (Chapter 1): When Mrs. G did infer, from the analyst's response (or his silence), that she may have hurt him by disagreeing with him, she became upset, anxious, less assertive, less insightful, and more defensive. She retreated temporarily.

Thus, this patient's movement in a particular direction was temporarily facilitated when the analyst's behavior was experienced by Mrs. G as disconfirming her pathogenic belief, and temporarily disrupted when the analyst's behavior was experienced by her as confirming that belief. The analyst, we infer, could influence her progress in a given direction, but he did not himself determine that direction. Moreover, during the period studied, the analyst did not know just where the patient was going. It is therefore unlikely that he could have pushed Mrs. G to go there.

Nor can Mrs. G's goal-directedness be explained readily by a blind play-of-forces hypothesis. Mrs. G became less anxious about both assertiveness and submissiveness; she gained increasing control over both kinds of impulses; she spontaneously (i.e., without interpretation) re-called significant new memories, including becoming conscious of a previously repressed sexual fantasy toward the analyst, and she did so calmly and without coming into conflict with or isolating the new material. In addition, she spontaneously acquired significant new in-sights into her relationship with the analyst and with her parents. The nature of these improvements suggests that the patient's behavior during this period was not driven by the automatic interaction of impulses and defenses, but was taking place under her own control.

EARLIER STUDIES OF MRS. C

Let us now examine research studies reported in Chapters 12, 13, and 14 that demonstrate in the case of Mrs. C what Weiss found in his informal study of Mrs. G. We will show that these studies are consistent with expectations based on the plan concept.

Mrs. C, according to our formulation of her plan (Chapter 10), suffered from a number of inhibitions and compulsions, which stemmed from the pathogenic belief that she would hurt her parents if she held ideas or values different from theirs, if she disagreed with them or op-posed their wishes, or if she were freer and happier than she believed they had been. We inferred that she would work, during the first period of her analysis (and most likely for several years), to change these beliefs, and to overcome the inhibitions and compulsions that stemmed from them. We predicted that she would work to change these beliefs in a number of ways: She would test these beliefs in relation to the analyst. She would evaluate the analyst's comments and interpretations by the criterion of whether they supported or disconfirmed her pathogenic be-liefs. She would think about and attempt to increase her understanding of her inhibitions and compulsions, and of the beliefs from which they stemmed.

We found, in the study reported in Chapter 14, that Mrs. C *was* thinking persistently throughout the first 100 sessions of analysis about a particular domain of ideas. This was the domain that we had identified, in our formulation of her plan, as of central importance to her, and that we assumed she would work to understand and control—namely, her pathogenic beliefs about hurting others, and the various symptoms to which they gave rise. Mrs. C, during the first 100 sessions, was not only persistently concerned with this domain, but made progress in her under-standing of it. We demonstrated, by a scale which was rated reliably by independent judges, that Mrs. C became increasingly aware, over the 100 sessions, of the extent to which she felt guilty toward other people, responsible for their problems, and afraid of hurting them by her thoughts and actions. We demonstrated, too, that she became somewhat more comfortable with feelings of power in relation to others, and that she began to think about the distinction between rational and irrational fears of hurting others.

These changes cannot have been due to compliance with the analyst's comments, interpretations, or suggestions. First of all, the analyst scarcely interpreted to the patient in this domain. Second, on the infrequent occasions in which he did so, his remarks *invariably* followed rather than preceded the patient's lead. Specifically, the patient acquired each new level of insight into this domain prior to *any* interpretation by the analyst at that level.

Moreover, as the reader will recall, Mrs. C was analyzed in another city by an analyst who was, at the time, entirely unfamiliar with our ideas. Indeed, our research did not begin until several years after Mrs. C had completed the first 100 sessions of her analysis. Much later still, when we discussed the analysis with the treating analyst *after its completion*, we discovered that the analyst had not considered important Mrs. C's irrational feelings of responsibility to others and her fears of hurting them. The treating analyst's own case formulation (see Chapter 10) and records also document this.

As Mrs. C gained insight into her irrational feelings of responsibility for others and her fear of hurting them, she made important changes in her behavior. She became more assertive to the analyst and others, she became friendlier and more cooperative to the analyst and others, she became freer sexually, and she became more capable of having pleasure. These behavioral changes took place without any increase in anxiety and with a significant reduction in feelings of drivenness (Chapter 13).

In addition, Mrs. C became aware spontaneously during the first 100 sessions of a number of mental contents that she had warded off previously (Chapter 12). She became aware of these contents without any increase in anxiety, experienced them vividly, and worked with them therapeutically.

This combination of changes cannot be explained readily by a blind-play-of-forces theory. While Mrs. C worked on and gained greater understanding of her irrational fears of hurting others, and as she became more able to express assertive and affectionate–sexual feelings, she felt less driven, displayed more control over her behavior, and was judged independently by two training analysts (who were not members of our research team) to be freer and more relaxed (Chapter 13).

This network of changes is explained most readily by the hypothesis that Mrs. C, during the period of her analysis we studied, worked persistently in a particular direction: to understand and change certain pathogenic beliefs (which we had identified in our formulation of her plan), and to overcome the inhibitions and compulsions that stemmed from them. She worked, as we shall see in Chapters 17 and 18, by testing these beliefs in relation to the analyst, and also by evaluating the analyst's comments and interpretations by the criterion of whether they confirmed or disconfirmed these beliefs (Chapters 19 and 20). She also worked by thinking about her inhibitions and compulsions and the beliefs from which they stemmed (Chapter 14). As certain of her pathogenic beliefs were partially disconfirmed, Mrs. C felt safe enough to recall certain warded-off contents (Chapter 12); to become more conscious of feelings of guilt and responsibility, more aware of her fears of harming others, more tolerant of feelings of power (Chapter 14); and more free to express warded-off strivings in her behavior (Chapter 13).

As we have seen, Mrs. C's persistence in working on a particular domain of ideas throughout the 100 sessions cannot convincingly be attributed either to a push in that direction by the analyst, nor to a blind play of forces. The research findings we reported in earlier chapters are most compatible with the hypothesis that the patient had certain goals and plans at the beginning of analysis, and worked steadily, during the sessions studied, to carry out these plans and to attain these goals.

THE PATIENT DEMONSTRATES FLEXIBILITY IN WORKING TOWARD GOALS

Further evidence that a patient's goal-directedness may indeed be purposeful and guided by higher mental functions is afforded by those instances in which the patient exhibits flexibility in pursuit of his goal. For example, the patient may shift his approach toward the goal in response to the particular therapeutic stance taken by the analyst.

I mentioned earlier that flexibility is a frequent characteristic of *conscious* planned behavior. A person acting in accord with a conscious plan often retains his goal but changes his course if the path he is following appears unnecessarily difficult or impassable. For example, in carrying out my plan to write this chapter, I am following an outline that indicates the topics I intend to take up, the order in which I shall discuss them, and the main lines of my argument. If, as occasionally happens, I discover that I cannot discuss topic N effectively until I have discussed another topic—say, topic X—which was not included anywhere in my outline, I modify the plan represented by the outline.

Flexible and adaptive behavior may also be observed frequently in behavior guided by *unconscious* plans, such as the behavior of the analytic patient in his treatment. I shall illustrate this with an example from the analysis of Mr. E, a case studied by Weiss from the analyst's process notes. Because this case was not described in Part I, I shall develop it fully here.

MR. E

Mr. E, according to Weiss's formulation, was guided by the unconscious goal during an early period of his analysis of bringing to consciousness and mastering his homosexual conflicts. Mr. E was tempted unconsciously to submit to the analyst and to develop an intense love for him as in childhood, he had submitted to his father and developed an intense love for him. Mr. E feared this temptation because he believed that if he yielded to it, the analyst would need his love and submission and would oppose his efforts to develop a life of his own, as he believed his father had in childhood.

Mr. E planned to work toward the goal of bringing his homosexual conflicts to consciousness and mastering them by first establishing a capacity to make himself important and to ignore the analyst. Once he could feel assured that he could maintain a life of his own independent of the analyst, he could safely bring to consciousness his temptation to submit to the analyst and to feel intense love for him. He could experience this temptation safely if he could maintain comfortably his own sense of importance and independence.

Over a period of weeks Mr. E emphasized his own importance and scarcely paid attention to the analyst. During this period, he occasionally, and only in passing, hinted at homosexual feelings toward male authority figures. After several months, the analyst interpreted that Mr. E was making himsellf important and ignoring the analyst in order to avoid certain feelings toward the analyst. Mr. E, because of his unconscious need to submit to the analyst, was unable to continue the pattern of acting important and neglecting the analyst. He feared he had threatened the analyst by this behavior. At the same time, because of his continuing fear of homosexual submission to the analyst, Mr. E could not investigate and so risk experiencing the feelings the analyst had suggested he was avoiding.

Mr. E then developed, Weiss inferred, a revised plan to enable him to bring his homosexual conflicts to consciousness safely. He attempted to establish a capacity to stubbornly withhold from the analyst. If he could do this comfortably, he could safely tolerate in consciousness his love for the analyst and his wish to submit to him. He could then resist the analyst if the analyst tried to prevent him from developing a life of his own.

For a period of months Mr. E was conspicuously withholding in his sessions. His associations became sparse, he was frequently silent, and he responded in a vague and noncommittal way to the analyst's attempts to clarify what was happening. Eventually the analyst interpreted the patient's behavior as defiance. Once again the patient, because of his unconscious need to submit, could not continue this behavior, for he believed it had threatened the analyst. At the same time, because he still felt endangered by homosexual submission, he could not safely bring to consciousness his homosexual temptations and conflicts.

Mr. E once again revised his plan of how to bring his homosexual conflicts safely to consciousness. He attempted to establish a capacity to be active heterosexually. If he could do so comfortably, he could feel assured that if he brought to consciousness his homosexual temptations, the analyst could not exploit his homosexual submission and prevent him from developing a life of his own.

Mr. E began to date a number of women and to have sex with many of them. He talked of his strong libidinal desires and of his wish to have numerous affairs. The patient inferred that the analyst approved of his heterosexual activity, for the analyst interpreted only inhibitions to Mr. E's sexual freedom and enjoyment. Mr. E continued this new pattern for a number of months, overcame to some extent his unconscious belief that the analyst might be threatened by his heterosexuality, and became increasingly comfortable with it.

After becoming comfortable with his heterosexuality, Mr. E spontaneously and calmly became conscious of homosexual fantasies toward the analyst, and began to explore and attempt to understand these fantasies and their childhood origins.

Not all patients are as flexible as Mr. E in devising new paths toward their goal when the analyst's attitude, as the patient perceives it, makes the initial path relatively impassable. Such patients may have to persist along a single path, in which case the success of the treatment may depend primarily on the analyst's eventual understanding and flexible response to the stalemate. However, cases such as that of Mr. E are by no means infrequent. They demonstrate the adaptive and flexible nature of the patient's behavior. Such cases lend strong if informal support to the hypothesis that the patient's behavior is guided by higher mental functions such as planning, anticipating the consequences of a course of action, assessing actual consequences, and modifying the course of action accordingly.

TESTING PATHOGENIC BELIEFS

One of the important ways in which the analytic patient works to overcome pathogenic beliefs, according to the plan concept, is by testing these beliefs in relation to the analyst. In testing, the patient makes use of trial actions. The patient may test a pathogenic belief by expressing certain impulses or seeking certain goals that, according to the belief, threaten his ties to the analyst and so put the patient in a situation of danger. If the patient infers from such trial actions that he does not affect the analyst as the belief predicts, he may become less anxious and take a step toward disconfirming the belief. If, however, the patient infers that his trial actions have affected the analyst as the belief predicts, he may temporarily become more anxious or defensive than he was before.

Testing implies the concept of planning, for, in order to test, a patient must plan a complex action, carry it out, and evaluate its outcome. The patient, in testing, is not simply repeating automatically an old pattern of behavior. This is demonstrated by Weiss's observation (Chapter 6) that if the patient, while testing the analyst, becomes afraid that the analyst will fail the test, he may coach the analyst on how to pass it.

Moreover, if a patient, in pursuit of a particular goal, tests the analyst and the analyst fails the test, the patient may carry out a more pointed test, which he assumes the analyst is likely to pass (Chapter 6).

PREDICTIONS DERIVED FROM THE TESTING HYPOTHESIS

These ideas about testing lead to certain formal predictions. I shall introduce and describe these kinds of predictions by reviewing an instructive sequence of events in the case of Miss P, the lawyer who set a deadline for terminating her analysis. I shall then describe the research study of Mrs. C's analysis by which we tested such predictions.

Miss P, as you will recall, unconsciously tested the analyst by setting a deadline for terminating analysis. She was testing whether the analyst would agree with her conscious termination plan and so reject her, as she unconsciously believed her parents had rejected her. When the analyst did not do so, but instead recommended that she continue and attempt to understand her wish to terminate, the patient, after a brief protestation, became less tense and more friendly. She then recalled, over several weeks, and with intense sadness, several new memories of childhood rejection by her mother. She developed considerably more insight into her feelings of rejectability. She also made progress toward her life goals; for example, she became more outgoing, more able to date, and more able to enjoy herself.

The sequence of events illustrated by this example may be stated as an hypothesis that can be investigated: If a patient tests a pathogenic belief in relation to the analyst, and if the analyst's responses are perceived by the patient as disconfirming that belief:

1. The patient is likely to become less anxious than he was before, for the danger he had anticipated has not been realized.
2. The patient may produce new memories about the traumatic situations in which the belief arose, for it is now safer for the patient to remember them (i.e., the patient is able to retrieve sad memories at the happy ending).
3. The patient may become conscious of the pathogenic belief or develop new insights about it.
4. The patient may make progress toward goals that he could not pursue earlier because the pathogenic belief he has now begun to disconfirm had warned him of the danger of pursuing these goals.

If, however, the analyst's responses to the patient's tests are perceived by the patient as confirming rather than disconfirming the pathogenic belief, the patient is likely to remain anxious, recover few new memories, and acquire few new insights. Indeed, he may even temporarily retreat from his goals.

A research study carried out on the first 100 sessions of Mrs. C's analysis and designed to test rigorously certain of these predictions is reported in detail in Chapter 17. First, *key tests* (i.e., tests central to the pathogenic beliefs the patient would work during this period of her analysis to disconfirm) were identified independently and reliably by analytic judges. Second, a new set of analytic judges, working independently of each other, rated reliably whether the analyst's responses to the patient's tests would be perceived by the patient as passing the tests, that is, as tending to disconfirm the pathogenic beliefs that she was testing. Finally, new judges, unfamiliar with the analyst's responses, rated brief segments of the patient's speech just before and just after the tests. These segments were presented to the judges in random order, and the judges did not know whether a segment occurred before or after the testing segment. These judges rated the segments for tension and anxiety, boldness in tackling problems, and involvement in the work of therapy.

The study demonstrated that the patient, immediately following a passed test, tended to become less anxious, more relaxed, more friendly, more involved in therapeutic work, and bolder in tackling problems. It provides evidence of the predictive power of the plan concept.

This study was designed to investigate the patient's immediate reactions to passed tests rather than her long-term reactions to them. (Examples of long-term reactions are the recovery of memories and the acquisition of insights.) When the results of this study, however, are combined with the results of the studies reported in earlier chapters, they support the conjecture that over the 100 sessions of Mrs. C's analysis there was a broad relationship between numerous passed tests, on the one hand, and the coming to consciousness of warded-off contents (including memories) and the acquisition of insight into pathogenic beliefs, on the other.

TESTING PATHOGENIC BELIEFS VERSUS SEEKING TRANSFERENCE GRATIFICATIONS

There is a situation which occurs frequently in psychoanalysis, and which is explained differently by two alternative psychoanalytic hypotheses. The situation is that the analytic patient makes a powerful implicit or explicit demand on the analyst for love, guidance, praise, special treatment, and so on. The classic example of this situation presented by Freud (1915) was of the woman patient who professes her love for the analyst and demands reciprocation from him.

Psychoanalytic theory offers two different explanations for the analytic patient's making such a demand. According to one explanation (based on the automatic functioning hypothesis), the patient, by making the demand, is attempting to gratify an unconscious wish. According to the other explanation (based on the higher mental functioning hypothesis proposed in Part I), the patient may be testing a frightening unconscious belief or expectation in relation to the therapist.

The two explanations make different predictions about how the patient will react if the analyst does not accede to his demands. According to the explanation based on the automatic functioning hypothesis, the unconscious wish will be frustrated and hence intensified, and the patient will come into more intense conflict with the wish. According to the explanation based on the higher mental functioning hypothesis, the patient will (in many instances) feel reassured, less anxious, and bolder and freer in tackling problems.

The two explanations—although both are contained within psychoanalytic theory, and although both are considered complementary by some analysts—are *competing* hypotheses rather than hypotheses that can be true simultaneously. Indeed, there are significant scientific disadvantages to the view that both hypotheses may be applicable to the identical situation:

1. The idea that the patient is, in any given instance, both testing the analyst and seeking to gratify a transference wish is not plausible, for the two activities are incompatible with each other. According to the one hypothesis, the patient is attempting to put his passions into action without regard to the real situation (Freud, 1912); according to the other

hypothesis, the patient is reality-testing. The one hypothesis characterizes the patient's behavior as a resistance to analytic understanding and progress (Freud, 1912), whereas the other characterizes this same behavior as unconscious progressive analytic work. The one hypothesis considers the patient's behavior to be determined by the interaction of powerful impulses and defenses outside of the patient's control, but the other hypothesis considers the patient's behavior to be a complex trial action, taking place under the patient's control and carried out in accord with an unconscious plan to test a pathogenic belief. The one hypothesis assumes that the patient is seeking to gratify an unconscious wish; the other hypothesis assumes that the patient is seeking to learn something about the reality of his unconscious anticipation of danger. In summary, it is not plausible that the patient's behavior, in a given instance, is taking place *both* automatically (outside of the patient's control, compelled, *and* as an attempt to put passions into action without regard to reality) *and* as reflecting a choice made by the patient, under his control, to carry out a trial action in accord with a plan, and to do so as a piece of reality testing.

2. There is a compelling empirical argument for considering the two hypotheses as competing rather than simultaneously true: The two hypotheses predict different behavior by the patient in the same situation. Predictions based on the automatic functioning hypothesis were well stated by the investigators in the Menninger Psychotherapy Research Project: "Patients whose neurotic needs are not gratified within the transference respond to this frustration with regressive and/or resistive reactions, and/or painful affects" (Sargent *et al.*, 1968, p. 85). In contrast, predictions based on the higher mental functioning hypothesis developed in Part I assume that in some instances the patient will be unconsciously pleased and reassured when the analyst does not accede to his transference demands. This hypothesis predicts that the patient will feel less anxious than he had been before, more relaxed, less defensive, and freer and bolder in tackling his problems.

We have carried out a study, reported in Chapter 18, that tests rigorously which hypothesis provides a better fit to data in the Mrs. C case. The method was straightforward and is described in detail in Chapter 18. It required us carefully to study a number of patient–analyst interactions that had the following characteristics: They would be conceptualized by analysts accustomed to thinking in terms of the automatic functioning hypothesis as interactions in which the patient unconsciously attempted to gratify a key (significant) unconscious wish and in which the analyst, using correct technique, frustrated this wish. They would, at the same time, be conceptualized by analysts accustomed to thinking in terms of the higher mental functioning hypothesis as interactions in which the patient unconsciously attempted to carry out a key test and in which the analyst, using correct technique, passed the test.

We obtained a number of such interactions. We thereby obtained a group of interactions that each hypothesis conceptualized in different terms, and about which each hypothesis made different predictions about how the patient would react when she experienced the analyst as not yielding to her unconscious demands. We could then test the explanatory power of the two hypotheses by finding out how the patient did react when she experienced the analyst as not yielding to her unconscious demands.

We found that when the analyst did *not* accede to the patient's key transference demands, she became less anxious, more relaxed, more flexible and spontaneous, more bold in tackling issues, and more positive in her attitudes toward others. These findings are not in accord with predictions derived from the automatic functioning hypothesis. They are in accord with predictions derived from the particular higher mental functioning hypothesis proposed in Part I.

This experiment in nature lends additional support to the plan concept, and suggests that it has greater explanatory power than concepts that account for the patient's behavior in terms of the dynamic interaction of impulses and defenses.

THE PATIENT'S RESPONSE TO INTERPRETATIONS

According to the plan concept, the analytic patient works during analysis to change certain pathogenic beliefs, to overcome the guilt, anxiety, and shame that stem from these beliefs, and to reach certain goals. The patient is likely to evaluate the analyst's comments and interpretations primarily by the criterion of whether he can use them as help in disconfirming the particular pathogenic belief (or family of beliefs) he is working to change, and thus whether he can use them to move in the direction he wishes to go.

The patient is likely *unconsciously* both to be pleased by and to benefit from comments and interpretations that he can use in his struggle to disconfirm those particular pathogenic beliefs. He may, in reaction to such interpretations, gain confidence in the analyst, produce confirmatory material, tackle his problems more boldly and insightfully, and bring forth previously repressed contents. A patient, as Weiss noted, may sometimes make effective use of an interpretation that is vague or off the mark. He may extract from it or attribute to it those ideas he can use in his struggle to change his pathogenic beliefs.

However, a patient is often set back unconsciously by an interpretation that impedes him in his struggle to overcome a particular pathogenic belief. He may temporarily become more defensive, less bold in tackling his problems, less confident in the analyst, and more anxious and less insightful.

The differential effects of interpretations that are in accord with the patient's plan versus interpretations opposed to it are illustrated by the case of Miss D (Chapter 5). The analyst's interpretations during the first 18 months of Miss D's analysis tended to confirm rather than disconfirm the pathogenic belief she was working to overcome. (This was the belief that if she were to become independent she would hurt her mother.) The patient made little progress during this period. Then, the analyst, after obtaining supervision, began to make interpretations that Miss D could use in her struggle to disconfirm the pathogenic belief that by becoming independent she would hurt her mother. She began then to make rapid progress.

This case, which is an experiment in nature, provides an introduction to the research studies to be presented in Chapters 19 and 20 and briefly described below. Our first step in carrying out the studies (reported in Chapter 19) was to have Mrs. C's unconscious goals and plans inferred by certain members of the research group. These inferences were replicated, with high interjudge reliability, by a second set of psychoanalytic clinicians working independently of each other (Chapter 16). The analyst's interventions were then classified reliably, by new judges, as likely to be facilitative (perceived by the patient as in accord with her goals and plans) or as likely to be hindering (perceived by the patient as in opposition to her goals and plans). The investigators then studied the immediate effects of the analyst's comments and interpretations on the patient's productivity. They found, in a pilot study, a clear relationship between how "pro-plan" an intervention of the analyst was rated and how boldly and insightfully the patient worked immediately following the intervention. Less definitive but partially supportive results were obtained in a replication study.

The final study of Mrs. C's responses to interventions (Chapter 20) was based on a formulation of her unconscious treatment goals and plans for the termination phase of her analysis. The analyst's interventions were then classified by independent judges as to their "plan compatibility" (the same kind of judgment as in the preceding studies). A new set of judges independently assessed the patient's progress toward termination following each intervention. The results in this study are similar to those obtained in the pilot study referred to above and provide strong support for the plan concept. (For another study that strongly supports the plan concept, see Chapter 22.)

THE RELIABILITY WITH WHICH A PATIENT'S UNCONSCIOUS PLAN MAY BE INFERRED

The studies in Chapters 17–20 all depend on the investigators being able reliably to infer the analytic patient's goals and plans. The reliability of a plan formulation is a measure of the degree to which two or more judges, working independently of each other, are in agreement about various aspects of the plan. The reliability is, therefore, a measure of the objectivity (i.e., the intersubjective agreement) with which the plan concept may be applied to the individual case. A high degree of reliability demonstrates that the patient's plans may be inferred with satisfactory objectivity, and therefore that the plan concept itself is amenable to systematic empirical research. For this reason, we have undertaken to demonstrate that the analytic patient's plan—specifically, that of Mrs. C—can be inferred reliably by independent judges (Chapter 16).

I should like here to present a few comments about how a patient's unconscious goals, purposes, and plans may be inferred. Though these comments are orienting, they are not a substitute for direct training and experience in the clinical use of these concepts. (The reader is also referred to Part I of this book for numerous examples of how a patient's goals, pathogenic beliefs, and ways of working in analysis may be inferred.)

A patient's unconscious plan may be inferred from his history, his psychopathology, his life situation, and his behavior with the analyst in the opening sessions.

The patient's childhood traumas provide important clues about the probable nature of his pathogenic beliefs, the dangers they foretell, certain life goals the patient may have relinquished in obedience to these beliefs, and how the patient may work in analysis to disconfirm these beliefs. For example, Mr. S, whose case was discussed by Weiss in Chapter 4, was left with relatives for several months when he was 2½ years old because his brother was ill with an infectious disease. His parents sent him away both to protect him from catching the disease and because they felt overburdened by caring for a sick child. Mr. S, however, was not told why he was sent away. He inferred, from various cues, that it was because he was a rowdy, energetic, and sometimes defiant boy. Shortly after being sent away, he became a model child: quiet, serious, and obedient. For this child, being sent away produced a trauma. Moreover, this trauma led to a powerful set of pathogenic beliefs which told him that if he asserted his will or was spontaneous, playful, or rowdy, he would be rejected. In his analysis, Mr. S gradually tested whether he would be sent away if he became rowdy, spontaneous, and defiant.

A clinician may infer a patient's pathogenic beliefs from chronic childhood strain traumas (which arise in a pathogenic relationship to a parent) as well as from acute childhood shock traumas, by asking himself what beliefs the patient is likely to have inferred from the early pathogenic experience. How a patient may infer a pathogenic belief from a trauma stemming from a pathogenic relationship is illustrated by the case of Miss D (Chapter 3). She inferred from her mother's chronic depression and listlessness (which she could alleviate to some extent by paying attention to her mother) that she was responsible for her mother's happiness. She also inferred from her mother's scolding her for her clinginess but ignoring her independent behavior that her mother did not want her to be independent. In general, as Weiss noted, a child is likely to infer that he is in some way responsible for any mistreatment or trauma to which he is subject, or for any trauma or suffering that his parents or siblings endure. Therefore, a clinician reviewing the patient's history may make some tentative inferences about how particular traumas are likely to have affected the patient.

Aspects of a patient's plan may also be inferred from the patient's symptomatology. For example, we inferred that Mrs. C, who suffered initially from feelings of *conscious* envy toward others, was warding off the unconscious pathogenic belief that her attractiveness and successes would cause intense envy in parents or siblings.

The patient's presenting complaints and current life situation may also imply particular pathogenic beliefs and goals. For example, a patient who enters analysis with the avowed aim of overcoming his inability to commit himself to his girlfriend and thereby becoming able to marry her may imply, both through his account of his history and by his behavior with the analyst, that he has been held back from competitive successes by Oedipal anxieties and guilt. In this case, the patient's avowed goal may well be congruent with his unconscious goal. If, however, the patient's history discloses difficulties based on guilt in separating from a possessive and depressed mother, and if the patient gives evidence that he is tied to his present girlfriend by an unconscious fear that he would hurt her if he left her, we may suspect that his unconscious goal is to free himself from his unconscious guilt to his mother and to his girlfriend, and so become able comfortably either to remain with his girlfriend or to leave her.

The patient's behavior with the analyst—in particular his ways of testing the analyst and his favorable or unfavorable reactions to the analyst's comments—typically provide important clues to the patient's childhood traumas, pathogenic beliefs, and goals.

16

THE RELIABILITY OF THE DIAGNOSIS OF THE PATIENT'S UNCONSCIOUS PLAN

JOSEPH CASTON

THE PURPOSE

The concept that the analytic patient devises an unconscious plan to overcome his difficulties with the help of the analyst was described by Weiss in Chapter 5 and was reviewed in Chapter 15.

A "plan" is a particular and complex kind of psychoanalytic formulation. In essence it delineates an unmastered problem area that the patient consciously or unconsciously shows a high priority to master. Specifically, it stresses the goals a patient is likely to pursue in the analysis, characterizes the dangers (from the ego's viewpoint) that impede the pursuit, specifies how the patient is likely to work in analysis, and how the analyst's interventions may facilitate or impede the process. *Although its terminology is somewhat different, the plan concept overlaps or is contained within the scope of classical psychoanalytic formulation, but differs by its greater emphasis on ego interests and on appraisals and reappraisals of internal dangers.*[1]

The studies in this section are almost entirely based on a formulation of the unconscious plan in the case of Mrs. C.[2] Such studies necessarily depend on the reliability with which such a formulation can be made, that is, on the extent to which independent, qualified clinicians are able to agree on the main features of the case in question. In this chapter I shall briefly discuss the problems of establishing reliability for complex

1. For an elaborate discussion of this thesis—leading to a somewhat different conclusion—see Chapters 2 and 5.

2. Studies by Caston (Chapter 19) and by Silberschatz (Chapters 17 and 18) also used measures derived from classical psychoanalytic concepts.

The author is grateful to Suzanne Gassner for her invaluable help in the preparation of the final version of this chapter.

clinical formulations in general and describe a method I developed as one solution to these problems. I shall then present applications of the solution to two psychoanalytic cases, one of which is the case of Mrs. C.

THE PROBLEM

Psychoanalytic and psychodynamic formulations have features that are hard to objectify and make the demonstration of reliability difficult. First, such formulations are narrative in character. They are, in effect, complex stories that describe a person's historical background, motives, defenses, and symptoms, and that propose more or less explicit connections between these elements or show how treatment may help resolve the patient's underlying psychological difficulties.

To compare two independent narratives about a given patient is not easy. The task is not unlike contrasting two paintings of the same landscape. There is often no uniformity in the topics covered, or how they are discussed. To what degree the two representations are similar is not a question that lends itself to precise quantitative answers. Clinical narratives, moreover, posit complex inferences grounded in tacit theoretical assumptions. It is rare for the narrator to distinguish between statements that are more descriptive rather than inferential, or between propositions to which he assigns high probability and those he would consider speculative.

As a result of these difficulties, psychotherapy researchers have rarely tackled the problem of evaluating the reliability of clinical formulations. They have instead studied simpler and for the most part isolated variables. Nevertheless, it is the *weave* of inferential variables in complex clinical case formulations that is the essence of a clinician's understanding of his patients.

PERTINENT LITERATURE

There has been no research undertaken prior to the present work whose purpose is to determine the reliability of the kind of complex case formulation that a clinician makes at the beginning of treatment, with the possible exception perhaps, of Seitz's study (1966), which is discussed below. There have been, however, several attempts to determine the reliability of formulations about one or several central psychodynamic features of a session or a group of sessions (Bellak & Smith, 1956; Knapp, 1963; Strupp, Chassan, & Ewing, 1966; Kernberg, Burstein, Coyne, Applebaum, Horowitz, & Voth, 1972; Sampson *et al.*, 1972; Horowitz *et al.*, 1975; Malan, 1976a, 1976b; Luborsky, 1976; Levine & Luborsky, 1981; Gassner *et al.*, 1982).

Seitz (1966) conducted the most extensive study of this sort. He worked with a group of five senior psychoanalysts who sought to develop a method that would enable clinicians to reach agreement about their interpretation of clinical data. The group eventually disbanded because of their inability to develop a reliable interpretive method.

Seitz's group approached the task of seeking consensus by having each individual member first make an independent formulation of some continuous case material obtained from the early treatment hours. They also assessed the meaning of specific segments of the case material, in particular, the patient's first reported dreams. The clinicians were asked to answer specific questions so as to identify the patient's focal conflict, the defenses against it, and efforts at its solution. There was a lack of agreement in these initial independent formulations.

As a second step, each clinician was given anonymous copies of every other clinician's initial formulation, and each was asked to revise his original formulation to allow synthesis with relevant ideas that others had generated. But even when the clinicians tried to reformulate the case by drawing on the additional ideas that each of the others had expressed, they were unable to agree. Seitz offered several explanations for his group's inability to achieve consensus.

One problem, apparently, was that each analyst focused on different aspects of the clinical picture. Seitz suggested that psychoanalytic assumptions concerning the overdetermination of mental events and the coexistence of opposite motives had led to the judges describing different and at times seemingly contradictory aspects of the case material. A second problem Seitz reported was that the clinicians were relying excessively on their intuitive impressions, without paying sufficient attention to how well these impressions accounted for the data at hand.

Finally, Seitz concluded that it is particularly difficult "to interpret material from relatively early phases of ongoing analyses, during which conflict and defense patterns were still very disguised and obscure. The dynamics of the analytic process are much clearer and more easily interpretable toward the end of the analysis, when the intensity of defenses has been reduced markedly" (1966, p. 215). The group concluded that it was not possible for clinicians to achieve consensus about drive–defense configurations early in treatment.

In my opinion Seitz's judges were in more agreement than he was able to show. His awareness of this is indicated by his observations that it was not the case that the several judges were "all wrong" in their judgments, but rather that each was "partly right." The high degree of overdetermination in clinically rich material expands the number of possible interpretations. The difficulty in achieving consensus was further compounded by the requirement that Seitz's judges' interpretations be virtually identical. As a result, Seitz did not attempt to measure the *degree* of similarity between various formulations. The stringency of a criterion such as Seitz's inevitably obscures how much agreement actually exists between different judges' formulations. I shall offer a solution to this problem below.

Generally speaking, research that has depended on clinical formulations has bypassed the step of establishing their reliability. For example, no effort to establish the reliability of clinical judgments had been undertaken in 17 of the 19 studies Meehl cited in his classic monograph, *Clinical and Statistical Prediction* (1954). The thesis of Meehl's work is that predictions based on psychometric measures are as accurate, or more so, than any that can be made by the clinician on a case-specific basis. No research has been undertaken, so far as I know, that compares the predictive power of clinicians' case-specific formulations, once they have been demonstrated to be reliable, to that of comparable predictions derived from actuarial measures. Undoubtedly, one reason for this is the dearth of methods for evaluating clinician consensus.

Various approaches have been used by research investigators who are aware of the difficulty in establishing the reliability of clinical formulations. Some investigators have demonstrated that once clinical formulations were arrived at by having judges confer with one another, these formulations could successfully be used to make meaningful predictions (Knapp, 1963). Malan (1976b), using a similar approach, asked judges to formulate the patient's basic neurotic conflict and the criteria for recovery. Like Seitz, Malan found that when judges worked independently they "imposed their own theoretical bias on the material, often producing hypotheses that had little in common with one another. The policy that we then needed to adopt in reaching a consensus became equally clear. The amount of theory had to be reduced to the point at which agreement could be reached, and the final result was the highest common factor among all the hypotheses that had been made independently" (1976b, p. 15).

Other researchers have demonstrated that clinician-judges working independently have been able to arrive at consistent judgments for single variables, once they have been provided with clear operational definitions of the concepts they are rating (Bellak & Smith, 1956; Bellak, 1958; Knapp, 1963; Fisher & Greenberg, 1977).

Strupp *et al.* (1966) found high reliability between judges who rated *descriptive* variables, but low reliability for judgments of *inferential* variables. They defined an inferential variable as one that cannot be evaluated directly by describing an observable event. Strupp *et al.* concluded that in order to establish reliability for inferential variables, it is essential that "the observer-rater be given specific and unambiguous criteria concerning the observational referents" for the concepts being rated (p. 367). He also concluded that unless judges are given extensive training, it is futile to seek reliability on dimensions that require a high level of inference. In this connection, we recall that Seitz's group had not initially been given any explicitly stated criteria to guide them in the empirical task of answering the questions they had been asked to evaluate.

There have been several studies in which clinician-judges, working independently, were able to rate reliably specific variables that require clinical inferences (Sampson *et al.*, 1972; Kernberg *et al.*, 1972; Horowitz *et al.*, 1975; Gassner *et al.*, 1982). Characteristically, these have been studies in which the theoretical variable has been well defined, and in which the judges had experience in making comparable inferences prior to completing the rating task.

Luborsky (1976) recently succeeded in developing a method whereby independent judges were able to rate reliably what he termed the patient's "core conflictual relationship" theme. The method is "based on the same basic inferential and interpretive processes used by the psychoanalytic clinician in drawing conclusions about the major conflictual theme or the main transference pattern, in a patient's free associations. This theme is the one which is most redundant across many examples of the patient's relationships" (Levine & Luborsky, 1981, pp. 502–503).

It is of interest that Luborsky and his collaborators have been better able to develop a method in which independent clinician-raters could reliably make clinical inferences than have most other investigators in this area. I will later return to this point and discuss the relationship of his approach to the one independently evolved here. But first I shall describe my research strategy and findings.

RELIABILITY OF CLINICAL FORMULATIONS: A SOLUTION

A three-step procedure, designed to establish the reliability with which independent judges could formulate the nature of a patient's unconscious plan, was used.

The first step was to dissect the concept of the "unconscious plan" into its component parts, so that the reliability of the clinical judgments required for each part could be later *separately* determined. The "plan" is a complex formulation, based on inference, which asserts propositions about a patient's goals (i.e., what he unconsciously seeks to accomplish in treatment); the obstructions (i.e., the unconscious irrational dangers that interfere with his ability to achieve his goals); and how the patient is likely to work in analysis (i.e., by testing the analyst, the analytic situation, or himself to reappraise and overcome these dangers). In the process of developing such a formulation, it is important to assess the effect of the interventions on the patient so as to derive a sense of what makes them plan-compatible or plan-incompatible. The components of such a plan formulation are explicitly interrelated; together they provide a coherent account of the patient's goals, his difficulties, and the way he is likely to work in an effort to overcome these difficulties.

Second, a series of separate clinical statements pertinent to each component of the plan was developed by proposition-generating judges, who were directed to discern and generate the fullest array of relevant clinical possibilities. These statements represented clinically plausible propositions for this case.

Third, a new group of judges was asked to rate the relative contextual importance and relevance of each of these statements. Rater-judges were thus not required to develop their own separate formulations, but were instead provided with a fixed, comprehensive, case-specific array of possible clinical propositions relevant to the first five hours of process notes. To have allowed rater-judges to have freely described their own assessments of the process materials might have produced idiosyncratic, difficult-to-compare formulations. Defining the task as was done allowed assessment of the degree of agreement that existed between judges. Each judge, blind to the others and having made scaled ratings on the fixed arrays of clinical propositions provided, was in effect developing a hierarchy for the degree of presence or relevance of those propositions under each component. Thus each judge generated his own *profile* of high- and low-rated clusters among the items. Whenever extensive similarities of profiles between judges were obtained, statistically reliable agreement could be demonstrated. One could thus avoid the difficulties in determining reliability that other researchers encountered when their judges were given the unstructured task of developing formulations independently and/or consensually.

In order to avoid artificially inflating or deflating reliability coefficients, an effort was made to include a range of statements for each component, such that each statement was clinically plausible for the given case. In particular, it was important to avoid the inclusion of clinically *ir*relevant items, which might have tended to produce spuriously high reliabilities.

For the purposes of this study I developed a manual (Caston, 1980) that defined the plan components and provided some directions and examples for assessing each component of the plan. The manual was designed to be used by clinicians who had *already* had clinical training and experience in applying the plan concept.[3]

Some of the essential features of the plan components may be described as follows:

1. *The patient's goals.* Goals refer to attitudes, mood states, or behaviors that the patient wants to become able to achieve or renounce. The patient's goals as defined here are realistic, adaptive human activities or states and usually represent a developmentally higher level of functioning than the patient currently exhibits. Judges were asked to separately rate "immediate" and "eventual" goals.

2. *Obstructions.* Obstructions refer to those unconscious attitudes and convictions that make it dangerous for the patient to pursue the goal. Examples of obstructions include irrational beliefs in one's power to hurt others, vulnerability to injured self-esteem, fear of retaliation, the danger of catalyzing a repetition of a previous trauma, or the fear of being overwhelmed by an affective state.[4]

3. *Tests and test power.* Tests are trial actions unconsciously carried out by the patient and are intended to confirm or disconfirm the above unconscious pathogenic convictions. Such tests also provide the patient with a basis for assessing how dangerous it would be for the relationship with the analyst to pursue a particular goal. The assumption is made here that the greater the likelihood that a test will generate clarifying information from the therapist regarding the relative danger or safety of the goal, the more powerful is the test.

4. *Test outcome and the plan compatibility of the intervention.* If the analyst's intervention (e.g., clarification, interpretation, silence) passes the test, the patient will show an advance in any one or more of the

---

3. The manual is a useful adjunct in understanding the diagnostic operations. However, it is hardly a complete basis for training in itself, and alone is not likely to be an effective and reliable instrument for the application of these concepts. Requests for the manual may be made to the Secretary of the Mount Zion Psychotherapy Research Group, Department of Psychiatry, Mount Zion Hospital and Medical Center, P.O. Box 7921, San Francisco, CA 94120.

4. The centrality of pathogenic beliefs in maintaining the patient's psychopathology was recognized by Weiss subsequent to the studies reported here; therefore, "obstructions" came to be specifically reconceptualized in terms of the patient's "pathogenic beliefs."

following ways: The patient may increasingly behave in ways consistent with his unconscious goals[5,6]; may become more generally flexible, bold, and relaxed; may expand on relevant material; may bring forth previously warded-off contents; or may become more exploratory or self-confronting. A retreat is characterized by opposite behaviors.

THE FIRST STUDY: MISS K

THE METHOD

The first study involved an analytic patient, Miss K, who had a predominantly hysterical character makeup. She tended to develop profoundly clingy and dependent relationships, was moody, and was often excessively compliant with regard to other people's wishes and expectations.[7] Her analyst took detailed process notes of the first five treatment hours. These notes included an extensive description of each of the themes the patient touched upon, and a near-verbatim account of the interventions the analyst made. All major silences and pauses were recorded, and the length of each silence was estimated. As an experienced psychoanalyst, I used these process notes to generate the rating materials that were used in this study. A list of 33 plausible goals, 22 possible obstacles, 11 patient tests and 19 analytic interventions (both actual and hypothetical) were presented to judges to rate on a 9-point scale. The contents of the rating materials were specific to the case under investigation.

Four judges who were unfamiliar with the case were provided with the detailed process notes from the first 5 hours of the analysis, the *Manual on How to Diagnose the Plan* (Caston, 1980), and the rating materials. The judges had had between 2 and 10 years of prior experience

---

5. An additional component I conceptualized was the formal "means" by which the patient attempted to master a problem. I identified various means such as "inching up on the problem," "counterphobically plunging into desired behaviors," and "identifying with the strength of others." However, because this aspect of plan formulation does not capture a dimension the clinician needs to use to formulate a case, and because a patient may vary in the means he uses, it was decided that it was unnecessary to ask judges to rate this component of the plan.

6. In those instances where the patient's unconscious goal is to acquire an increased capacity to fight or oppose, it is a difficult task to evaluate the test outcome. In such instances an "advance" may be demonstrated by the patient's becoming, for instance, more stubborn, superficial, or silent, in the sense that he was previously *unable* to choose to be or not be that way.

7. This thumbnail description of the patient was not given to the judges in this study.

with case application of the concept of unconscious plans. The judges reported that they did not find it a difficult task to complete the ratings, and no formal training seemed necessary for them to apply the instructions in the manual to the case material.

What follows is more detailed information about the rating materials the judges were given.

The Immediate and Eventual Goals

The statements used in this study expressed unmastered goals that the patient might possibly want to attain, either immediately or eventually. The judges were asked to rate each statement with regard to whether it was viewed as an immediate or eventual priority of the patient's. A rating of "1" indicated that the item had no importance or priority as an immediate (or eventual) goal; a rating of "9" indicated that the item had an extremely high degree of importance or priority.

A Summary Statement of the Overall Goal

The judges were also given a list of five possible goal statements (shown below) and were asked to choose which statement best expressed the patient's overall goal. The judges were told:

From the following summary descriptions of possible *immediate* goals, choose the one you believe is the most likely one operative in this case (closest to your own formulation).

1. The patient wishes to be able to recognize, manage, and renounce her Oedipal attachment to her father and her envy of men.
2. The patient wishes to be able to become independent from, and reject if necessary, various important others.
3. The patient wishes to recognize and manage her attachment to her mother and the homosexual strivings that have developed from it.
4. The patient wishes to be able to express and enjoy deep feelings of closeness to significant others.
5. The patient wishes not to be so subject to a loss of control in her hostile urges toward men and her brother.

Obstructions

The statements that referred to obstructions describe either what makes the goals dangerous, or what the defensive behaviors are that are used to ward off the dangers. Judges indicated on a 9-point scale the degree to which they inferred that a particular obstruction was operative.

Test Power and the Plan Compatibility of the Intervention

Based on the raters' choices of what constituted the patient's overall goal, they were asked to use a 9-point scale to rate the power of the patient's test and the plan compatibility of the analyst's response to the test. In addition to actual instances of tests and interventions, possible hypothetical examples were also included, which had the following form: "At point X, what if the patient (or analyst) had instead said Y?" There were 11 test items and 19 intervention items.

FINDINGS

As can be seen in Table 16-1, the reliability coefficients for the components of the unconscious plan ranged from .72 to .92. The level of reliability obtained is remarkably high, and it contrasts to the lack of consensus in previous research of this type.

The four judges were unanimous in their choice of the patient's overall goal. They selected the goal statement that "the patient wishes to become independent from and reject if necessary various important others."

Because the results of the study indicated that the method used was one that could solve the "consensus problem," the same kind of materials were given to a different group of clinical judges, whose task it was to diagnose Mrs. C's unconscious plan.

Table 16-1. The Reliability Coefficients in the First Study (Miss K)

Plan component	Number of items	Reliability coefficients
Immediate goals	33	.87
Eventual goals	33	.72
Obstructions	22	.91
Test power	11	.85
Plan compatibility of interventions	19	.92

THE SECOND STUDY: THE CASE OF MRS. C

THE METHOD

Mrs. C had been diagnosed as obsessive–compulsive. She tended to be plagued with feeling tense, self-critical, overcontrolled, and distant. She had come into treatment because of her difficulty enjoying sex and being comfortable with intimacy. (See Chapter 10 for a fuller description.)

As in the previous study, a highly experienced psychoanalyst, working with the detailed process notes of the first five hours of Mrs. C's analysis, generated a list of plausible goals, obstructions, tests, and therapist interventions (actual and hypothetical), which were given to judges to rate.[8] An effort was made to construct rating materials whose content would be specific to the case of Mrs. C.

The four judges in this study were all advanced psychoanalytic candidates. They had all had at least some brief exposure to the concepts that comprise the components of the unconscious plan. They were less experienced at applying these concepts to the task of plan formulation than the judges in the first study. None of the judges had any knowledge of the case they were studying, other than that provided by the detailed process notes of the first five sessions. They were also given the *Manual on How to Diagnose the Plan* (Caston, 1980) and the rating materials (see Appendix 7).

The Immediate and Eventual Goals

In the study of Mrs. C, judges were given 33 goal statements to rate on a 9-point scale (see Appendix 7). Judges were asked to rate how likely it is that each of these statements represents an immediate and an eventual goal. Judges were instructed to rate the propositions in a forced *Q*-sort with a bell-shaped distribution over the 9 points. The *Q*-sort method was not used in the previous study but was introduced here because it compels judges to differentiate items more sharply than is required by ratings of individual items.

---

8. Two steps were used in the generation of these items. In the first step, Abby Wolfson developed a questionnaire consisting of a series of multiple-choice items covering various aspects of the case, and had these items filled out (as part of a separate study) by 22 analysts in another city. Owen Renik then used the results of Wolfson's questionnaire to identify relevant items for our own reliability study. He also added a number of items that he considered useful, from his own evaluation of the case.

A Summary Statement of the Overall Goal

Judges were given five different summary descriptions of Mrs. C's immediate goal and were asked to choose the one they believed was closest to their own formulation. The statements read as follows:

1. The patient wishes to be able to confront the sources of her envy and jealousy without shame so that she can feel less compelled toward self-defeating competitiveness.
2. The patient wishes to be able to attenuate her unrealistic perfectionism without anxiety so that she can be more able to be satisfied with herself.
3. The patient wishes to be able to be stubborn, separate, and aggressive without guilt so that she can be more comfortable being close.
4. The patient wishes to be able to bring forth and explore her unconscious homosexuality without anxiety so that she can more freely enjoy a heterosexual relationship.
5. The patient wishes to be able to master her feelings of being messy and defective without anxiety so that she does not always have to maintain tight control of herself.

Obstructions

The judges were given a list of 20 possible obstructions and asked to use a 9-point scale and to rate the degree to which they inferred that a particular obstruction was operative.

Test Power and the Plan Compatibility of the Intervention

Judges were asked to use a 9-point scale to indicate how plan-relevant and powerful a test was. As in the prior study, both hypothetical and actual instances of tests were included. Examples from the materials written for the case of Mrs. C are as follows:

An example of an actual test: The patient asks about the people in the front office leaving, and about how the analyst would know that she was there waiting.

An example of a hypothetical test: The patient refers to having been late during the last sessions and asks what she should do.

Both actual and hypothetical instances of analyst interventions were also used.

An example of an actual analyst's intervention: After patient asks if she should force herself to say things, even if she is not ready, analyst responds by asking patient if she remembers the rule.

An example of a hypothetical analyst's intervention: In reference to the item above, what if the analyst has said instead, "You are implying you need me to tell you what to do."

There were 21 test items and 18 intervention items used.

FINDINGS

The reliability coefficients for the components of the unconscious plan are generally quite high. As can be seen from Table 16-2, with one exception, they range from .69 to .92. We found that not all of the judges were able to apply reliably the concept of obstructions. However, two of the four judges correlated highly with each other, and these ratings also correlated significantly with my ratings. When the ratings of only these two judges were used, their reliability coefficient was .80, in contrast to the .14 correlation coefficient obtained by using the ratings of all four judges. The two judges who were unable to achieve reliability on the obstructions component of the plan were nevertheless able to achieve agreement on all of the other plan component ratings.

The four judges were unanimous in their choice of the patient's overall goal. The summary statement which the judges chose was: "The patient wishes to be able to be stubborn, separate, and aggressive without guilt so that she can be more comfortable with being close." This statement agrees with the case formulation of our research group, which had been based on studies of the first 10 hours of the process notes (see Chapter 10). The agreement between the research group and the four judges, who were independent of the research group, is further evidence for the reliability with which a patient's broadly stated immediate goal can be identified.

Table 16-2. The Reliability Coefficients in the Second Study (Mrs. C)

Plan component	Number of items	Reliability coefficients
Immediate goals	33	.89
Eventual goals	33	.69
Obstructions		
Four judges	20	.14
Two judges	20	.80
Test power	11	.76
Plan compatibility of interventions	19	.92

SUMMARY AND DISCUSSION

The preceding two studies demonstrate that high levels of interrater reliability may be obtained for psychoanalytic case formulations which are complex, inferential, and unique to the specific patient.

The general method of the present investigation consists of (1) the dissection of underlying clinical concepts from the given formulational paradigm so as to simplify the relevant tasks for judges; (2) the development by proposition-generating judges of comprehensive, *fixed* arrays of clinical propositions (under each component) about the specific case; (3) and the rating of these propositions by individual judges from a second team. Elimination of the use of unstructured formulations from the task thus facilitated the comparison of agreement between rater-judges. The strength of this method lies in allowing the overlap of clinicians' agreements to be statistically captured by a correlational approach.

In its application to the formulation of the unconscious plan, the plan paradigm was first broken down into components such as "goals," "obstructions," and "tests"; then proposition-generating judges prepared concise clinical statements or items for each component. After reading the clinical material, independent rater-judges evaluated each proposition for its pertinence or priority to the case of Mrs. C.

This method permits but does not guarantee demonstrating agreement for clinical formulations. We should keep in mind that some kinds of psychoanalytic formulations may be more difficult to establish reliability for, and some individual cases may be more difficult to formulate under a given approach. It might be the case, for instance, that it is relatively easier to establish adequate reliability for a *plan* formulation. If so, it would likely be due to the relative uniformity and degree of definition of the components of a plan formulation, which, although inferential, may be closer to observation than other kinds of psychoanalytic concepts. In classical terms, plan goals are equivalent to *ego interests*, and obstructions are closely equivalent to the components of *resistances*. It may be easier to reliably identify where a patient "wishes to go" (his goals) from early sessions than to reliably identify his relevant impulse-defense configurations at that point in time. Since the development of concepts derived from the theory of the unconscious plan has tended to be tied to *operationalized* research paradigms, they may be more explicitly connected to observables.

However, *which* kinds of psychoanalytic concepts are more reliably identifiable is an empirical question. The general method presented here will allow an examination of such an inquiry, and it is eminently applicable to assessing the reliability of clinical variables based on classical psychoanalytic theory, such as resistances, transference configurations, and conflicts.[9]

In this connection, Luborsky (1976) and Levine and Luborsky (1981) have been able to obtain high reliabilities for assessments of the "core conflictual relationship theme" in 15 different patients, a single variable that they believe is homologous with the basic enduring transference pattern in the patient. The task is to identify (1) a central and recurrent close-to-the-surface wish in terms of some object relation, and (2) the real or imagined consequence of the wish. To do so they used a method which is akin to the one presented in this chapter; it involves a focus on concrete episodes in the text, the use of a standard arboreal schema for the elaboration of possible themes, and the use of two separate judge-teams to carry out the two-step procedure. They have concluded that independent rater-judges can successfully infer such a theme, which, though complex and patient-specific, is "sufficiently reproducible and measurable to provide a basis for clinical research" (Levine & Luborsky, 1981, p. 519).

The power both of the general method presented in this chapter and of Luborsky's method to generate reliability for such complex variables very likely depends on their related features. On the other hand, whenever clinical formulations are built up from *several* interwoven concepts, such as the ones presented here, each needs to be operationalized, an unnecessary step for single-variable studies. In addition, the nature of most components of multifaceted clinical formulation demands a wider array of plausible items or propositional choices than the highly redundant themes of Luborsky's study.

As the reliability of the diagnosis of the unconscious plan in the case of Mrs. C is now established, the requisite first step for the studies of the succeeding chapters has been accomplished. This will permit the testing of hypotheses based on this formulation of Mrs. C's unconscious plan, comparison with other hypotheses, and other experimental attempts at validation of the plan concept.

9. I have recently undertaken a study of the reliability of *classical* psychoanalytic formulations.

17

TESTING PATHOGENIC BELIEFS

GEORGE SILBERSCHATZ

This chapter reports an empirical investigation of the explanatory power of an important hypothesis proposed by Weiss in Part I: that the analytic patient works unconsciously throughout his analysis to disconfirm pathogenic beliefs by testing them in relation to the analyst (see Chapters 5 and 6). If the analyst's response to the patient's test is perceived by the patient as disconfirming that belief, the patient may behave as follows (see Chapter 15):

1. The patient may become less anxious, for the danger he had anticipated (on the basis of the pathogenic belief) has not been realized.
2. The patient may also, over a period of time, produce new memories about the traumatic situation in which the belief arose, for it is now safer to remember them.
3. The patient may, over a period of time, become conscious of the pathogenic belief, or develop new insights about it, for it is now safer to become aware of the belief and to think about it.
4. The patient may make progress toward goals which he could not pursue earlier because the pathogenic belief had warned him of the danger of doing so.

If, however, the analyst's response to the patient's test tends to confirm rather than disconfirm the pathogenic belief, the patient is likely to remain anxious. He is unlikely to recover new memories or to gain new insights into his pathogenic beliefs and their consequences. He may even temporarily retreat from his goals.

The present study tested rigorously some of these predictions. It identified *key tests* during a period of Mrs. C's analysis, that is, tests

The author is very grateful to Robert Holt, Hartvig Dahl, Thomas Kelly, Marshall Bush, and Suzanne Gassner for their valuable contributions to this work.

The work presented in this chapter was supported in part by the Chapman Research Fund.

judged to be central to the pathogenic beliefs that the patient, according to our plan formulation, is likely to work to disconfirm. It examined the *immediate effects* of the analyst's "passing of the test," that is, of the analyst responding to the test in a way the patient perceives as disconfirming the belief the patient is testing. The immediate effects are unlikely to include the recovery of memories and the development of new insights. (Miss P, as described in Chapter 1, recalled previously repressed memories several hours after the passed test.) However, our hypothesis predicted that the patient would, immediately following a passed test, become less anxious, more relaxed, more positive toward the analyst and the analysis, more involved in the therapeutic work, and bolder in tackling problems.

It is this prediction that was investigated in the present study. If this prediction is confirmed, it would lend support to our hypothesis and provide a demonstration of its explanatory power.

METHOD

OVERVIEW OF METHOD

The method to test this hypothesis involved three basic steps: (1) the reliable identification of the patient's key tests; (2) reliable judgments of whether or not the analyst's responses to these tests would be perceived by the patient as disconfirming the belief the patient was testing; and (3) independent and reliable assessments of the patient's behavior and affects just before and just after the tests, in order to determine whether the patient changed in the predicted directions.

Before describing how each of the three steps was carried out, we shall briefly remind the reader of Mrs. C's pathogenic beliefs, which were identified in the plan formulation.

REVIEW OF PATHOGENIC BELIEFS

According to the plan formulation (Chapter 10), Mrs. C, during her childhood, perceived her parents as fragile, unhappy, and vulnerable. Her mother seemed grim, joyless, and unable to protect herself. Her father seemed to her to be in danger of losing control, to require constant reassurance, and to be unable to tolerate (without feeling hurt or angry) his children having ideas or values different than his own. Moreover, her parents did not seem affectionate toward each other, and both were possessive toward her. She unconsciously thought that her parents and siblings envied her attractiveness, social skills, and successes.

Mrs. C's pathogenic beliefs included the idea that she could devastate her father and cause him to lose control if she disagreed with him, criticized him, or held values different from his. She believed also that she would hurt both parents and make them envious if she were less burdened and joyless than they were—if she had fun, were outgoing, were close to other people, loved her husband, and wanted and enjoyed sexual relations with him. She also believed that if she were independent and strong she would make her parents and siblings envious.

We assumed that Mrs. C would attempt to test and disconfirm these beliefs in relation to the analyst. We thought it likely that she would test first whether the analyst would be hurt or angry if she were to disagree with him, not submit to him, and have opinions of her own.

SELECTING KEY TESTS

The selection of key tests (i.e., tests connected to central pathogenic beliefs) involved two steps.

The first step was the selection, from the verbatim transcripts of the first 100 sessions, of a pool of *possible* tests. Nine graduate students in psychology were instructed to select transcript episodes in which the patient seemed to be pulling, explicitly or implicitly, for some response from the analyst. I assumed that many tests would have this form, and that such instructions would help judges with limited clinical training to select a large pool of potentially relevant test episodes. Each judge read a different portion of the 100 hours and selected instances that he or she deemed relevant. Each hour was read by at least two raters independently, thus minimizing the systematic biases of any one judge, and also generating a maximum number of instances. The result of this first step was a deliberately overinclusive pool of 87 incidents considered relevant by one or more raters. Typescripts of the 87 segments were then prepared. They included the patient's transference pulls (e.g., seeking approval or guidance or affection), and the analyst's responses (which in some instances was silence). In addition to these 87 targeted segments, 15 interchanges not selected by any of the judges were also included for control purposes.

The second step made use of three psychoanalytically trained judges who were familiar with the clinical use of the concept of testing. They read a short case formulation prepared by senior clinicians, and then identified which of the pool of 87 incidents (plus the 15 control segments) represented attempts by the patient to carry out central or key tests.

The following case description was given to the judges:

Mrs. C, a married social worker in her late 20s, had been diagnosed as having an obsessive–compulsive character structure. Her major complaints were a general sense of inhibition, chronic tension, an inability to relax and enjoy herself, and sexual frigidity.

Mrs. C was the second child of a comfortable, middle-class family. She was raised in a small midwestern community. She had an older sister and a younger sister and brother. Her father was a successful businessman. She characterized him as unable to tolerate disagreement or criticisms, and as requiring frequent reassurances that he was right. Occasionally he lost control of himself and would rage at or physically strike her or other members of the family. Mrs. C characterized her mother, who was a housewife, as driven, joyless, bound by duty and feelings of obligation, and unable to relax. Her mother did not fight back against her father's domination and criticisms, and the patient remembered also an occasion in early childhood when *she* had hit her mother, and her mother did not defend herself but doubled up in pain and went weeping to her room.

In the first two sessions of her analysis, Mrs. C presented certain perspectives on her problems and her goals. She made clear that she would like to be able to enjoy herself more. She mentioned difficulty in disagreeing with her parents, who insisted that their way is right. Her parents, perhaps especially her father but also her mother, would feel criticized if they knew she was in analysis. She noted her tendency to take blame for what happens to other people, and she implied that she feels guilty irrationally even when she has not done anything wrong. Moreover, when she makes mistakes, even minor ones, she has to suffer for doing so. She also made evident that she would like to be considerably more daring, more self-assertive, and less preoccupied with other people's approval or disapproval, and that she would like to think for herself. She feared that analysis might make her dislike her family.

The three psychoanalytic judges also received an abbreviated formulation of the patient's plan[1]:

Mrs. C was very inhibited. It was inferred that her immediate difficulties were caused by unconscious guilt based on the omnipotent belief that if she asserted herself with other people, she would hurt them seriously. Because of this guilt, she was in danger of submitting in a close relationship, and of allowing herself to be criticized, put down, humiliated, and dominated. In order to avoid these

---

1. Later studies done on the case of Mrs. C employed a more complex plan formulation; the later formulations subsume the earlier version within a more comprehensive exposition.

dangers, she had to avoid feelings of closeness, including feelings of sexual closeness and responsiveness.

It was also inferred that Mrs. C had developed an unconscious plan to reduce her fears about hurting others, and to reduce her guilt and her omnipotence. Thus, she would attempt to test the analyst to see whether he was hurt when she disagreed with him, criticized him, or found fault with him. More generally, she would work in various ways to develop the capacity to fight with others in addition to the analyst. When she developed this capacity, she would then feel safe enough to risk feelings of closeness, including feelings of sexual pleasure with her husband. She would feel safe enough to experience sexual pleasure with him, if she could feel able to fight back if he should attempt to exploit her guilt in order to make her submit.

A sample of 46 segments was selected by all three judges as instances of key tests. The reliability of these ratings was as follows: $r_{ll} = .63$, $r_{kk} = .82$.

CLASSIFYING THE ANALYST'S RESPONSE TO THE TESTS

The next step used four other psychoanalysts who were familiar with the clinical application of the testing concept. They were asked to rate on a 7-point scale (shown in Appendix 11) the extent to which the analyst passed the 46 key tests. The reliability of their ratings was as follows: $r_{ll} = .58$, $r_{kk} = .89$.

In order to provide a sense of the kind of clinical task which these judges were given, we shall present two of the items that they were asked to judge. In the first example, the judges rated the analyst as passing the patient's test; in the second instance, they rated the analyst as failing the patient's test:

Example 1

PATIENT: Thinking back on your question just a little while ago, I think probably my—after initially reacting when I was talking in here, then I thought back on the remark about my stirring up things, and I think probably my first inclination was to think, now which way did you mean it, did you mean it as something I shouldn't do or is it all right for me to do it? (*Pause.*) And perhaps one reason why I get feeling sort of panicked when I have nothing to say is that I feel you'll feel very impatient that I'm not saying anything, or even disapprove. (*Silence.*)
ANALYST: When you think I'll be impatient or disapprove if you don't say anything, what do you imagine could happen then?

The judges assigned this example a mean rating of 6.0 on a scale of 0 to 6; that is, it received the highest possible rating.

Example 2

PATIENT: Is it better to force yourself to say something that you feel sort of not ready to say?

ANALYST: Well, what was the rule I told you? Or what did I say was your job?

The judges assigned this example a mean rating of 0.5 on the 0 to 6 scale.

These examples can be understood as instances in which Mrs. C tests whether the analyst will be upset if she questions his authority and his rules by not complying immediately with his expectations. As we have noted, Mrs. C believed she would devastate her father if she disagreed with him or did not fulfill his expectations of her.

The analyst's response in Example 1 was judged to be passing the test because his neutral investigatory stance would be unlikely to confirm the patient's pathogenic belief that she would hurt the analyst were she to proceed on her own terms. By contrast, in Example 2, the analyst's response would be unlikely to disconfirm Mrs. C's belief that were she to behave autonomously she would harm the analyst. The judges rated the analyst as, in this instance, failing the test.

BEFORE AND AFTER PATIENT MEASURES

The patient's behavior immediately before and after the analyst's interventions was assessed on several patient measures. Each measure was scored by a different group of judges. The segments were approximately 6 minutes of patient speech. These were presented to the raters in random order, and without any context. Moreover, the raters were unaware whether the segment occurred before or after the testing segment. In addition, all judges were unaware of the aims of the research. The measures were as follows:

The Experiencing Scale

Derived from a Rogerian client-centered framework, the Experiencing Scale (Klein *et al.*, 1970) assesses the extent to which a patient focuses on his feelings while simultaneously reflecting about these feelings for problem-solving purposes. This 7-point scale is thought to tap such constructs as insight, lack of resistance, and high-quality free association (Kiesler, 1973). At the low end of the scale, the patient is abstract, impersonal, and minimally involved; he is remote from his feelings and unable to understand their implicit meanings. At the high end of the scale he is aware of his feelings and internal processes; he is involved in his experience and is able to articulate and explore it.

The Experiencing Scale is designed to measure 2- to 8-minute segments of psychotherapy interviews. It has been found to be "sensitive to shifts in patient involvement . . . making it useful for microscopic process studies, for example . . . to assess the productivity of different topics . . . it can pinpoint special moments or phases in therapy" (Klein *et al.*, 1970, p. 1). Detailed training procedures as well as an extensive review of the relevant research literature are presented in the authors' research and training manual (Klein *et al.*, 1970), which includes 90 training segments from therapy interviews. Two kinds of ratings are made for each segment: The modal score characterizes the overall level of the segment, while the peak score is given to the highest scale level reached during the segment. The Experiencing Scale can be applied equally well by either clinically naive or sophisticated judges, with interjudge reliability (r_{kk}) approximately .80 or above (using three or more judges).

Three undergraduate psychology majors and one advanced graduate student in clinical psychology participated in the standardized training procedure described in Klein *et al.*'s (1970) research and training manual. After completing the 16-hour training program, the judges rated all of the pre- and posttransference-pull segments.

The Boldness Rating Scale

The Boldness Scale, developed by Caston, is a 5-point rating scale that assesses the degree to which the patient is able to confront or elaborate "nontrivial material" (see Chapter 19), that is, the extent to which he boldly tackles issues or retreats from them. At the low end of the scale, the patient is anxious, is generally inhibited, and may express dissatisfaction about his handling of the material. At the high end of the scale the patient seems able to plunge ahead and confront a variety of issues even if they are painful and distressing. Caston has reported (Chapter 19) a reliability (r_{kk}) of .82, with four judges (psychology interns) rating 15 segments of psychoanalytic sessions. In addition, he has presented a correlation of .93 between ratings of boldness and insight.

Two clinical psychologists were given the 15 segments that Caston's raters had scored and were asked to rate them for training purposes.

Following Holt's recommendation (1965), Caston's 5-point integer scale was expanded to a 5-point continuous scale (resulting in a 40-point scale). The modified continuous scale was used for rating the training segments and the segments used in this study.

The Relaxation Scale

This scale measures the patient's degree of freedom and relaxation in the psychoanalytic session. At the high end of the scale the patient is able to associate freely, easily, and flexibly; to be playful with ideas and to explore the connections between his thoughts in an uninhibited, spontaneous manner; and to experience and explore his feelings freely and undefensively. At the low end of the scale the patient is defensive, constricted, or narrow in his associations; he is halting, timid, or bothered by his train of thoughts, and his associations come with great difficulty; in general, he seems tense, rigid, tight, or grim. The 5-point scale, originally described as the Freedom versus Beleaguerment Scale, was recently developed by Mayer, Bronstein, and F. Sampson (see Chapter 13) to rate entire sessions for the degree of patient relaxation.

Three advanced graduate students in clinical psychology familiarized themselves with the scale by rating five sample segments on this 5-point continuous scale. They then rated the segments used in this study.

Affects

The patient's emotions were categorized according to an affect classification system developed by de Rivera (1962) and modified by Dahl and Stengel (1978) and by Dahl (1979). We used four affect categories: love, satisfaction, anxiety, and fear.[2]

An attempt was made to include as many manifestations of these affects as possible. Thus, any reference to these emotions was scored: word labels for an affect (e.g., I feel anxious), metaphorical expressions, denial of affect, representation of emotions in actions, and the attribution of affect to another person. Each sentence within a segment was scored. A sentence could contain multiple scores for one category (e.g., several manifestations of fear), or scores for several affect categories simultaneously (e.g., two fear scores, one anxiety score, one satisfaction score). If a

---

2. This work was part of a larger study of Mrs. C's affects. Information about the patient's expression of those affects not pertinent to the hypothesis that this study was testing is available from Dr. George Silberschatz, Department of Psychiatry, Mount Zion Hospital and Medical Center, P.O. Box 7921, San Francisco, CA 94120.

Table 17-1. Reliabilities for Experiencing, Boldness, Relaxation, and Affect Measures

Rating scale	Number of judges	r_{ll}	r_{kk}
Experiencing Scale			
Mode	4	.55	.83
Peak	4	.58	.84
Mode + peak	4	.64	.88
Boldness	2	.47	.64
Relaxation	3	.45	.72
Love	2	.69	.82
Satisfaction	2	.82	.90
Fear	2	.46	.63
Anxiety	2	.88	.94

sentence contained no scorable affect, it was tabulated in a "lack of affect" category. We calculated the sum of the scores across sentences for each emotion category in every segment. Two undergraduates, who had undergone extensive training with Dr. Dahl, scored all of the segments. Reliabilities on the four affects ranged from .63 to .94 (see Table 17-1).

RESULTS

Table 17-1 shows how reliably judges were able to make ratings on the patient measures: the Experiencing Scales, the Boldness and Relaxation Scales, and Dahl's Affect Measures.[3] In all instances, the reliability of these patient measures was satisfactory.

The correlations between the analyst "passing the test" ratings and the patient measures for the key tests are presented in Table 17-2. They were *all* in the direction predicted by our hypothesis, and six of the seven

3. Reliability data for these ratings—as well as for all of the other measures—are in terms of the intraclass correlation (Ebel, 1951; Guilford, 1954) using the residual mean square as the error term (i.e., mean differences in judges' ratings are not regarded as error). Two figures are reported: r_{ll} = the estimated reliability of the average judges, and r_{kk} = the estimated reliability of the mean of K judges' ratings. For an overview of the various methods of computing interrater reliability, see Tinsley and Weiss (1975). For a more comprehensive treatment of reliability theory, see Cronbach, Gleser, Nand, and Rajaratnam (1972). Intercorrelations of all of these measures are presented in Appendix 12.

correlations were statistically significant. How well the analyst passed the test correlated significantly ($p < .05$) with changes in the patient's level of experiencing, boldness, relaxation, and love. There was a significant negative correlation ($p < .05$) between how well the analyst passed the test and changes in the patient's level of fear and anxiety. These results suggest, as predicted, that the analyst's passing of the patient's tests is associated with the patient becoming less anxious, more friendly to the analyst, more productive in the analytic work, and more relaxed.

SUMMARY AND DISCUSSION

The present study supports our hypothesis about the patient's testing of the analyst, and shows that this hypothesis has significant explanatory power. It is interesting, moreover, that there are demonstrable *immediate* effects of a passed test. The clinical observations of passed tests we have reported (e.g., Miss P in Chapter 1) sometimes involve more long-term effects. For example, Miss P, many days after a major test which the analyst passed, recovered significant new memories. She continued to recall new memories related to the passed test for several weeks, and, more or less simultaneously she both developed a number of new insights about her pathogenic beliefs and made progress toward her goals outside of the analysis. In addition, our clinical observations indicate that these long-term therapeutic effects are typically the result not of a single, discrete passed test but rather of a prolonged series of tests of the analyst.

Table 17-2. Correlations between the Degree to Which the Analyst Passed the Patient's Tests and Changes in the Patient Measures for the Key Tests ($N = 46$)

Measure	r
Experiencing	.33*
Boldness	.32*
Relaxation	.35*
Love	.37*
Fear	−.34*
Satisfaction	.15
Anxiety	−.29*

*$p < .05$, two-tailed test.

The results of the present study suggest there also are lawful *immediate* effects of passing or failing tests. Caston (Chapter 19) and Bush and Gassner (Chapter 20) also found significant immediate effects following pro- and anti-plan interpretations.

Although the present study was not designed to investigate longer-term effects of passed tests, combining the results of this study with the studies reported in previous chapters suggests that there is a broad association between a series of numerous passed tests and other progressive changes over a longer time period. As we have seen, Mrs. C, during the first 100 hours, became conscious, without interpretation, of previously warded-off contents (Chapter 12), including memories. She began to acquire more insight into her pathogenic beliefs (Chapter 14), and her behavior became more assertive, affectionate, and sexual (Chapter 13). This pattern of results is consistent with our view that Mrs. C did begin to disconfirm pathogenic beliefs during this period of her analysis, in part through testing these beliefs with the analyst, and that the analyst's passing tests enabled her to feel safe enough to change in the various ways we have described.

18

TESTING PATHOGENIC BELIEFS VERSUS SEEKING TRANSFERENCE GRATIFICATIONS

GEORGE SILBERSCHATZ
HAROLD SAMPSON
JOSEPH WEISS

In this chapter we shall present an experiment in nature that casts light on the accuracy and explanatory power of competing hypotheses, which are based on the automatic functioning and the higher mental functioning concepts. We shall refer to these hypotheses as the AF (automatic functioning) hypothesis and the HMF (higher mental functioning) hypothesis.

The opportunity to test these hypotheses against each other arises from the fact that they explain a particular therapeutic situation in distinctly different ways, and make different predictions about the behavior of the patient in this situation.

The situation is a familiar one in psychoanalysis: the patient often makes a powerful unconscious transference demand of the analyst. He may, for example, invite the analyst's approval, or praise, or love; he may invite the therapist to nurture him, or to treat him as special, and so forth. The AF and HMF hypotheses explain the patient's transference demand differently, account differently for the therapeutic value of the analyst's

Portions of this chapter are adapted from J. Weiss and H. Sampson, Testing alternative psychoanalytic explanations of the therapeutic process. In J. H. Masling (Ed.), *Empirical studies of psychoanalytical theories* (Vol. 2). Copyright 1986 by Lawrence Erlbaum Associates, Inc. Adapted by permission of the publisher.

Portions of this chapter are also adapted from H. Sampson and J. Weiss, Testing hypotheses: The approach of the Mount Zion Psychotherapy Research Group. In L. S. Greenberg and W. M. Pinsof (Eds.), *The psychotherapeutic process: A research handbook*. Copyright 1986 by The Guilford Press. Adapted by permission of the publisher.

The authors wish to acknowledge the valuable contributions of Hartvig Dahl, Robert Holt, Suzanne Gassner, and Thomas Kelly.

The work presented in this chapter was supported in part by the Chapman Research Fund.

not acceding to the patient's demand, and make different predictions about how the patient will behave if the analyst indeed does not accede to the demand.

According to the AF hypothesis, the patient makes the transference demand in order to gratify an unconscious transference impulse. The impulse is frustrated by the analyst's neutrality. The impulse then becomes intensified and so pushes to consciousness. According to the HMF hypothesis, the patient may, in making a transference demand, be testing the analyst to ensure himself against a certain danger, which stems from a pathogenic belief. The analyst, by his neutrality, passes the test. The patient is reassured, and decides that he may safely bring forth an unconscious content that he had been warding off.

According to the first explanation, as, for example, in the theory set forth by Freud in his *Papers on Technique* (1911–1915), the broad meaning of the patient's behavior, in making a powerful transference demand, is unequivocal. The patient's behavior is primarily an expression of unconscious wishes seeking gratification without regard to reality. These imperious wishes "endeavor to reproduce themselves in accordance with the timelessness of the unconscious and its capacity for hallucination. Just as happens in dreams, the patient regards the products of the awakening of his unconscious impulses as contemporaneous and real; he seeks to put his passions into action without taking any account of the real situation. . . . This struggle . . . is played out almost exclusively in the phenomena of transference" (1912, p. 108).

The patient's behavior, in making a transference demand, is, according to the AF hypothesis, also serving as a powerful resistance: The patient is repeating rather than remembering infantile material; moreover, the demand serves as an *agent provocateur* (1915, p. 163), which puts the analyst in an awkward position. In response to a patient's demand, the analyst should, according to Freud, frustrate it in a neutral and investigatory manner. The analyst must be "proof against every temptation" (1915, p. 166). If a woman's "advances were returned it would be a great triumph for her, but a complete defeat for the treatment. She would have succeeded in what all patients strive for in analysis—she would have succeeded in acting out, in repeating in real life, what she ought only to have remembered, to have reproduced as psychical material and to have kept within the sphere of psychical events" (1915, p. 166). Analytic technique "requires of the physician that he should deny to the patient who is craving for love the satisfaction she demands. The treatment must be carried out in abstinence" (1915, p. 165).

How, according to this hypothesis, does a patient respond when the analyst does not reciprocate his transference demands? The answer is again unequivocal: The patient's unconscious transference wishes are frustrated, his unconscious longings are intensified, his instinctual conflicts are further mobilized, and, over time, there is "an acute revival of his pathogenic conflict" (Weinshel, 1971, p. 74). The patient may manifest this intensified conflict along with regression, or he may manifest instead intensified efforts at defense. The libido of the instinctual wishes, frustrated by the analyst, may flow back to the infantile memories and lead to their emergence; in such a case, the repressed memories will emerge because of their instinctual thrust, and the patient will be in conflict about their emergence.

The investigators in the Menninger Psychotherapy Research Project (Sargent et al., 1968) agreed with this hypothesis as to how a patient will respond when he expresses a powerful transference demand, and the analyst does not accede to it. Their conclusion was stated in this formal prediction: "Patients whose neurotic needs are not gratified within the transference respond to this frustration with regressive and/or resistive reactions, and/or painful affects" (Sargent et al., 1968, p. 85).

Let us now consider the second explanation for a patient's making a powerful transference demand on the analyst, namely, that the patient may do so to test a pathogenic belief. This explanation offers a different rationale of why the analyst should respond in a neutral and investigatory manner; and it predicts certain significant differences in how the patient will respond when the analyst does not accede to the transference demand.

According to this explanation, a patient, in making a powerful pull or demand in the transference, may unconsciously be carrying out a trial action designed to test an unconscious infantile belief. For example, a patient may invite the analyst to reciprocate his professed love to test his unconscious belief that if he were sexual or affectionate toward a parental figure, he would seduce him. If the analyst maintains his analytic stance, the patient may take a step toward disconfirming the belief.

According to this explanation, a patient's behavior in making a transference demand may be a complex trial action unconsciously planned and carried out to test an unconscious pathogenic belief (as it pertains to the patient's relationship with the analyst) and thus to determine whether an unconscious conviction of danger (about how the patient may affect the analyst) is justified. The patient's behavior may then be a part of the patient's reality testing. The patient is motivated to work, by testing the belief, to disconfirm it; for the belief is frightening to him and has caused him to renounce important goals, institute defenses, and develop inhibitions and symptoms.

The analyst, in not acceding to the patient's demand, may disconfirm the patient's unconscious conviction of danger and thus reassure the patient rather than frustrate him. According to this theory, the patient should feel unconsciously reassured and pleased, more confident of the analyst and the analysis, and more relaxed, and he should show reduced defensiveness and increased freedom and boldness in exploring his problems.

Because the two theories differ in their predictions about certain aspects of the patient's response in a particular situation, it should be possible to test which theory better fits observation. We, as well as our colleagues, have carried out this test informally in the course of clinical work. Our observations have supported the HMF hypothesis. In order to compare the two hypotheses more rigorously, systematically, and objectively, Silberschatz devised a formal research study that controlled for a number of possible sources of bias.

OVERVIEW OF METHOD

To provide a fair comparison of the AF and HMF hypotheses, it was necessary to find instances of the phenomenon—a patient making implicit or explicit transference demands—that fit the criteria of *both* hypotheses. Such instances would be ones that psychoanalysts accustomed to applying AF concepts would identify reliably as instances of the patient seeking to gratify a key or central unconscious wish, *and* that psychoanalysts accustomed to applying HMF concepts would identify reliably as instances of the patient carrying out a key or central test of the analyst. Only such overlapping instances, selected as appropriate by both AF and HMF judges, are appropriate to test the alternative hypotheses. The several steps involved in identifying these overlapping instances will be described subsequently.

The analyst's response to the patient's transference pull or demand was rated by AF psychoanalyst judges for the degree to which it frustrated, in a neutral manner, the patient's unconscious wish, and by HMF psychoanalyst judges for the degree to which it passed or failed the patient's unconscious test. A passed test is one in which the analyst's response is likely to disconfirm the pathogenic belief which the patient is testing; and, conversely, a failed test is one in which the analyst's response is likely to confirm that pathogenic belief.

Finally, the patient's behavior prior to the analyst's response was compared, in terms of several patient measures, to the patient's behavior following the incident. Each patient measure was scored by different groups of judges. Then, changes in the patient's behavior following the analyst's interventions were compared to the predictions of each theory.

STEP 1: INITIAL IDENTIFICATION OF PATIENT'S TRANSFERENCE DEMAND

The purpose of this initial step was to identify a large pool of instances that might meet the criteria of each of the two theories. The method was precisely that described in the preceding chapter. Nine raters, graduate students in clinical psychology, read through the verbatim transcripts of the first 100 hours of Mrs. C's psychoanalysis and were asked to identify all instances in which she was making a transference demand of the analyst. Each rater read a different portion of the 100 hours. Each hour was read by at least two raters independently, thus minimizing the systematic biases of any one judge, and also generating the maximum number of instances.

The result of this step was a pool of 87 incidents which one or more raters considered to be instances of a patient making a demand of the analyst. Among the instances included were attempts by the patient to elicit reassurance, approval, affection, love, guidance, more active participation by the analyst, permission (to be critical, angry), or punishment. In addition to these 87 incidents, 15 random segments not identified by any of the judges were included as control segments.

Typescripts of each of the 102 segments were then prepared. They included the patient's transference pull or control segment and the analyst's response, which in some instances was silence.

STEP 2: RATINGS OF THE 102 INSTANCES

Two independent groups of judges (psychoanalysts and advanced candidates in psychoanalytic training) were asked to read a brief description of the patient, including her presenting problems and relevant historical data. The judges were then given the typescripts containing the transference demands (*and controls*) and the analyst's interventions. Five analysts accustomed to applying AF hypotheses in their clinical work rated the degree to which in each instance the analyst's response (which might be silence) was a neutral nongratification of the patient's transference wish. Similarly, four analysts accustomed to applying HMF hypotheses in their clinical work rated the extent to which the analyst passed or failed the patient's test. Each group of judges made their respective ratings on a scale of 0 to 6 (see Appendix 9).

STEP 3: SELECTING KEY TESTS AND KEY FRUSTRATIONS

The 87 instances of a transference demand selected by graduate students in Step 1 were not all of equal salience to the patient, nor of equal pertinence to the hypotheses being tested. In order to compare only instances that clearly conformed to the theoretical issues, Silberschatz used two new sets of psychoanalyst judges. The first set consisted of three AF judges. Their task was to identify those instances, within the pool of 102, in which the patient was seeking to gratify a key (i.e., centrally important) unconscious wish. The second set consisted of three HMF judges. Their task was to identify instances in which the patient was carrying out a key (i.e., centrally important) test of the analyst. Each judge was to make his judgment on the basis of a brief case formulation written from his own perspective. AF judges were presented with the following case formulation prepared by the treating analyst and a senior colleague of his who had followed the case throughout the analysis:

After the birth of her brother the patient, who was 6 years old at the time, detected a marked change in her parents' (especially her father's) attitude toward her. She felt that her parents immediately began to value the baby boy more than they valued her and that her father's interest and love had shifted away from her to her brother (her father's first and only son). She attributed the change in her father's attitude to the fact that her brother had a penis and that she did not. This fantasy gave rise to the idea that her lacking a penis would forever doom her to an inferior position in life. The patient's central unconscious wish was to redress her "castrated state." The patient would attempt to do so by trying to get a penis of her own and/or by getting rid of penises altogether, thereby obliterating differences between the sexes.

The HMF or "testing" judges were presented with a brief case formulation prepared by senior clinicians in our research group. This formulation has already been described in Chapter 17.

The AF judges identified reliably, on the basis of this case formulation, 59 of the 102 instances as attempts to gratify *key unconscious wishes*. The "testing" judges identified reliably 46 segments as *key tests*.

STEP 4: THE POOL OF OVERLAPPING INSTANCES

We now identified those instances that the AF judges rated as key frustrations and the HMF judges identified as key tests. There were 34 such overlapping instances. These instances had already been rated (in Step 2) for the analyst's interventions. In the comparisons to be reported subsequently, we used only the overlapping instances, which were selected to meet the requirements of both hypotheses.

STEP 5: BEFORE AND AFTER PATIENT MEASURES

The patient's behavior before and after the analyst's intervention was assessed on several patient measures. Each measure was scored by a different group of judges. The segments were approximately 6 minutes of patient speech. These were presented to the raters in *random order*, with the judges unaware of whether the segment was a "pretransference demand" segment or a "posttransference demand" segment. The measures used were the Experiencing Scale, the Boldness Scale, the Relaxation Scale, and a measure of the patient's level of fear, anxiety, love, and satisfaction (see Chapter 17).

RESULTS

Table 18-1 shows that each group of judges achieved satisfactory reliability. The 7-point scales the judges used are presented in Appendices 8 and 10. On the basis of the case formulation the AF judges were given, 59 of the 102 segments were identified as attempts to gratify key unconscious wishes. These judgments yielded an r_{11} reliability of .54 and an r_{kk} of .86.[1] Judges who used the testing formulation identified 46 of the 102 segments as key tests. These judgments yielded an r_{11} of .42 and r_{kk} of .75. Judgments by the AF judges of how well the analyst avoided gratifying the patient's unconscious wish yielded an r_{11} correlation of .35 and an r_{kk} correlation of .74. The testing hypothesis judges' ratings of how well the

---

1. Reliability data for these ratings—as well as for all of the other measures—are in terms of the intraclass correlation (Ebel, 1951; Guilford, 1954) using the residual mean square as the error term (i.e., mean differences in judges' ratings are not regarded as error). Two figures are reported: r_{11} = the estimated reliability of the average judges, and r_{kk} = the estimated reliability of the mean of K judges' ratings. For an overview of various methods of computing the interrater reliability, see Tinsley and Weiss (1975); for a more comprehensive treatment of reliability theory, see Cronbach *et al.* (1972).

Table 18-1. Reliabilities for the Patient and Analyst Scales

Rating scale	Number of judges	r_{11}	r_{kk}
Key Unconscious Wishes Scale (AF)	5	.54	.86
Key Unconscious Test Scale (HMF)	4	.42	.75
Analyst Passing the Test Scale (HMF)	4	.47	.78
Analyst Frustrating the Wish Scale (AF)	5	.35	.74

analyst passed the patient's test yielded an r_{11} reliability correlation of .47 and an r_{kk} correlation of .78.

As had been expected, there was considerable agreement between the AF judges and the HMF judges in the ratings of the analyst's interventions. There were 34 segments that were rated as key tests and key frustrations, and for this sample the correlation between the two groups' ratings of the analyst's interventions was .81 ($p < .001$). This means that those interventions viewed by one group as passing a test tended to be viewed by the other group as frustrating a wish; and similarly, what was viewed by one group as failing a test tended to be viewed by the other as gratifying a wish. The significant positive correlation between these two sets of ratings indicates that both theories recognize the patient's transference demands as important, and both agree that in many instances the analyst should not yield to a patient's pull for a response.

The agreement between the predictions made by each theory and the data are presented in Table 18-2. This table shows the correlations for the 34 overlapping instances, between passing key tests and changes in the patient's measures. For each of the seven measures, the correlation is in the direction predicted by the HMF model and is opposite to the direction predicted by the AF model. Four of the seven correlations are statistically significant.

DISCUSSION AND CONCLUSIONS

In this study we compared two competing theories about what a patient will feel and do when the analyst responds neutrally to a transference demand. According to one theory, such a sequence would be likely to frustrate the patient's powerful unconscious infantile wishes; the patient would be expected to respond with tension, anxiety, conflict, and resistive or regressive reactions. According to the other theory, if analytic neutrality signified passing the patient's test, the patient should respond to the analyst's neutrality with a greater sense of confidence and an increased capacity to work progressively in the treatment.

We identified 34 instances of patient–analyst interchanges that were pertinent to both theories. These segments were understood by the "frustration hypothesis" judges to exemplify the patient seeking to obtain from the analyst gratification of a key infantile wish. At the same time, these interchanges were understood by the "testing hypothesis" judges to be instances of key tests. Both theoretical positions recommend approximately the same response by the analyst. The theories contrast sharply, however, in their account of what the patient's response should be.

Our findings indicate that when the analyst did not accede to the patient's key transference demands, the patient became significantly less anxious; more relaxed, flexible, and spontaneous; more bold in tackling issues; and more positive in her attitude toward others. These findings are, of course, immediately comprehensible if the patient's transference demands were a test of a pathogenic belief, and if the analyst's not acceding to the demands was therefore a reassurance against a danger associated with the pathogenic belief. These findings would not be expected if the patient's transference demands were powerful unconscious

Table 18-2. Correlations between Ratings of the Therapist's Behavior and Changes in the Patient Measures for Segments Identified as Both Key Frustrations and Key Tests ($N = 34$)[a]

	Results obtained	Predicted by AF	Predicted by HMF
Experiencing	+ .23	−	+
Boldness	+ .41*	−	+
Relaxation	+ .35*	−	+
Love	+ .36*	−	+
Satisfaction	+ .15	−	+
Fear	− .31	+	−
Anxiety	− .34*	+	−

[a]The correlations were virtually identical when made between frustrating a wish and changes in the patient's measure, and there are no changes in the significance tests.

*$p < .05$, two-tailed test.

wishes and the analyst's not acceding to them was therefore a frustration of these wishes. For according to the frustration hypothesis, "patients whose neurotic needs are not gratified within the transference respond to this frustration with regressive and/or resistive reactions, and/or painful affects" (Sargent *et al.*, 1968, p. 85).

The results of the present study, then, lend support to the "testing hypothesis" (HMF) in comparison to the "frustration hypothesis" (AF). But what of a theory that combines AF and HMF concepts? Is it possible that Mrs. C was *both* frustrated *and* reassured when the analyst did not accede to her major transference pulls and demands? There is certainly no evidence of Mrs. C's frustration in the results we have obtained. However, for reasons mentioned previously, such a combined theory is difficult to disconfirm conclusively, for its predictions in any given situation are not definitive.

A limitation of this study should be noted: Whereas there is much evidence for the reliability of the case formulation that the testing judges used, there was no comparable demonstration of the reliability of the case formulation provided to the AF judges. This latter formulation represents the understanding of the case of Mrs. C shared by the treating and supervising analysts. It is therefore a significant formulation. Nonetheless, it is possible that other analysts who formulate cases in terms of wish–defense constellations might have inferred that different infantile wishes were of central importance.

It should be noted that the concept of passing a patient's test is broader than the concept of analytic neutrality. Although in this study analytic neutrality was understood to coincide with the kinds of responses that would pass this patient's key tests, there are instances in which passing a patient's test would, according to the AF hypothesis, provide unconscious gratification.

Overall, this study represents an important initial step in submitting competing clinical theories to rigorous empirical investigation. The results show that the HMF model is better able to predict and explain the data than the AF hypothesis. Replication of this study on other patients as well as on later phases of therapy would strengthen the results. Such replication studies are currently underway.

19

THE IMMEDIATE EFFECTS
OF PSYCHOANALYTIC
INTERVENTIONS

JOSEPH CASTON
RUTH K. GOLDMAN
MARY MARGARET McCLURE

.

The investigations reported in this chapter were designed to study the immediate effects of the analyst's verbalized interventions on the patient. An immediate effect is positive, according to generally held psychoanalytic concepts, if the patient's associations progress in the direction of lessened defensiveness (Brenner, 1955; Fenichel, 1941). Two hypotheses regarding psychoanalytic interventions were studied:

1. The first was a case-specific hypothesis derived from the higher mental functioning theory: The immediate effect of an intervention depends on its compatibility with the patient's unconscious plan. The plan concept assumes that if a conviction about an unconscious or conscious danger can be overcome, the patient may be free to pursue a goal that was previously inhibited by that conviction. The plan concept is psychoanalytic in its methods of discovery and formulation of such danger; however, the application of the plan concept to making interventions in a given case focuses on such inferred goals and dangers.

2. The second hypothesis derives from the ubiquitous clinical finding that immediate effects depend on the psychoanalytic interpretiveness of the analyst's interventions. "Psychoanalytic" refers to clinical inference, which is bound both to contents of the patient context and to

The authors are grateful for the help of Paul Ransohoff in the early phase of the replication study, and for the help of Suzanne Gassner in the preparation of this chapter.

While this chapter is largely concerned with the main theme of this book (the testing of the higher mental functioning hypothesis), it also takes up a topic that does not bear on this theme (the effect of analytic "interpretiveness"). In this chapter as in others, the wishes of the principal authors were respected (JW and HS).

general conventions regarding defensive behaviors, developmental sequence, and Oedipal/pre-Oedipal dynamics. In this view, the direct *or* preparatory action of interpretiveness facilitates a lessening of warding-off processes in the patient (Fenichel, 1941; Greenson, 1967).

The way in which these two aspects of interventions intertwine is a crucial matter. For example, the first hypothesis would base what makes interpretiveness effective entirely on the plan compatibility of an intervention. The alternative posits *multiple* factors and themes as contributing to immediate effects. The interpretiveness hypothesis is so significant in psychoanalysis and in the experimental literature that it is valuable to attempt to separate the two hypotheses or clarify how they overlap.

In these investigations we followed Bachrach's lead (1980) in his review of studies relating analyzability to analytic outcomes. He clarified that for patients selected as "analyzable," standard technique does not *in itself* predict good outcome; so far, the few variables that predict success (e.g., good ego functioning) account for a small portion of the variance. He concludes that empirical studies of *the details of the analytic process* are more likely to shed light on what makes for good results.

THE PERTINENT LITERATURE

Beneficial factors in interventions that theorists have considered pertinent are rather numerous, and include moderateness of interpretive depth, completeness, accuracy, causal or linkage-making explanation, transference-centeredness, and resistance-centeredness (Freud, 1912, 1914; Strachey, 1934; Fenichel, 1941; Kris, 1951, 1956a; Loewenstein, 1957; Greenson, 1967; Brenner, 1976; Compton, 1975), as well as timing, dose, tact, economy, degree of analytic neutrality, empathy, and "working alliance" (Greenson, 1967; Ornstein & Ornstein, 1975; Dewald, 1976, 1978).

Clinical observations of psychoanalytic process have gone far to illuminate theory of technique, but few *controlled* experiments have attempted to do so. Of these, most have focused on some general aspect of psychoanalytic interpretiveness. Three studies investigated aspects of interpretive complexity in tape-recorded cases. Either the relative *depth* of interpretation or the relative *complexity* of psychoanalytic explanation was assessed. Speisman (1959) tested and confirmed Fenichel's hypothesis that moderately deep versus very deep or superficial interpretations are more immediately therapeutically effective. Garduk and Haggard (1972) found that explanatory, linkage-making interpretations of unconscious material were associated with significantly more affect, insight, defensive associations, and transference-related responses as compared with noninterpretive interventions. Colby (1961) found that interventions that interpreted causal linkages were followed by more free association than were questions.

These research designs tend to assume that any interpretation is as accurate or timely as any other, thus implicitly trusting in the acumen of the treating analysts. Whether or not such a view is naive, these studies do demonstrate an aspect of lawfulness in the realm of immediate effects of psychoanalytic interventions.

Other experimental work has related interpretive aspects of patient–therapist interaction to ultimate treatment outcome. Luborsky, Bachrach, Groff, Pulver, and Christoph (1979) found a parallel between patients' immediate "positive" responsiveness to transference interpretations and final treatment outcome ($N = 3$, all psychoanalyses). Malan (1976a, 1976b) found significant positive correlations between the mean density of interpretations of the "transference–parent" link throughout the treatment, and final outcome ($N = 14$–30 in brief/longer psychotherapies). He has also clinically noted positive *immediate* responses to this type of interpretation.

Malan's "focality" (1976a) is a case-specific measure of the therapist's (and patient's) ability to stick to a theme that he has singled out within a session. Focality in early hours correlates positively with final treatment outcome. While focality depends on the formulation of the therapist's plan *for* the case, it is likely that interactions with high focality may often contain plan-compatible interventions.

PILOT STUDY ON THE PROCESS NOTES

OVERVIEW

The pilot study was undertaken to explore our questions about the two hypotheses. Caston developed several scales to study these questions. The Plan Compatibility Scale is a patient-specific scale that measures interventions according to their likely facilitation of the patient's unconscious plan. The second scale, Psychoanalytic Interpretiveness, measures interventions according to the degree to which they interpret, focus on, or are preparatory to the interpretation of an unconscious defense. Scales to evaluate immediate effects were also developed. In each case the investigation involved two steps:

1. The analyst's interventions were evaluated along a continuum of either plan compatibility or psychoanalytic interpretiveness, using separate groups of judges for each variable.
2. To observe the effects of either dimension, we evaluated the patient's verbal productions before and after the analyst's intervention in terms of *general* measures of insight and self-confrontation.

RATIONALES FOR RATING INTERVENTIONS AND EFFECTS

Plan Compatibility

The earliest version of the formulation of the unconscious plan in the case of Mrs. C was used. The reliability of this formulation is discussed in Chapter 16. This formulation emphasized the patient's goal of establishing an ego-syntonic capacity to be flexibly oppositional.

Guidelines about what would constitute pro- and anti-plan interventions specific to this case were provided. "Pro-plan" characterizes those interventions or interpretations that would likely facilitate Mrs. C's overcoming her defensiveness against independence from the analyst and others. Interventions not opposing the patient's withholding from, disagreeing with, or criticizing others are also identified as pro-plan. Anti-plan interventions were identified as those that Mrs. C would likely perceive as encouraging her dependence and submissiveness, as implicitly guilt-provoking, or as reflecting a defensive, mocking, or indifferent stance toward the patient's oppositionalness.

Psychoanalytic Interpretiveness

Interventions are considered psychoanalytically interpretive to the extent that they directly elucidate unconscious associative or causal linkages, name warded-off states or relations, or provide a preparatory focus on material proximal to that being warded off. Such interventions have been observed to be followed by patient productions that are or lead to further verbalized understandings (Fenichel, 1941; Greenson, 1967). Since there are no restrictions on the nature or range of what is warded off, a sampling from the full spectrum of interventions is indicated, rather than a sampling keyed to selected thematic features, as with plan compatibility.

Construction of the Psychoanalytic Interpretiveness Scale extended and refined features of scales from Speisman's (1959) and Garduk and Haggard's (1972) studies.

Immediate Effects

In evaluating effects, we felt it was insufficient to show that the patient was merely following the lead of the analyst. Achievement of insight and overcoming of neurotic inhibitions within the psychoanalytic process may sometimes *depart* from the immediate or apparent focus of the analyst's intervention. This assessment therefore required a *general* rather than a highly specified range of patient productions.

Effects were grouped in two overlapping types of patient response. Level of *insight* with respect to significant associative or causal linkages represented one dimension, and *self-confrontiveness* (a demonstrated tackling of issues, including the bold addressing of relevant affects, experiences, and topics) represented a second dimension. The assessment measured the productivity of the patient's responses following the intervention versus prior to the intervention.

SELECTION OF EXCERPTS TO BE RATED FROM PROCESS NOTES

Fifteen items meeting predetermined formal criteria were found through a random search of the first 100 hours of process notes. The criteria were devised to provide sufficient context, natural process configurations, and manageable excerpt size, as well as to maintain a relative uniformity among units and avoid selection bias. Each excerpt consisted of process material containing the intervention that was the "target" of ratings for the independent variables. Excerpts met four criteria:

1. *The nonrated analytic intervention prior to the target.* Each excerpt began with an intervention that was not to be rated, which oriented the judge to the nature of the interaction in which the target intervention was embedded.
2. *The patient context segment.* Between 7 and 26 typed lines of uninterrupted patient speech followed the analyst's prior intervention and preceded the target intervention.
3. *The target intervention.* This was the comment or interpretation to which the ratings of the independent variables were applied.
4. *The patient effect segment.* The target intervention was followed

by 7–26 typed lines of uninterrupted speech ending at some natural cleavage such as before another analytic intervention or a silence.

THE RATINGS

Protocols for these ratings are presented in Appendices 13, 14, 17, and 18.

Judges

Different sets of judges were used for each variable studied. Four were used for rating plan compatibility, two for psychoanalytic interpretiveness, four for the effect variables (insight and boldness), and two for the preintervention levels of the effect variables. Judges were clinicians from the mental health disciplines of psychiatry, psychology, and social work. Professional experience ranged from advanced trainee to practitioner with many years of clinical experience. All had had psychoanalytically oriented training.

Rating Target Interventions on the Plan Compatibility Scale

Four judges were asked to evaluate the analyst's interventions on a 5-point pro-plan/anti-plan dimension. They were given a guide to rating the analyst's interventions, which contained a description of the patient and her presenting problem, a brief formulation of the patient's plan, and guidelines for describing the kinds of interventions that would be expected to be pro- and anti-plan, with hypothetical examples.

The judges rated 15 random interventions from different hours. Each excerpt included the analyst's "prior" intervention, which was not to be rated; the patient's context segment, which followed the latter; and the target intervention itself, which was rated for plan compatibility. Judges were blind to the patient's actual responses.

The four judges' averaged ratings were used as the measure for the prediction. Its reliability was .72 (Spearman–Brown coefficient).

Rating Interventions on the Psychoanalytic Interpretiveness Scale

Two judges were asked to evaluate the analyst's interventions on a 6-point scale for the degree of psychoanalytic interpretiveness. Each was given a guide to rating interventions for psychoanalytic interpretiveness. This guide is applicable to any case and provides no formulation specific to the given patient. It presents a hierarchy of levels of interpretiveness, with hypothetical examples. The judges were told, "The interventions are judged in the light of the immediately preceding production by the patient. How far beyond the patient's material the cognitive content of the intervention reaches is, of course, one consideration in the assessment." An intervention with a complex interpretive form would be rated lower if it is merely a paraphrase of what the patient has just expressed than if it goes beyond.[1]

1. Two judges, both psychoanalytically oriented clinical psychologists, applied the Psychoanalytic Interpretiveness Scale to 22 psychoanalytic interventions in items consisting of a brief patient speech followed by the analyst's intervention; the patient's postintervention responses were not included. The source of the excerpts was the process notes from the case of Mrs. C. An interjudge reliability of .82 was achieved (Spearman r); the reliability of the average of the two judges' ratings was .95 (Spearman–Brown prediction).

In order to validate this scale we asked whether psychoanalytically informed clinicians who were *uninstructed* with respect to the Psychoanalytic Interpretiveness Scale would be likely to order interventions in a similar way for judges using this scale. In doing so the former would have to rely on their individual assimilation of psychoanalytic principles as refined by practice. Three judges carried out this task; they included a psychoanalytic candidate who was a practicing psychiatrist, a psychologist, and a psychiatric resident in the last year of training. They were given the same 22 items and asked to evaluate how "psychoanalytically interpretive" the analyst's interventions appeared to be, in several graded steps. The first task required the judge to record whether each intervention was or was not a psychoanalytic interpretation, or in between. They were then required to rank all interventions by Q-sorting over a 7-point spectrum with a bell-shaped distribution. Finally, all interventions were rank-ordered within each level; a completely rank-ordered list of the 22 interventions was thus generated. The reliability among the three uninstructed judges was .84 ($p < .001$, Kendall). The average of the three judges' rankings correlated with the scores from a different set of judges using the Psychoanalytic Interpretiveness Scale (.82, $p < .001$). We believe this to be a highly satisfactory indication that the psychoanalytic conventions that underlie the scale are generally similar to those acquired in professional psychoanalytically oriented training.

We also obtained validating support from high correlations between the present measure and related instruments. Although Garduk and Haggard (1972) used a method of distinguishing between interpretations and "noninterpretations" to carry out their main studies, a measure based on finer distinctions can be developed from their discussion in the appendix to their work: a 5-point scale which recognizes three levels of interpretation and two levels of noninterpretation. Applying such a scale with Garduk and Haggard's descriptions correlates .85 with our scale. Correlation with Harway et al.'s (1955) Depth of Interpretation measure, for those 17 items in our set of 22 that are rankable by their system, yields a value of .79.

It is significant that items that our "uninstructed" psychoanalytic clinicians strongly agreed were psychoanalytic interpretation yield an average of 3.7 on our Psychoanalytic Interpretiveness Scale. On this scale a level of 3 represents interventions that select from what is relatively manifest in the patient's productions without *explicitly* pointing to what is warded off, whereas interpretative linkages between manifest content and what has been inferred to have been warded off are clearly made at level 4 and above. This indicates to us that psychoanalytic clinicians conceive of interpretation as beginning at a level somewhat simpler than the level of explicit interpretation of *connections* with what is warded off.

Judges rated target interventions from the same 15 excerpts as above, with the actual responses to the target intervention removed. The reliability of the average of two judges' ratings on these items was .90.

Rating the Patient's Postintervention Material for Effects

Four judges rated the patient's material for immediate effects following the intervention, using two scales. They reviewed entire excerpts with the target intervention removed. The ratings were carried out on the effect segment *in the light of* the preintervention patient material, which meant that shifts in the level of boldness or insight were taken into clinical consideration by judges.

The Boldness Scale measures the degree to which the patient pursues a deepening self-confrontation of significant personal issues. At the high end of the scale the patient plunges ahead and at the low end retreats.

The Insight Scale was used to rate the degree to which the patient is developing nontrivial insights. The judge combines several factors in making this rating: the significance of themes, the extent of the patient's insight, and the degree to which she integrates material.

The same judges evaluated the material on both scales. The correlation between boldness and insight was so high (.93) that the scores were combined into a single scale, "boldness/insight," for the purpose of the pilot study. The reliability of this combined measure was .82.

An additional pair of judges evaluated the patient's level of boldness/insight for the preintervention material *only*, blind to the rest. We used this variable to explore the extent to which the patient's preintervention state might itself be used to predict the postintervention state.

RESULTS

This small sample yielded several findings that were in the predicted direction, and enabled refinements in method for the replication on the verbatim transcripts. (See Table 19-1.)

Plan Compatibility

Ratings of the plan compatibility of the analyst's interventions correlated significantly with the boldness/insight ratings for the postintervention segment of patient speech (.48, $p < .05$). This indicates a significant

Table 19-1. Pilot Study: Correlations between Dependent and Independent Measures (*N* = 15)

	Psychoanalytic interpretiveness	Boldness/insight (context)	Boldness/insight (effect)
Plan compatibility	.32	.07	.48*
Psychoanalytic interpretiveness			.28
Boldness/insight[a] (context)			.50*

[a]Boldness and insight were combined and analyzed as a single dependent variable in both the context and effect measures.

*p < .05.

relation between the plan compatibility of the interventions and the patient's immediate responsiveness in terms of levels of insight and self-confrontation.

Boldness/Insight

We correlated the patient's baseline level of boldness/insight (*before* the target intervention) with the level *after* ($r = .50, p < .05$). This indicates a moderate tendency in the patient to persist at the same level of productiveness after an intervention as before it.

There was virtually no correlation ($r = -.07$) between the patient's level of boldness/insight preceding the target intervention and the level of plan compatibility of the analyst's intervention following it. Thus, each of these two variables contributed *independently* to the patient's postintervention level of responsiveness, and together account for half the variance which is surprisingly large. However, unless the remainder of the variance is entirely due to error, it is likely that other factors are also involved in postintervention effects.

Psychoanalytic Interpretiveness

Ratings of the psychoanalytic interpretiveness of the analyst's interventions correlated with the boldness/insight ratings of the postintervention segments in the predicted direction (.28, N.S.). Ratings of psychoanalytic interpretiveness and of plan compatibility of the analyst's interventions were correlated (.32, N.S.). Given the small sample size, we regarded these positive correlations as nonetheless important and suggestive. If this magnitude of correlation held in a large-scale replication, both values would achieve statistical significance, and it would be crucial to separate the effects of the two independent variables.

METHODOLOGICAL CONSIDERATIONS
FOLLOWING PILOT RESULTS

The pilot study demonstrated the need to control for baseline levels of preintervention boldness and insight, and for the levels of psychoanalytic interpretiveness and plan compatibility with respect to each other. Despite overlap, we believed that boldness and insight were concepts distinct enough to use separately, but that separate sets of judges would be required to minimize halo effects.

Findings by Silberschatz led us to consider the possible influence of transference focus and the power of the patient's testing on immediate effects as modifiers of our main hypotheses (see Chapters 17 and 18). His method differed in significant ways from ours, but one aspect of his study was homologous with our plan compatibility experiment—the degree to which the analyst responded to the patient's "tests" of him in a way that was compatible with her unconscious plan. Silberschatz found that "passing the test" correlated significantly with the postintervention segment boldness rating ($r = .41$, $p < .05$).

Because of different experimental goals, criteria for item selection were restricted in Silberschatz's work to excerpts that show the patient both (1) making transference demands *and* (2) presenting issues relevant to the patient's unconscious plan, that is, "testing." These were called "key tests." Thus, in his study, the prediction regarding plan compatibility holds true for a particular group of events rather than for all events sampled randomly.

In contrast, our studies proposed to explore the plan compatibility hypothesis for interventions not preselected for presence of testing or transference in interactions. As we were interested in the effects of plan compatibility across the full range of interventions, we did not restrict the material by type of content. Study of the interpretiveness hypothesis also required that the subject matter be "wide open" rather than limited to only oppositionalness and guilt.

For the purposes of the pilot study, we assumed that the ego appraises the safety or danger of interventions regardless of the degree of the patient's efforts to actively "test" the therapeutic atmosphere. The pilot results at this point appeared to indicate that the plan compatibility hypothesis holds true for interventions in general; in that light, Silberschatz's study implied that testing and/or transference might enhance the immediate effects of interventions.

THE REPLICATION STUDY ON
THE VERBATIM TRANSCRIPTS

In the light of pilot findings, we undertook a replication on a larger sample from verbatim transcripts, using refined strategy and measures. We asked whether the following would hold:

1. Would the plan compatibility of interventions correlate positively with immediate effects in the patient's responses as measured by boldness and insight scales?
2. Would the psychoanalytic interpretiveness of interventions correlate positively with immediate effects?
3. Would the patient's *pre*intervention level of responsiveness correlate positively with immediate effects?
4. Would plan compatibility and psychoanalytic interpretiveness correlate positively with immediate effects when the overlap between them was statistically removed?
5. Would the patient's testing and transference increase the positive correlation between plan compatibility and immediate effects?

The method was similar to that of the pilot except for three major changes: (1) Criteria for selecting units of excerpted text material no longer required the initial orienting analyst's comments, and context and effect segments were considerably longer. (2) Judges were given more training to increase uniformity of ratings. (3) A Test Power Scale was introduced to measure the patient's preintervention material in relation to her unconscious plan. Protocols for these ratings are presented in Appendices 13–19.

SELECTING THE UNITS TO BE STUDIED
FROM THE TRANSCRIPTS

Eighty-one excerpts, each with an analytic intervention, were randomly selected from the first 100 hours of the transcripts on the basis of formal criteria.

1. *Patient context segment.* This segment contained 15–35 typed lines, representing about 2 minutes of uninterrupted patient speech. A silence might occur at the beginning or end, but no silence greater than

one minute was embedded *within* the excerpt; work by Marshall Bush and Suzanne Gassner (personal communication) suggested that embedded silence can represent a "test" different from that of the patient's speech.

2. *Target intervention.* The analyst made a verbal statement following the patient context segment. In some cases a negligible amount of patient speech was interspersed within the analytic intervention.

3. *Patient effect segment.* A target intervention was followed by patient speech (about 2 minutes long) ending at a natural cleavage such as silence or a subsequent intervention.

Training of Judges

The judges were clinicians of experience and sophistication similar to those of the pilot study. Different sets of judges were trained to use the different scales. Invented texts were used, and the basis for ratings explored; practice items were rated and discussed.

Rating the Target Interventions on Plan Compatibility and Psychoanalytic Interpretiveness

These scales are described above. Plan compatibility was now expanded to 9 points. Four judges were used for plan compatibility, and two for psychoanalytic interpretiveness. The judges were given 81 excerpts in random order, each consisting of only a patient context segment followed by its target intervention.

Rating the Target Interventions on Test Power

This 5-point, patient-specific scale measures the likelihood that the patient's statement will generate interventions by the analyst that clarify how safe the goals of the patient's unconscious plan are. Two judges evaluated test power, using *only* the patient's preintervention speech (patient context segment) from the 81 excerpts. The judges were blind to the target intervention and the patient effect segment. They were told: "In this material which just precedes the analyst's intervention, is there evidence that the patient is testing the analyst, and if so, how powerful is the test?" They were given a copy of Mrs. C's plan formulation and the *Manual on How to Diagnose the Plan* (Caston, 1980), which describes this concept.

Rating Immediate Effects

Two groups of judges were used; one group of three judges evaluated boldness, and one group of four assessed insight. We determined boldness and insight effect measures in two main ways. First, ratings of effect segments for either boldness or insight would be statistically adjusted (*residualized* by a multiple regression technique) based on the ratings of their respective preintervention context segments. Unadjusted ratings would come from the 162 randomized pre- and postintervention segments rated blindly as to order or association. Second, a *clinical* judgment of the shift from the pre- to postintervention state would be rated separately on matched (before-and-after) pairs following the first rating procedure; this latter method was conceptually close to that of the pilot study.

THE BOLDNESS SCALE

The scale used in the pilot was now expanded to 9 points. Judges rated 162 randomly distributed patient speech segments, half consisting of speech prior to the target intervention and half of speech after it. Judges were unaware of the ordinal placement of the segments and were blind to the interventions.

THE BOLDNESS SHIFT SCALE

The judges rating boldness made a further clinical assessment after completing the rating of the 162 items: They now compared the patient segment immediately preceding the intervention with that following, and rated the degree of positive or negative shift in the patient's boldness, using 81 matched pairs of the before-and-after patient speeches without the intervention. The pairs were presented in randomized order. The scale used $+/-$ 3-point ratings with a middle no-change category (effectively 7 points). (See Appendix 20.)

THE INSIGHT SCALE

The scale used in the pilot was now expanded to 9 points. A different set of judges was used than for boldness; other than applying the insight scale, the procedure parallels that for rating boldness.

THE INSIGHT SHIFT SCALE

The judges rating insight made a further clinical assessment after completing the rating of the 162 items. Except for the content, the scale structure and method of administration is like that of boldness shift (see Appendix 20).

RESULTS OF THE REPLICATION STUDY

Results of the pilot study were partially confirmed by those of the replication study: In brief, the findings supported the psychoanalytic interpretiveness hypothesis and did not support the plan compatibility hypothesis.[2]

The reliability of the ratings made for each of the scales in this study was calculated using intraclass correlations. The reliability correlations, shown in Table 19-2, were lower than those found in the pilot study; they are nonetheless satisfactory. In the pilot, reliability coefficients were .72–.90; the comparable reliability coefficients in this study are in the .60–.66 range.

As in the pilot study, we found that the patient's levels of boldness and insight preceding the analyst's intervention correlated significantly with boldness and insight following the analyst's intervention. On the

Table 19-2. Replication Study Scale Reliabilities ($N = 81$)

Variable	Number of judges	Cronbach's α
Plan compatibility	4	.64
Psychoanalytic interpretiveness	2	.69
Test power	3	.60
Boldness (context)	3	.70
Insight (context)	4	.67
Boldness (effect)	3	.66
Insight (effect)	4	.64
Boldness shift	3	.65
Insight shift	4	.66

2. Further studies of the hypothesis that pro-plan interventions produce immediate patient progress have supported this hypothesis (see Chapters 20 and 22).

Table 19-3. Replication Study Intercorrelations among Nonresidualized Dependent Measures ($N = 81$)

	Insight (context)	Boldness (effect)	Insight (effect)	Boldness shift	Insight shift
Boldness (context)	.53**	.48**	.33*	−.20	−.05
Insight (context)		.35**	.31*	−.07	−.08
Boldness (effect)			.49**	.31*	.33*
Insight (effect)				.17	.60**
Boldness shift					.40**

*$p < .005$.
**$p < .001$.

Insight Scale this correlation was .31 ($p < .005$); on the Boldness Scale, the correlation was .48 ($p < .001$). Table 19-3 shows the correlations between the patient context and effect segments.

In calculating the correlations between the independent variables and postintervention effects, we statistically removed that portion of the variance from postintervention boldness and insight scores that is attributable to the preintervention levels of boldness and insight (see Table 19-4). This is comparable to adjusting the postintervention effect levels to what they would have been, by prediction, if the baseline levels of boldness and insight had been constant.

We employed a stepwise multiple regression procedure to determine both the partial and combined effects of the independent variables

Table 19-4. Pearson Product–Moment Correlations between Major Variables and Residualized Postintervention Measures of Boldness and Insight in the Replication Study

	Psychoanalytic interpretiveness	Test power	Boldness (residualized)	Insight (residualized)
Plan compatibility	.08	.03	−.04	−.01
Psychoanalytic interpretiveness		.28*	.19	.30**
Test power			.05	.10
Boldness (residualized)				.39**

*$p < .01$.
**$p < .001$.

(Table 19-5). By this means, we were also able to determine whether there were any interactions among the independent variables themselves.

The major finding of the pilot study—that the plan compatibility of the target intervention correlated significantly with the measure of boldness/insight—was not upheld by the present findings. Also, when the effect of psychoanalytic interpretiveness was statistically removed from plan compatibility, significant correlations of plan compatibility with the effect variables still did not emerge. Further investigations beyond this replication, involving *post hoc* statistical analyses, demonstrated significant effects associated with plan compatibility; these analyses, and those that evaluate the role of test power, are taken up in the Discussion.

The correlation of psychoanalytic interpretiveness with the insight effect was .31 ($p < .01$), and with insight shift .28 ($p < .05$). When plan compatibility effects were removed from psychoanalytic interpretiveness, these last two correlations remain significant.

The statistical interaction (area of overlap only) between the two independent variables—plan compatibility and psychoanalytic interpretiveness—correlates significantly with boldness (.22, $p < .04$). In this instance, plan compatibility, which did not show an independent correlation, does contribute to the effect when conjoined with psychoanalytic interpretiveness.

Table 19-5. Replication Study Comparison between Residualized and Nonresidualized Plan Compatibility and Psychoanalytic Interpretiveness[a]

Independent variables	Dependent variables			
	Boldness (residualized)	Insight (residualized)	Boldness shift	Insight shift
Plan compatibility	−.04	−.01	.03	.06
Plan compatibility (residualized)	−.04	.04	.10	.13
Psychoanalytic interpretiveness	.19	.31**	.18	.28*
Psychoanalytic interpretiveness (residualized)	.19	.28*	.13	.24*

[a]Plan compatibility residualized to remove effect of psychoanalytic interpretiveness; psychoanalytic interpretiveness residualized to remove effect of plan compatibility.

*$p < .05$.

**$p < .01$.

Other statistical analyses were undertaken to determine whether any unpredicted relationships occurred between the independent variables and preintervention patient context measures. No significant findings emerged.

DISCUSSION AND FURTHER DATA ANALYSIS

THE PLAN COMPATIBILITY HYPOTHESIS

Only the pilot study revealed the predicted correlation between plan compatibility and immediate effects. We were not able to replicate this finding using verbatim transcripts in the second study. To attempt to understand this discrepancy, we considered several factors and carried out additional data analyses.

Did differences in method between the pilot and the replication account for the failure of this hypothesis? In fact, the two studies did differ in several aspects. In the pilot each segment of patient speech preceding the target intervention was preceded by an unrated intervention. The resulting form was a few minutes of patient speech sandwiched between two analyst's interventions and followed by another patient speech. These excerpts therefore represent a dense period of analyst–patient interaction, and clinical reexamination shows that most were marked by transference or testing of the analyst—a characteristic we had not sought. In the filtering effect of writing process notes, the treating/recording analyst may have unwittingly retained details of such active episodes over others.

Our retrospective opinion is that the pilot study likely confirms the plan compatibility hypothesis, not for the general case but for a narrower sector of events, close to that of Silberschatz's study on the verbatim transcripts: those in which the patient is in a transference mode and is powerfully testing the safety of what is as yet unmastered (cf. Footnote 2).

Further investigation supports these ideas. Using test power ratings of the preintervention segments, we narrowed the random sample of verbatim items to those containing the *highest third* of test power ratings, then narrowed the latter group further by limiting it to items that were also *transference-referent*. As shown in Table 19-6, the correlations of plan compatibility with effect scores rises into a range (.33) comparable to other findings in the study, although the shrunken N does not yield significance.

Table 19-6. Replication Study Correlations of Plan Compatibility with Insight Effect

Sector of items	N	r
Entire sample	81	.06
Sector of sample with highest test power ratings of patient preintervention speech	27	.15
Sector of sample with highest test power ratings and overt transference focus	16	.33

We would conclude, thus far, that while these findings do not confirm the plan compatibility hypothesis for the full spectrum, support pertinent to narrower sectors of events was obtained in our pilot study, in Silberschatz's work, and in Bush and Gassner's recent work on termination.

Did the scale for plan compatibility contain a flaw? Our conceptualization and instructions for evaluating plan compatibility may have been more adequate in its upper ranges than in its lowest. One clue came from Thomas Kelly's (personal communication) independent work on Silberschatz's data; correlations between the "passing-the-key-test" variable and immediate effects increased in magnitude (.4 to .7) when items rated lowest for the former were deleted. It was as if the patient reacted predictably to passed tests, and unpredictably to failed tests.

Following Kelly's lead, we looked for whether such a pattern was operative in our data. The basic correlations of the replication study were repeated, but with the sample altered by excluding the third of items rated lowest for plan compatibility ($N = 54$); items now fell within rating points 4–8 of the original 9-point spectrum (mildly anti-plan to highly pro-plan). Results are reported in Table 19-7.

These post hoc *results were strikingly in line with the original predictions: Statistically significant, positive correlations were obtained between plan compatibility and three of four immediate effect variables.* In addition, correlations remained significant when plan compatibility scores were adjusted to exclude overlapping effects of the psychoanalytic interpretiveness variable. Review of the test power data showed that there was not a preponderance of powerful preintervention tests by the patient on the analyst in this narrowed sample; therefore heightened testing was not a likely explanation for these new findings.

These results cannot yet claim lawfulness for plan compatibility over the general spectrum of interventions. According to these results the patient appears to have differentiated between pro-plan and mildly anti-plan interventions. Several explanations may be considered: (1) a complex and peculiar rather than simple relationship holds for the ego's appraisal of anti-plan interventions in general; (2) there was an idiosyncratic relation in this area for this patient; or (3) our instructions to judges were in error in this range.

Clinical reexamination revealed that for *mispredicting* items rated low for plan compatibility, the analyst appeared neither to follow the patient's immediate *conscious* focus nor some aspect of her unconscious, plan-related goals as inferred. We originally instructed judges to lower ratings whenever the analyst appeared to be "pushing for" his own focus versus the patient's own, reasoning that a patient who needed to master oppositionalness would perceive his action to mean that the analyst would not be tolerant of it.

This supposition was clearly wrong. The patient appeared to have merely regarded such interventions as investigative or supportive of the general therapeutic enterprise. In order to retrospectively realign this set of behaviors with the plan compatibility hypothesis, one would have to say that this patient perceived such "off-track" investigations by the analyst to be in her own behalf.

The analyst's so-called off-track investigations might yield immediate benefits based on another principle, however, one which holds that

Table 19-7. Correlations of Items Scored for Upper Two-Thirds of Plan Compatibility (PC) Scale: PC × Dependent Variables $(N = 54)^a$

Variable	Plan compatibility (psychoanalytic interpretiveness retained)	Plan compatibility (psychoanalytic interpretiveness removed)
Boldness (residualized)	.24*	.14
Boldness (effect)	.11	.04
Boldness shift	.37***	.34**
Insight (residualized)	.40***	.32**
Insight (effect)	.30**	.22*
Insight shift	.47***	.39***

[a]One-tailed test of probability.

*$p < .05$.

**$p < .01$.

***$p < .005$.

the analyst's tacks relate to his recognition of a specific unconscious relationship in the material, and that these interventions are helpful *because* they focus on, are preparatory to, or are interpretive of a conflict-related defense *other* than that specified in the diagnosis of the unconscious plan. Accordingly, this would require that a hypothesis other than that of plan compatibility is *also* operative.

THE PSYCHOANALYTIC INTERPRETIVENESS HYPOTHESIS

The replication study on the verbatim transcripts confirms the hypothesis that immediate positive effects depend on the psychoanalytic interpretiveness of the analyst's interventions over the *general* spectrum of interventions. This relationship appears to be independent of plan compatibility, based on the statistical adjustment of psychoanalytic interpretiveness scores to exclude the overlapping effects of the plan compatibility variable. *It would therefore appear that both of these variables can operate independently of each other, and both contribute to immediate positive effects in the patient's productions.*

Although plan compatibility has been minutely characterized, the nature of psychoanalytic interpretiveness has been barely laid out. Validation of this measure in our study included correlations with scales for depth of interpretation and complexity of psychoanalytic explanation (Speisman, 1959; Harway, Dittimar, Raush, Bordin, & Ringler, 1955; Garduk & Haggard, 1972), and significant correlation with ratings by "uninstructed" (blind to our scale) clinicians who were guided only by psychoanalytic conventions of interpretive technique. The average rating on the Psychoanalytic Interpretiveness Scale given to interventions that uninstructed clinicians agreed *are* interpretations was 3.7 on a 6-point scale (see Footnote 1). This is a simple level of interpretation but more than a mere echo of the patient, and more effective, according to our findings. The studies in the literature also show greater effectiveness for moderate levels of depth of complexity of interpretations.

Psychoanalytic interpretiveness is not limited to a single genre, as with plan compatibility, but originates from a diverse body of possible ideas or patterns outside awareness for which evidence obtains. What is interpreted may be variously organized (e.g., resistance-centered, transference-centered, reconstruction-centered).

It is doubtful that the mere *degree* of interpretiveness in itself could be beneficial. Clinical experience bears out that irrelevant, prematurely deep, or bizarre interpretations are generally ineffective. In order to make sense of this variable, one would have to assume that the treating analyst carefully undertook to make evidence-based inferences close to the patient's material. Perusal of the transcripts of the first 100 hours shows that Mrs. C's analyst listened carefully and was not premature; his interventions did not tend to be overly complex, long, or widely sweeping.

What does psychoanalytic interpretiveness represent when it has been statistically adjusted to remove the overlapping influence of plan compatibility? The rubric originally encompassed an unrestricted range of possible topics, *some* of which related to the plan (as when the analyst commented on conflicts involving guilt, stubbornness, and omnipotence). With the effects of plan compatibility removed from the psychoanalytic interpretiveness ratings, it is as if the focus of planfulness had been kept *constant* for all the interventions. The adjusted measure of interpretiveness then represents the variation of interpretiveness over the *remainder* of subject matters of conflict—especially those *not* relevant to the plan.

Fenichel has elaborated: "The motive for a pathogenic defense is . . . an estimate of the danger of an aroused instinct," which remains exempt from correction until interpreted and worked through (1941, pp. 16–18). But the myriad expressions and defensive alterations of the instincts signified for both Freud and Fenichel a broad band of warded-off processes.

Present findings regarding the effectiveness of psychoanalytic interpretiveness support a *broad span of multiple unconscious dangers* in the neurotic patient, each of which requires mastery; following Hartmann (1958), these are likely ordered as a hierarchy of priorities. If it is the case that the subject matter of the patient's unconscious plan represents the highest priority for mastery and therefore for interpretation, our findings indicate that there are nonetheless other priorities to address.

TEST POWER AND SALIENCY IN THE THERAPEUTIC PROCESS

We have reported a trend in which positive effects tend to increase following plan-compatible interventions when the patient is in a transference and/or testing mode. To this finding we add another, more striking one: Whereas the original correlations of psychoanalytic interpretiveness and insight are of a .3 magnitude, when the sample is narrowed to include only items for which the preintervention patient context segments are rated highest in terms of test power ($N = 27$), the new correlation jumps to .54 ($p < .05$). It appears that if the patient is in a mode of intense testing, the predictive relation between the independent variables and immediate effects increases. It is interesting that this effect is observed even though psychoanalytic interpretiveness is a general measure and test power is meant to be plan-relevant. Thus, the presence of a testing mode in the patient may add *saliency* to that juncture, and the patient may more clearly discern the implications of the analyst's intervention. Is it the case that, although the ego is probably "always" appraising danger and safety, it is more highly attuned when the patient can be observed to be testing?

CONCLUDING COMMENT

Findings so far indicate that plan compatibility is predictive of immediate positive effects, not across all interventions, but at least for those that take place during heightened analyst–patient interactions, particularly when the patient tests issues relevant to his unconscious plan and/or is in a transference mode. Our inability to confirm the prediction for plan compatibility across a general sampling of interventions may relate to a deficiency in our ability to correctly identify interventions that are very "anti-plan."

Psychoanalytic interpretiveness, on the other hand, is significantly predictive of positive immediate effects in the patient's productions, confirming the findings of previous experimental investigators. Moreover, it does so independently of the planfulness dimension. We understand this to mean that the psychoanalytic interpretiveness of that which is warded-off *beyond* what is plan-relevant demonstrates its own positive effects. If we consider this finding in terms of the theory of higher mental functioning, we would have to consider that there are other priorities for mastery beyond that diagnosed as the "unconscious plan" of the patient. If we consider this finding in terms of classical psychoanalytic theory, we would say that our finding is consistent with the proposition that the interpretable domain of the derivatives of unconscious conflicts is wider than—and encompasses—the domain of derivatives that pertain to the unconscious plan.

We raise this issue based on our study of verbatim transcripts; these findings account for a modest portion, at best, of the variance in these correlations, as do most findings in this genre of research. We adduce that *multiple* factors contribute to the immediate effects of psychoanalytic interventions. Fully exploring these factors is a matter for future explication and research.

20

THE IMMEDIATE EFFECT OF THE ANALYST'S TERMINATION INTERVENTIONS ON THE PATIENT'S RESISTANCE TO TERMINATION

MARSHALL BUSH
SUZANNE GASSNER

BROAD OBJECTIVES

This study had two broad objectives: (1) to demonstrate the power of the plan concept for predicting the immediate effect of analytic interpretations, and (2) to apply the higher mental functioning hypothesis developed in the first part of this book to an understanding of Mrs. C's resistance to termination[1] and the manner in which it was resolved.

METHODOLOGICAL CONSIDERATIONS

The design of this study was guided by several methodological considerations that we believe to be important in successfully carrying out this type of clinical research.

Particular care was taken to ensure that the interventions we studied were highly relevant to the patient's plan and spanned a wide range of

---

1. From the perspective of the higher mental functioning hypothesis, these resistances were manifestations of the ego's unconscious defensive activities within the therapeutic setting. The ego's defensive operations are regulated by considerations of safety and danger as defined by the individual's unconscious pathogenic beliefs. Resistances function to protect the individual from unconsciously feared dangers that may arise in relation to the therapist. Complex behavior patterns, such as the constellation of behaviors usually encompassed by the rubric "resistance to termination," may serve both defensive and testing functions, or may contain elements of defense and elements of testing.

This research was supported by a grant from the Chapman Research Fund.

examples on the dimensions of interpretiveness and plan compatibility. Lack of plan relevance or a restriction in range on the dimensions of interpretiveness or plan compatibility in a set of interventions can make it difficult if not impossible to test hypotheses about the immediate effect of analytic interventions on patient behavior meaningfully.

A special effort was made to give our judges a high degree of clinical orientation by providing them with (1) an extensive amount of clinical context for the purpose of making plan compatibility ratings and (2) a plan formulation that was expressly tailored to their specific rating task. In our earlier research judges were given only a global plan formulation, which they had to adapt to the portion of the analysis being studied and to the rating tasks they were asked to perform. In this study judges were given a plan formulation that specifically focused on the patient's goals for the phase of the analysis being studied and on the particular pathogenic beliefs that the patient was actively working to disconfirm.

This study used a different type of outcome measure than was used in previous research. Previous studies assessed the patient's immediate reaction to analyst interventions or to passed and failed tests through the use of general measures of patient functioning, such as changes in insightfulness, boldness, and anxiety. In this study the outcome measure used to assess the immediate effect of analyst interventions was derived from and was highly specific to the patient's immediate therapeutic objectives.

REASONS FOR STUDYING MRS. C'S RESISTANCE TO TERMINATION

We had several reasons for deciding to study Mrs. C's resistance to termination from the perspective of the higher mental functioning hypothesis presented in the first part of this book. First, we wanted to see whether the general plan formulation derived from the first 10 hours of Mrs. C's analysis would still apply during the termination phase. Second, we wanted to find an important therapeutic phenomenon that would be explained in strikingly different ways by the higher mental functioning hypothesis and by the automatic functioning hypothesis contained in classical psychoanalytic theory. Lastly, we wanted the higher mental functioning explanation of that phenomenon to lead to testable predictions as to how the patient should respond to the analyst's interventions.

The resistance to termination was well suited to meet these aims for a variety of reasons: (1) It occupies a position of strategic importance in the psychoanalytic theory of therapy. (2) The way it seemingly arose and was overcome in the case of Mrs. C corresponded perfectly to the automatic functioning explanation of that resistance. (3) The treating analyst understood and analyzed Mrs. C's resistance to termination in the manner prescribed by the automatic functioning hypothesis. (4) The patient's gradual resolution of her resistance to termination, and the confirmatory associations she produced in response to the analyst's termination interventions, appeared to validate the analyst's interpretations. (5) The higher mental functioning hypothesis provided a markedly different explanation of the development and resolution of Mrs. C's resistance to termination. (6) The explanation provided by the higher mental functioning hypothesis led to predictions that could be tested by a rigorous research methodology and that would not ordinarily be made on the basis of the automatic functioning hypothesis.

RESISTANCE TO TERMINATION ACCORDING TO THE AUTOMATIC FUNCTIONING HYPOTHESIS

The concept of resistance has a position of pivotal importance in the psychoanalytic theory of therapy. There is no doubt that Freud (1904, 1913, 1914, 1917) considered the overcoming of resistances to be the essential purpose of and curative factor in analytic therapy. Contemporary analytic theorists (e.g., Weinshel, 1983) continue to define the psychoanalytic process in terms of the interpretation of resistances and the patient's subsequent reaction to such interpretations.

According to the automatic functioning hypothesis, resistances are automatically regulated by the pleasure principle, and the overcoming of a resistance is inherently associated with some reexperiencing of the anxiety (or other painful affect) which formed the motive for the resistance (Freud, 1920; Nunberg, 1937; Fenichel, 1941; Dewald, 1971). It is for this reason that patients resist the analysis of their resistances.

The resistance to termination holds a position of special importance in the psychoanalytic theory of therapy because it is an impediment to the resolution of the transference neurosis. A successful and enduring analytic cure can only be achieved if the transference neurosis is satisfactorily analyzed and resolved. Overcoming the resistance to termination is a final and a crucial step in resolving the transference neurosis (Glover, 1955; Calef, 1968; Dewald, 1971).

The psychoanalytic theory of therapy contains a prototypic explanation of the resistance to termination based on Freud's early assumptions about the etiology of neurosis, the structure of the mind, the patient's unconscious motives and activity in psychoanalysis, and the biphasic nature of analytic treatment. The resistance to termination is primarily considered to be an id resistance in that it is rooted in the patient's instinctual fixations, in his unconscious wish to have his childhood instinctual impulses gratified in the transference, and in his desire to avoid the pain involved in (1) mourning the loss of the analyst as a love object, (2) accepting the ultimate frustration of one's most cherished infantile wishes, and (3) renouncing the use of gratification through fantasy as a means of preserving those wishes (Ferenczi, 1927; Reich, 1950). It is because the termination process in a successful analysis involves painful experiences of anxiety, frustration, renunciation, separation, loss, and mourning that it evokes such powerful resistances to a final ending of the treatment and a complete resolution of the neurosis.

One commonly noted specific resistance to termination is a resurgence of symptoms, which serves the purpose of trying to convince the analyst that one is not yet ready to terminate (Reich, 1950; Glover, 1955; Dewald, 1971). Many other manifestations of resistance to termination have also been noted. "The patient's reactions to the looming up of ultimate frustration of transference wishes may include, in addition to symptomatic exacerbations, all manner of cynical comments about proffered interpretations, depreciation of the analyst, skepticism about the worth of the analytic work, wishes to terminate immediately, seeking of substitute objects, explosions of rage, anxiety, and mournful sadness" (Firestein, 1978, p. 245).

The final outcome of the therapy is considered to hinge upon the degree to which a patient experiences and completes the difficult tasks of renunciation and mourning.

The patient in the termination phase of psychotherapy who is experiencing sadness or grief over the loss of the therapist must similarly go through the process of mourning and grief-work to resolve this loss. The more that the patient consciously experiences and elaborates the sadness, depression, anger and helplessness at the loss, the greater is the possibility of his working through to a resolution of his transference relationship. The more that the patient avoids the experience of grief, the greater is the potentiality for an unresolved and persistent transference relationship, and thus a failure to achieve the full benefit of insight-directed therapy as well as the possibility of subsequent neurotic disturbance in the future. (Dewald, 1971, p. 281)

Dewald (1972) suggested that during termination the degree of structural change that has occurred may be assessed in the following way:

During the termination phase, assessment of structural change involves evaluating the extent to which there is a resolution of the transference neurosis through a voluntary renunciation of the infantile drives and objects, with accompanying grief and mourning, and without cathecting substitute infantile objects. The emphasis is on the degree to which the patient himself accepts the inevitability of the frustration of his infantile drives and recognizes the benefits of the reality-principle and the needs for such renunciation. The more that such renunciation and awareness must be actively stimulated or fostered by the analyst, the less extensive has been the degree of structural change. (p. 322)

MRS. C'S RESISTANCE TO TERMINATION

Mrs. C's behavior closely conformed to the automatic functioning explanation of the termination process. After nearly 5 years of analysis, she began to tentatively express thoughts about ending her treatment. (The actual termination took place more than a year later, after another few hundred hours of analysis.) The patient first introduced the notion of termination at a very appropriate point in her analysis. She had overcome her presenting symptoms, she was able to function much more independently and assertively in her dealings with other people, a strong transference neurosis had developed and was extensively analyzed, her infantile neurosis had been reconstructed in detail, and the patient was able to relate to her husband in a more mature and sexually satisfying way.

Shortly after the analyst showed his concurrence with Mrs. C's desire to terminate, by suggesting that they discuss a specific date for ending, she began to display a very strong resistance to the idea of termination. She became very anxious and depressed, and experienced a resurgence of symptoms. Her conscious attitude toward the idea of termination turned extremely negative. She complained that she was no better off than when she started. She angrily accused the analyst of turning away from her, pushing her out, and cruelly abandoning her to a life of despair. She had thoughts about killing him and made vague references to feeling suicidal. She expressed great worry and pessimism about her future. She felt empty, unprotected, and unfulfilled. She insisted that she was not cured and could not function on her own. Her life would be meaningless without the analyst and no one could ever replace him.

She stated her refusal to give up her wish to acquire a penis and to win the analyst's love. She expressed a strong desire to become pregnant. She wanted to avoid thinking about a final ending and instead proposed that she continue to see the analyst once a week after the termination of her analysis. For several months Mrs. C avoided setting a specific termination date even though the analyst had invited her to do so.

Several examples of how Mrs. C expressed her resistance to termination are presented in Appendix 23. They illustrate how well her expressions of resistance support the automatic functioning explanation of the prototypical resistance to termination.

Over the course of the last 114 hours, Mrs. C gradually became less resistant to the idea of termination, more confident of her ability to solve problems on her own, and less fearful of the future. By the end of the analysis she consciously felt sad about leaving the analyst but also felt ready to terminate. The ending of her analysis closely conformed to Ferenczi's (1927) description of an analytic cure:

One might say that the patient finally becomes convinced that he is continuing analysis only because he is treating it as a new but still a fantasy source of gratification, which in terms of reality yields him nothing. When he has slowly overcome his mourning over this discovery he inevitably looks round for other, more real sources of gratification. . . . The renunciation of analysis is thus the final winding-up of the infantile situation of frustration which lay at the basis of the symptom-formation. (p. 214)

THE ANALYST'S RESPONSE TO MRS. C'S RESISTANCE TO TERMINATION

The analyst was very active in interpreting Mrs. C's resistance to termination. It was clear from his interpretations that he believed those resistances were primarily stemming from her anger, anxiety, and despair over having to accept the ultimate frustration of her most important infantile Oedipal wishes, having to renounce the fantasy gratification of those wishes, and having to separate from the analyst and to mourn the loss of the transference relationship, with its attendant gratifications.

The analyst attempted to bring about the fullest possible acknowledgment by Mrs. C of her deepest infantile transference wishes so that she could renounce and mourn them in the most definitive way. Similarly, he tried to get her to face the full magnitude of her grief and anxiety over separating from him so that she could fully mourn the loss and achieve a final resolution of the transference relationship and the transference neurosis. He repeatedly interpreted her attempts to manipulate him into postponing her termination date, and he held firm to the date she had initially set. He also interpreted Mrs. C's desire to ward off the work of mourning by becoming pregnant.

We inferred from the analyst's interventions that he held the following views about Mrs. C's neurosis and the termination process of her analysis:

1. He believed that the patient's neurosis stemmed primarily from the frustration of her Oedipal strivings to win her father's love, to be his favorite, to have his baby. He believed that Mrs. C developed intense penis envy and a strong castration complex after she suffered a traumatic loss of her father's love at age 6. At that time her mother became pregnant and gave birth to her younger brother.
2. He believed that the patient unconsciously wanted him to oppose the idea of her terminating as a way of demonstrating she was his favorite and that he could not bear to lose her.
3. He believed that he was frustrating her Oedipal transference wishes and thereby eliciting her resistances to termination when he concurred with her expressed desire to terminate, when he prompted her to set a specific termination date, when he refused to change that date, and when he showed confidence in the patient's readiness to terminate and ability to function on her own.

The analyst's views were highly consistent with the automatic functioning theory of neurosis and therapy.

Some typical examples of how the analyst understood and interpreted Mrs. C's resistance to termination are presented in Appendix 24. These interventions, which were excerpted from the analyst's process notes of the last 114 hours, illustrate how closely his understanding of Mrs. C's termination dynamics follows the traditional theory explanation of the termination process.

HOW MRS. C'S RESISTANCE TO TERMINATION WAS CONCEPTUALIZED FROM THE HIGHER MENTAL FUNCTIONING HYPOTHESIS

Our plan formulation for the termination phase of Mrs. C's analysis was derived from a detailed study of the analyst's process notes from the first 10 hours (hours 1015 through 1024) of the last 100 hours (hours 1015 through 1114). Our formulation is presented in Appendix 25. It is highly consistent with the plan formulation derived from a clinical assessment of the first 10 hours of the analysis, and it demonstrates the continuity of the patient's own work and therapeutic goals across the entire analysis.

Our formulation took for granted the appropriateness of both the patient's initial desire to consider termination and the analyst's decision to support that wish by suggesting they consider a specific date. However, our view of Mrs. C's termination phase differs markedly from the analyst's in terms of how we conceptualized the origin and function of the powerful resistances to termination which subsequently arose.

In contrast to the automatic functioning explanation of the termination process, which assumes that the patient in a successful analysis will be primarily struggling with very painful conflicts around loss and renunciation, our view was that Mrs. C was primarily struggling with very intense unconscious guilt, of the kind described by Modell (1965) and Loewald (1979), about wanting to establish her independence from the analyst. It should be noted that we do not assume that every patient will have the same termination dynamics as Mrs. C, although her case is not atypical.

We did not believe, as did the treating analyst, that Mrs. C unconsciously wanted to preserve or to gratify her infantile wishes to win the analyst's love, to have his baby, to acquire a penis, or to remain forever in analysis. We believed instead that Mrs. C was retaining her infantile transference wishes and attachments out of unconscious loyalty and guilt, and that she unconsciously wanted to be able to renounce them, rather than to gratify them, so that she could be free to fully invest herself in an intimate love relationship with her husband and to pursue other important life goals. Consequently, we did not view Mrs. C's resistance to termination as a defense against experiencing the loss and the frustration involved in not having her infantile transference wishes fulfilled, in having to renounce those wishes, and in having to give up the analyst as a transference love object.

Our understanding of Mrs. C's resistance to termination was that it primarily stemmed from her unconscious pathogenic beliefs about her power to devastate the analyst by making him feel unimportant, excluded, rejected, and jealous. Mrs. C was reluctant to terminate because of her fear of hurting the analyst. Her thoughts about his dying and her killing him were not expressions of her anger over feeling rejected by the analyst. They were expressions of her worry that the analyst might die if she no longer needed him and if she ended their relationship. Her resistances to termination were primarily motivated by unconscious guilt, which stemmed from her belief that she was abandoning a weak and needy father figure.

We did not think that Mrs. C's pathogenic beliefs in her power to hurt the analyst were serving either a significant defensive or gratification function. We saw them as having been directly engendered by traumatic childhood experiences in which her father had seemed extremely possessive, jealous, pathetic, insecure, violently out of control, and narcissistically needy and fragile. Her father's narcissistic vulnerability was manifested in such behaviors as asking the children for constant reassurance that all of his actions and ideas were right; wanting his family to share all of his preferences, even for the same flavor of ice cream; needing to viciously demean anyone who was not like him; and being moved to tears when he recounted, as he frequently did, a notable expression of approval and loyalty from one of his children. Mrs. C believed that her father desperately needed to feel admired and envied by others, and to have his children demonstrate their loyalty by deferring to his authority, by modelling themselves after him, and by having him be the central and most important figure in their lives.

We assumed that Mrs. C would work to overcome her resistance to termination by repeatedly testing the analyst in order to disconfirm her pathogenic beliefs in her power to hurt him (1) by no longer wanting his love or needing his help; (2) by having confidence in her own insights and judgment; (3) by functioning well independently of him; (4) by not being preoccupied with his approval and opinions; (5) by taking pride in her femininity and not wanting to be a man—like the analyst; (6) by not preferring the analyst to her husband as a love object; and (7) by enjoying being sexual and emotionally intimate—things her father did not approve of and could not tolerate in himself and others. A clinical illustration of how Mrs. C tested the analyst during the 10 sessions (hours 1015 through 1024) from which we derived our plan formulation is presented in Appendix 26. Other clinical examples of how patients may test the analyst during termination are described by Buxbaum (1950).

Put in slightly different terms, we thought that Mrs. C's primary therapeutic goal during the termination period of her analysis was to overcome the unresolved aspects of her transference neurosis, and especially of the father transference. She unconsciously feared that the analyst was like her father in terms of being narcissistically needy and vulnerable to being hurt by her. She had taken his penis envy interpretations to mean that he needed her to admire him, to feel inferior to him, and to want to be just like him. She had similarly taken his interpretations about how desperately she wanted her father's love—and now wanted his love—as an indication that he needed to feel irreplaceable. She feared that the analyst wanted her to feel helpless, empty, unprotected, and bereft at the thought of termination, and that her termination was actually going to be a very painful loss for him.

According to our view, the anguish and despair Mrs. C expressed about termination unconsciously served four basic functions: (1) It served as a self-punishment that relieved her guilt about wanting to terminate. (2) It represented an attempt to protect the analyst's narcissism by reassuring him of his importance to her. (3) It served an important testing function in that it was intended to elicit further information about how much the analyst needed to feel that he was irreplaceable. (4) It served an important defensive function in that it allowed Mrs. C to feel like she was being victimized by the analyst instead of victimizing him.

THE HYPOTHESIS WE TESTED ABOUT HOW MRS. C OVERCAME HER RESISTANCE TO TERMINATION

The basis hypothesis we tested was that Mrs. C's progress in overcoming her resistance to termination would be directly affected in either a positive or negative way depending on whether the analyst's interventions supported or opposed the patient's unconscious plan for mastery during the termination period. We predicted that plan-compatible interpretations would lead to an immediate decrease in her resistance to termination, while plan-incompatible interpretations would have the opposite effect. Plan-compatible interventions would be ones that tended to disconfirm the patient's pathogenic beliefs about the analyst's vulnerability and her power to hurt him. Plan-incompatible interventions would be ones that lent credence to the patient's pathogenic beliefs.

We assumed that Mrs. C would actively work throughout the termination phase of her analysis to overcome the pathogenic beliefs responsible for her resistance to termination so that she could terminate in a relaxed, confident, and optimistic manner. We expected her to feel relieved and reassured, and therefore to exhibit increased feelings of readiness for termination, following interpretations that suggested to her that the analyst supported the idea of her terminating and was able to let her go. Examples of such interventions would be ones that questioned the patient's claims of unpreparedness for termination or that pointed out her overvaluation of the analyst's real power and importance in her life. Conversely, we expected her to feel more guilty and worried, and therefore to express more resistance to the idea of termination, following interventions that suggested to her that the analyst was possessive and needed her to make the termination process into a painful ordeal of mourning and renunciation in order for him to feel assured of his importance. Examples of such interventions would be ones that emphasized the analyst's preeminence in her emotional life, her wishes to win the analyst's love and to have his child, and her desire to have the analyst demonstrate his favoritism toward her by opposing or postponing her termination.

Since the analyst was working within a theoretical frame of reference different from our own, we expected him to inadvertently make a variety of plan-compatible and plan-incompatible interpretations. We also assumed, from the fact that Mrs. C gradually did overcome her resistance to termination, that his interpretations would become increasingly more pro-plan over time.

Although our theory about Mrs. C's termination dynamics and the automatic functioning theory of the termination process provide competing explanations of the resistance to termination in this particular case, our study was designed to test only the predictions made by the higher mental functioning hypothesis. It is, however, worth noting that there is at least one point where the two theories do predict different outcomes. We predicted that interventions which implied the analyst's support for the idea of termination and his lack of possessiveness would be unconsciously reassuring to Mrs. C and would lead to an immediate decrease in her resistance to termination. The automatic functioning hypothesis predicts that such interventions should frustrate the patient's unconscious transference wishes, increase her sense of loss and rejection, and lead to an intensification of her resistance to termination.

METHOD

OVERVIEW OF METHOD

The purpose of this study was to test the hypothesis that the analyst's termination interventions would have an immediate and predictable effect on the patient's resistance to termination, according to whether they supported or opposed the patient's own unconscious plan for the termination phase of her analysis.

The design was similar to that used for the studies reported in the previous chapter. It involved two broad steps: (1) an independent evaluation of the analyst's termination interventions on the dimension of plan compatibility; and (2) an independent assessment of the patient's attitude towards termination preceding and following the analyst's interventions, to see how that attitude was affected by each intervention.

THE DATA

Portion of the Analysis Studied

This study was originally intended to encompass the last 100 hours of Mrs. C's analysis, which is why the plan formulation was based on a clinical assessment of the first 10 of the last 100 hours. We subsequently discovered that the analyst made a number of termination interventions in the preceding 14 sessions (hours 1001 to 1014), so those hours were also included in the study. Hence, the interventions we used were drawn from the last 114 hours of Mrs. C's analysis.

Use of Process Notes

This study was carried out on process notes because verbatim transcripts were not available. We knew that the analyst was an extremely conscientious and reliable reporter. We also assumed that any inadvertent bias in his notes would tend to work against our predictions, since the analyst would organize the material in terms of his own theory.

The Selection of the Units of Study

We selected clinical segments for measuring Mrs. C's attitude toward termination in the following way. Two graduate students independently read through the process notes and identified and blocked out all references Mrs. C made to termination. If two or more references to termination occurred without an intervening interpretation, they were treated as a single unit. If only a single reference to termination occurred before or after an interpretation, then that reference alone made up the unit of study.

The same students also identified all analyst interventions that bore on termination or on a termination theme. All items identified by either student as being a reference to termination by the patient or the analyst were eligible for inclusion in this study.

We selected for study all interventions that were followed by one or more references to termination by the patient. There were 112 interventions that met this criterion. They will be referred to as the target interventions. In 93 instances those interventions were preceded as well as followed by some patient reference to termination. In other words, 83% of the target interventions were cued by some mention of termination by Mrs. C. This finding is consistent with our clinical observation that Mrs. C's expressions of resistance to termination, in addition to expressing a genuine resistance, were also partly serving a testing function, which was to solicit information about the effects of her impending termination on the analyst.

MEASURES

The Analyst Scale

A 7-point Plan Compatibility Scale was used to assess the target interventions in terms of the patient's unconscious plan for termination. The high end of the scale, a rating of +3, was defined as follows: "The therapist's intervention is *strongly and unambiguously supportive* of the patient's current efforts at mastery. *It is very pro-plan.*" The low end of the scale, a rating of −3, was defined in a parallel way: "The therapist's intervention *strongly and unambiguously opposes* the patient's current efforts at mastery. *It is very anti-plan.*" The analyst scale is presented in Appendix 21. The judges used the Plan Compatibility Scale in conjunction with the plan formulation presented in Appendix 25.

Two experienced therapists, who were knowledgeable about the higher mental functioning paradigm but unfamiliar with the specific hypothesis we were attempting to test, applied the Plan Compatibility Scale to the 112 target interventions. Their task was to assess how the patient would hear each intervention in light of the pathogenic beliefs she was trying to disconfirm. They were given as immediate context for making each rating all the material from the beginning of the session through the target intervention.

In an attempt to study the effect of providing a judge with *complete* context, that is, with all available clinical material, one judge was asked to continue reading the process notes for the remainder of the session *after* rating each target intervention. The other judge did not read past the target interventions.

Before making their final ratings, the judges participated in a training session in which they made practice ratings of termination interventions that could not be used in the actual study because they were not followed by any reference to termination on the patient's part. They found the plan formulation relatively easy to apply and showed good agreement in their practice ratings.

The reliability coefficient[2] for the mean of the two judges' plan

2. Reliability estimates are expressed in terms of intraclasss correlations (Ebel, 1951; Guilford, 1954) which use the residual mean square as the error term (i.e., mean differences in judges' ratings are not regarded as error). The figures reported are the estimated reliabilities for the mean of the judges' ratings.

compatibility ratings was .65. To our surprise the ratings made by the judge who did not read past the target interventions correlated more highly with our outcome measure (which is described in the following section) than did the ratings made by the judge who did. We attributed this difference to the fact that the judge who did not read past the target interventions had considerably more experience in applying the higher mental functioning hypothesis in his clinical work. We also inferred that having judges read just the clinical material from the beginning of the session up to the target intervention provided sufficient context for making valid and reliable ratings.

In order to increase the reliability of the mean plan compatibility ratings we added two more judges to the study. They were given the same training procedure the first two judges received, and they made their ratings without reading past the target interventions. The reliability coefficient for the mean plan compatibility ratings made by the two new judges was also .65. The reliability coefficient for the plan compatibility score based on the mean of the ratings made by all four judges was .80. This mean score was the one we used in the data analysis.

The Patient Scale

A 5-point Attitude toward Termination Scale was constructed to measure the patient's expressed feelings of resistance to or readiness for termination. Judges gauged the intensity of Mrs. C's resistance to termination from the following behaviors: (1) The patient seems uncomfortable, conflicted, apprehensive, or despairing in referring to termination. (2) The patient seems unable to accept the idea of termination, and she is either defiantly angry or anxiously depressed (as opposed to appropriately sad) about it. (3) The patient feels extremely helpless, dependent, and unsure of her ability to handle conflicts on her own. (4) The patient feels worried and pessimistic about the future. (5) The patient feels she cannot replace the analyst or be happy without him.

An attitude of readiness for termination was inferred from the following behaviors: (1) The patient appears to be comfortable and matter-of-fact in referring to termination. (2) The patient seems accepting of the idea of termination and feels appropriately sad (as opposed to anxiously depressed) about it. (3) The patient feels confident of her ability to handle conflicts on her own. (4) The patient feels optimistic about the future. (5) The patient feels that she can find healthy replacements for the functions that the analyst and the analysis have been serving.

The complete patient scale is presented in Appendix 22. It was used to assess the immediate impact of the target interventions on Mrs. C's attitude toward termination, and to track changes in her resistance to termination over the last 114 sessions.

In the 93 instances in which a target intervention was preceded as well as followed by a patient reference to termination, separate scores were obtained for the preintervention and the postintervention segments. Shift scores were then derived using a regression technique recommended by Cohen and Cohen (1975) which removes the effect of the preintervention scores from the postintervention scores. Through the use of this technique, the postintervention scores were statistically adjusted to take account of the patient's baseline level of functioning prior to each intervention. The scores produced by this procedure are referred to as residualized gain scores. They have been demonstrated to be more reliable than difference scores arrived at through simple subtraction. These residualized gain scores were used to assess the immediate effect of the target interventions on the patient's resistance to termination. In the 19 instances in which the target interventions were not preceded by a patient reference to termination, the scores for the postintervention material alone were used to assess the immediate effect of the analyst's intervention.

Two judges, both advanced graduate students in clinical psychology who were unfamiliar with the hypothesis we were attempting to test, were trained in the use of the Attitude toward Termination Scale. The training procedure involved having them first become familiar with the psychoanalytic literature on the resistance to termination, and then make practice ratings on segments of patient material that could not be used in the study proper because they occurred in sessions where the analyst made no termination interventions. During the training session the judges agreed highly with each other and encountered few problems in applying the Attitude toward Termination Scale to the practice segments.

In making their final ratings, the judges were instructed not to read the analyst's interventions, unless the patient's material was unintelligible without knowing what the analyst had said. There were only a few instances in which the judges needed to refer to the analyst's intervention in order to clarify the meaning of the patient's response.

The reliability coefficient for the mean of the judges' ratings on the Attitude toward Termination Scale was .83. There was a significant correlation of .48 between the mean preintervention and the mean postintervention scores on the Attitude toward Termination Scale. This finding is consistent with those reported by Caston, Goldman, and McClure in Chapter 19 with respect to the relationship between preintervention and postintervention measures of patient functioning. It indicates that the degree of measurable effect an intervention can have immediately on the patient's level of functioning is usually constrained by the level of the patient's behavior on the relevant dimension prior to the intervention.

RESULTS

THE IMMEDIATE EFFECT OF THE TARGET INTERVENTIONS ON THE PATIENT'S ATTITUDE TOWARD TERMINATION

The data analysis was based on the previously described mean ratings for which we reported reliability coefficients. All reported significance levels are for two-tailed tests.

The immediate effect of the target interventions on Mrs. C's resistance to termination was measured by the correlation between the plan compatibility scores and the postintervention residualized gain scores on the Attitude toward Termination Scale. In those 19 instances where there was no preintervention score to be partialled out, a score equivalent to the raw postintervention score was used. The obtained correlation was .44 (significant beyond $p = .0001$).

Thus, the analyst's termination interventions had a demonstrable immediate effect on the patient's resistance to termination in the manner predicted by our hypothesis. Pro-plan interventions tended to be followed by a more positive (or less negative) attitude toward termination, and anti-plan interventions by a more resistant attitude.

We performed a few additional analyses in an attempt to more fully understand the relationship between the analyst's termination interventions and subsequent shifts in the patient's attitude toward termination. We did separate data analyses for those 19 interventions that were not preceded by a patient reference to termination and for the remaining 93 interventions that were. This comparison was prompted by the finding that there was a small but significant correlation of .21 ($p < .05$) between the preintervention patient scores and the plan compatibility scores in the 93 instances where the analyst's interventions were preceded by a patient reference to termination. We interpreted this finding to mean that the analyst showed some tendency to follow the patient's lead in making pro-plan and anti-plan interventions. In other words, he would be somewhat more likely to make a pro-plan intervention when the patient was expressing a positive attitude toward termination and an anti-plan intervention when the patient was expressing a negative attitude toward termination.

We found a striking difference between the results obtained from the separate analyses of 19 interventions that were not preceded by a patient reference to termination and the 93 interventions that were. With regard to the former set of interventions the correlation between the plan compatibility scores and the postintervention patient scores was .80 ($p < .0001$). With regard to the latter set of interventions the correlation between the plan compatibility scores and the residualized gain scores was .35 ($p < .001$). Thus, the target interventions that had not been cued by a patient reference to termination seemed to have a greater immediate impact on the patient's attitude toward termination than did the target interventions that were so cued.

We interpreted this finding in the following manner. We inferred that one of the ways in which Mrs. C tested the analyst was indirectly to suggest either a pro-plan or an anti-plan interpretive theme and then to observe whether the analyst agreed or disagreed with what she was saying. One limitation of this type of testing strategy is that the patient remains uncertain about whether the analyst is just following her associations or whether he is stating a strongly held position of his own. The difference between a solicited and an unsolicited interpretation may be compared to the difference between a solicited and an unsolicited compliment or insult. The unsolicited comment, whether positive or negative, tends to have a greater impact on the recipient. We assume that the analyst's unsolicited termination interventions had a stronger impact on the patient because she took them as a truer reflection of his feelings about her impending termination.

We also did separate data analyses for the 14 interventions that occurred in the block of 10 sessions from which we derived our plan formulation (hours 1015 through 1024) and for the remaining 98 interventions that occurred outside that block of sessions. Our reason for analyzing the data this way was to rule out the possibility that the overall results could be accounted for by a particularly strong relationship between the plan compatibility scores and residualized gain scores in the 10 sessions we had clinically studied. We found that the correlation between the intervention scores and the patient scores in sessions 1015 through 1024 was .24 (N.S., $N = 14$), whereas it was .44 ($p < .0001$) for the remaining sessions (hours 1001 through 1014 and hours 1025 through 1114 combined). Thus the relationship between the intervention scores and the patient scores was weaker in the 10 sessions we clinically studied than it was in the rest of the last 114 sessions. We attributed this difference to the fact that Mrs. C seemed to be actively testing the analyst during sessions 1015 through 1024 in a way that allowed him to pass her tests by simply not responding to her demands and complaints (see Appendix 26 for a description of her testing during this period). In other words, the primary therapeutic transactions in that group of hours were occurring in response to what the analyst did not say rather than in response to what he did say.

CHANGES IN THE PLAN COMPATIBILITY OF THE ANALYST'S INTERVENTIONS AND IN MRS. C'S ATTITUDE TOWARD TERMINATION OVER TIME

In order to examine the relationship between the plan compatibility aspect of the analyst's interventions and changes in Mrs. C's attitude toward termination over longer time spans, we grouped data across blocks of six sessions each. That created 19 equal time intervals within the last 114 sessions. The correlation between the pooled scores for the therapist's interventions and the pooled scores for the patient's attitude toward termination (including both preintervention and postintervention scores) was .66 ($p < .01$). Hence, there is strong evidence that changes in the patient's attitude toward termination over time are related to changes in the plan compatibility aspect of the analyst's interventions.

Smoothed curves[3] for the ungrouped intervention scores and for the mean of the ungrouped pre- and postintervention patient scores are presented in Figures 20-1 and 20-2. Both of the curves are upward-sloping and display a rough correspondence in their wide fluctuations. They show that over time the analyst's interventions became more pro-plan and Mrs. C's attitude toward termination became less negative.

The general correspondence between the two curves conforms to our clinical understanding of how Mrs. C overcame her resistance to termination. It was our impression that she unconsciously found a way to accommodate her testing strategy to the analyst's theory so that she could enlist his support in disconfirming her pathogenic beliefs about her power to hurt him. She did this by subtly encouraging the analyst to shift his interpretive focus from the magnitude of the loss she was experienc-

---

3. The smoothing technique employed in preparing the curves presented in Figures 20-1 and 20-2 uses a compound smoothing procedure based on running medians. It is described in Velleman and Hoaglin (1981, pp. 171–173).

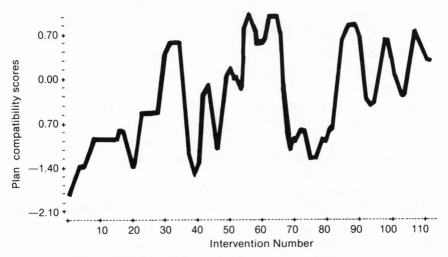

Figure 20-1. Smoothed curve for the plan compatibility scores.

ing in contemplating termination to the exaggerated quality of the special power and prerogatives she attributed to men because they have penises. The analyst's interventions became increasingly more pro-plan when he shifted away from interpreting her frustrated transference wishes and began to interpret the irrationality of her penis envy and castration complex. Although he never interpreted the patient's worries about hurting him, just the above shift in the nature of his interventions was

Figure 20-2. Smoothed curve for attitude toward termination scores.

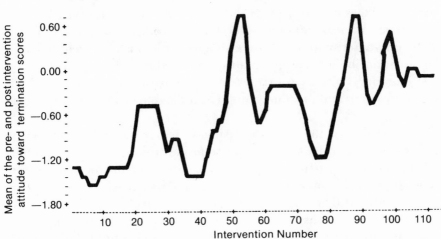

sufficient to help Mrs. C overcome her worries about his narcissistic vulnerability and his need for her love, admiration, and dependency.

The following is an example of this type of pro-plan intervention. It occurred in the session before her last. It received the highest mean plan compatibility score (+2.12) of all the target interventions, and it triggered an immediate shift in the patient's attitude toward termination from a preintervention score of −.75 to a postintervention score of +.75. Just prior to this intervention the patient was expressing worry that she would not be able to understand important things if she did not have the analyst to explain them to her. The analyst responded: "So again you're afraid that you can't think since you're not a male. But, in fact, you have been thinking, and you've been talking with your husband about things that you never have talked with him about. You've understood things without my saying anything. So you have been thinking, all without a penis."

COMPARISON OF RESULTS OBTAINED FROM VERBATIM TRANSCRIPTS AND PROCESS NOTES

At the time this study was done we were not aware that verbatim transcripts were available for three randomly selected sessions out of the last 114 hours. Two of those sessions each contained one target intervention, while the third contained two target interventions. Thus, for four interventions, we could compare the results obtained from process notes ratings with results for new ratings made from comparable segments of the verbatim transcripts.

Three months after our study was completed, we recalled the two judges who had made the attitude toward termination ratings and two of the four judges who had made the plan compatibility ratings. We had them repeat the original rating procedures on comparable portions of the verbatim transcript for the three sessions in question. They were given no information about the original ratings they had made from process notes. All four interventions contained in the verbatim transcript had both preintervention and postintervention attitude statements about termination.

We evaluated the effects of using verbatim transcripts instead of process notes by calculating comparable statistics for both the original ratings and for the new ratings made on the same four interventions. In other words, we compared how well our judges agreed with each other using the two different sources of data, and we made a similar comparison of the correlations between the mean ratings of the target interventions and the mean ratings of the patient's subsequent attitude toward termination. In each case, the correlations were higher using ratings made from the verbatim transcripts.

In terms of the plan compatibility ratings for the four interventions in question, the correlation between the original ratings made by the two judges was .40. When those judges made the same ratings from comparable portions of the verbatim transcript, the correlation was .97. For the attitude toward termination ratings made on the four preintervention segments and the four postintervention segments, the correlation between the original eight ratings made by the two judges was .58. When those judges made the same ratings from comparable portions of the verbatim transcript, the correlation was .71. In terms of the correlation between the four mean intervention scores and the four mean postintervention attitude scores, the one obtained for the original set of ratings was .66. The comparable correlation for the ratings made from the verbatim transcripts was .91.

It is, of course, not possible to draw any conclusions from a sample of four. Nonetheless, this small comparison of the results obtained from process notes and the results obtained from the verbatim transcripts leads us to expect that were the entire study performed on the basis of verbatim transcripts, our judges would have agreed more closely with each other and our findings would have been stronger.

DISCUSSION AND CONCLUSION

Our findings provide clear support for our hypothesis. Pro-plan interventions tended to be followed by an immediate decrease in Mrs. C's resistance to termination, whereas anti-plan interventions had the opposite effect. Moreover, a significant relationship between the plan compatibility of the analyst's interventions and Mrs. C's attitude toward termination was found to exist over blocks of sessions.

We found that the plan formulation derived from the first 10 sessions of the analysis was highly consistent with our plan formulation for the last 114 sessions. This finding implies the existence of a strong continuity in the patient's unconscious goals and manner of working across the entire analysis.

The results support our explanation of the primary unconscious determinants of Mrs. C's resistance to termination and of the way it was overcome. They are consistent with the hypothesis that the patient used the analyst's pro-plan interventions to help disconfirm the pathogenic beliefs responsible for that resistance. In our clinical assessment of the material we observed that the analyst also passed several key tests by holding firm to a fixed termination date. We believe that his pro-plan interventions in conjunction with his passing of important tests enabled Mrs. C to overcome her resistance to termination successfully.

More broadly, our findings contribute to the evidence for the practical and the theoretical usefulness of the plan concept. In this study the plan concept provided a coherent explanation of the termination phase of Mrs. C's analysis and enabled us to predict the immediate effect of the analyst's interventions on a clinically significant resistance.

Our explanation of Mrs. C's resistance to termination was markedly different from the one held by the treating analyst. The predictions we made would not have been made on the basis of the automatic functioning hypothesis and in some instances were contradictory to what that hypothesis would have predicted.

One of the crucial differences between the two theories may be summarized as follows: According to the automatic functioning hypothesis, the patient's resistances to termination in a prototypic analysis primarily stem from instinctual fixations, which are expressed in a libidinal attachment to the analyst and in infantile transference wishes that the patient unconsciously wants to gratify and perpetuate. According to our view, Mrs. C's infantile attachment to the analyst and expressed transference wishes did not represent an instinctual fixation and were not things she unconsciously wanted to gratify or perpetuate, but rather were things she unconsciously wanted to relinquish. Her attachment was maintained not by a wish for gratification, but by unconscious guilt stemming from her pathogenic beliefs about her power to hurt the analyst if she separated from him in a mature, independent, and self-confident way. Put more simply, the primary cause of Mrs. C's resistance to termination was not a wish for infantile transference gratifications but her unconscious fear of hurting the analyst.

It would have been difficult, if not impossible, to test our hypothesis without the use of a rigorous research methodology. The patient's material appeared to strongly corroborate the analyst's interventions and to support the automatic functioning explanation of the termination phase of analysis. Only a detailed empirical analysis of subtle changes in the patient's behavior following the target interventions could substantiate the predictions made by an alternative set of explanatory principles. This study provides further evidence for the vital importance of empirical research in testing competing psychoanalytic propositions.

PART III

A BROAD LOOK AT THE THEORY AND THE RESEARCH

21

A BROAD LOOK AT THE THEORY

JOSEPH WEISS

In this chapter I shall discuss the theory of the mind proposed in this book in order to put it in certain broad contexts. (In the next and last chapter Harold Sampson and I will do the same for the research.)

THE THEORY IS BOTH FREUDIAN AND NEW

The theory proposed here, as pointed out earlier, is both Freudian and new. It is Freudian in that its basic ideas are derived from concepts either developed by Freud or implied by his ideas. The theory is new in that it relies on certain of Freud's ideas and not on others. It relies on certain ideas that Freud introduced in his ego psychology and that assume the unconscious use of higher mental functions. It systematically applies such concepts both to the psychoanalytic theory of psychopathology and to the psychoanalytic theory of therapy and technique.

This theory is in the mainstream of psychoanalytic advance. It continues a trend, perhaps the predominant trend, in Freud's theorizing and in the theorizing of a number of analysts since Freud: This trend is away from concepts based on the automatic functioning hypothesis and toward concepts based on the higher mental functioning hypothesis.

I shall use the example of pathogenic belief to show how the theory proposed here relies on and indeed develops certain of Freud's ideas while being incompatible with others. Since the concept of pathogenic belief is based on the higher mental functioning hypothesis, it is not compatible with the main thrust of the theory of the mind that Freud presented in *The Interpretation of Dreams* (1900). According to that theory, a person is not able unconsciously to develop pathogenic beliefs. He is not able unconsciously to think or to infer beliefs from experience. He is unable unconsciously to face painful experiences, much less develop beliefs about them. Indeed, he turns away effortlessly (automatically) from such experiences.

Nor is it possible to assimilate the concept of unconscious patho-genic belief to Freud's early theory of the mind by equating pathogenic belief to a key concept of the early theory, namely, fantasy (as Freud defined fantasy in, say, *Formulations on the Two Principles of Mental Functioning* [1911].) Pathogenic beliefs and fantasies bear certain re-semblances to each other. Both play an important part in unconscious mental life, and both are related to experience. Both, viewed objectively from the vantage point of the adult, may appear to be farfetched. How-ever, pathogenic beliefs are not fantasies. Though fantasies and beliefs may appear similar to the adult, they are from the perspective of the child (and in the unconscious mind of the adult) quite different things. A child unconsciously derives pleasure from fantasies but not from pathogenic beliefs. Indeed, a child may be unconsciously terrified or weighed down by pathogenic beliefs. In producing a fantasy, a child ignores the fright-ening, frustrating aspects of reality, or he changes reality so as to perceive it as the fulfillment of various wishes. However, in producing a patho-genic belief, a child faces reality. He infers a pathogenic belief from the frightening, grim, traumatic aspects of reality, as he perceives it. In producing a pathogenic belief, the child attempts, albeit inadequately, to grapple with the dangers and frustrations of reality.

The concepts presented here about pathogenic beliefs are, of course, highly compatible with and indeed derived from certain of Freud's for-mulations about the part played by castration anxiety in the development of psychopathology in the male. Freud assumed that it is from fear of castration that a boy represses his Oedipal motivations and so develops a proclivity to neurosis. Freud also implies (he almost stated) that castra-tion anxiety arises from a belief. He wrote on a number of occasions of the male's "belief in castration" or his "conviction of the danger of castration" and only on a few occasions about his fantasy of castration. In *Inhibitions, Symptoms and Anxiety* (1926a) Freud stated that castration anxiety is acquired from experience by normal processes of thought and that it represents a real or perceived danger to the boy who suffers from it.

The concepts about pathogenic beliefs proposed here, while derived from Freud's views, develop and extend them. They are organized in an explicit theory about pathogenic beliefs. This theory assumes that psy-chopathology may arise from any of a number of pathogenic beliefs, including beliefs about the dangers stemming from a variety of motives, not just Oedipal motives. It assumes, too, that pathogenic beliefs play a crucial part in the development and maintenance of all psychopathology, not just of neuroses and perversions. In addition, the concepts proposed here extend Freud's ideas about the part played by pathogenic beliefs in the analytic process. Freud did assume that the male patient, in order to get well, must become aware of and change his belief that he will be castrated as a punishment for his Oedipal impulses. Freud assumed, too, that the female patient must change her corresponding pathogenic beliefs. Freud, however, did not point to the centrality in the therapeutic process of a patient changing his pathogenic beliefs. Nor did he point to the need of the patient in some instances to change beliefs other than those opposing his Oedipal impulses. The views proposed here extend Freud's views by assuming that a patient may need to change a variety of pathogenic beliefs, not just those opposing Oedipal impulses. The views presented in this book also extend those proposed by Freud by assuming that the patient's changing his pathogenic beliefs is the *essential* process of therapy.

THE THEORY PROPOSED IN PART I PRESENTS A UNIFORM, COHERENT CONCEPTION OF PSYCHOPATHOLOGY

The theory proposed in Part I provides a uniform approach to the study of psychopathology. According to this theory, all kinds of psychopathology are rooted in pathogenic beliefs. Pathogenic beliefs are the essential element, the *sine qua non*, of psychopathology, and variations in psychopathology reflect variations in pathogenic beliefs.

A particular kind of psychopathology reflects the kind of pathogenic belief underlying it. Also, the most fundamental way of describing a problem is in terms of its underlying pathogenic beliefs. It may be useful, in describing certain kinds of psychopathology, to consider such attributes as the capacity to develop object relations, the capacity to maintain transferences, and the capacity to repress. However, such attributes are themselves reflections of underlying pathogenic beliefs.

A pathogenic belief contains at least four components: (1) the attitudes, impulses, or goals with which it is concerned; that is, the attitudes, impulses, or goals it assumes are dangerous; (2) the kinds of dangers it foretells; (3) the kinds of remedies, such as repression or withdrawal, which it enjoins; and (4) the strength of conviction with which it is held. It is possible, by varying these four components, to derive the pathogenic beliefs underlying any kind of psychopathology.

For example, a patient with intense survivor guilt may assume that he scarcely has a right to live. He may condemn himself for feeling happy or becoming successful. He may risk experiencing intense guilt if he becomes relaxed, happy, or successful. He may attempt to avoid this guilt by leading a life of suffering similar to that of the person he has survived. If he is completely convinced that he has no right to a good life, he may remain chronically depressed. If this conviction is lightly held, on the other hand, he may suffer only occasional feelings of depression.

For another example, a person, as a consequence of his belief in castration as a punishment, may assume that if he permits himself to feel sexual excitement he will be castrated. He may attempt to avoid castration by repressing his sexual impulses. If he is deeply convinced of the danger of castration he may develop severe inhibitions. If he holds this belief lightly, he may simply experience mild anxiety about sex or occasional sexual difficulty.

HOW AN EXTERNAL CONFLICT BECOMES INTERNALIZED

The concept of pathogenic belief permits a particularly clear formulation of how an external conflict becomes internalized. It helps to pin down and make explicit the elusive concept of internalization: The child's conflict originally is with his parents. The conflict is between a wish and a fear. The child wishes to satisfy certain impulses (or to reach certain goals) in relation to his parents, but he fears his parents' reactions to his attempts to do so. His conflict is external in that he experiences the fear as coming from without and as real. The child, by internalizing the conflict (or more precisely the fears or dangers) does two things: (1) He infers and so acquires a pathogenic belief that links his wishes to the dangers. (2) He carries out certain actions that are enjoined by the belief (he represses, he withdraws, he becomes wary).

This acquisition by the child of a pathogenic belief is truly an act of internalization. By acquiring a pathogenic belief a child adds an important element to his unconscious mental life. This belief is a product of his own thoughts and perceptions; it encapsulates crucial formative experiences; and it is a powerful source of motivation. By developing a pathogenic belief, the child shifts the source of danger from without to within.

A UNIFIED VIEW OF THE THERAPEUTIC PROCESS

The theory proposed in Part I permits certain broad generalizations not only about psychopathology but about the therapeutic process as well. It assumes that psychopathology is developed and maintained in accordance with pathogenic beliefs. It also assumes that the therapeutic process is in essence a process by which the patient becomes conscious of and changes his pathogenic beliefs. This formulation of the therapeutic process applies to the treatment of various kinds of psychopathology. It also applies to a variety of processes that take place during the course of any psychoanalytic treatment.

THE FORMATION AND RESOLUTION OF A TRANSFERENCE

In the familiar formulations based on the automatic functioning hypothesis, the formation and resolution of a transference are conceptualized as separate and distinct. The formation (expression) of a transference is conceptualized as a dynamic process that takes place more or less automatically from an intensification of a repressed transference, which is pushing to the surface, and a weakening of the defenses opposed to its coming forth. The transference is intensified by the analyst's neutrality, which denies it the gratifications it seeks. The defenses are weakened (undermined) by the analyst's interpretations. The resolution of a transference, however, is conceptualized as taking place by quite a different process. In this process the ego is helped by analytic interpretations to gain insight into the transference. The ego, as a consequence of such insight, recognizes the transference as an irrational repetition of childhood experiences and abolishes it.

The theory proposed here differs from the familiar view outlined above in its conceptions both of the formation of a transference and of its resolution. According to this theory, both processes take place along a continuum in which the patient progressively disconfirms his pathogenic beliefs and so progressively gains control over the unconscious transference. As the patient, from testing and from the assimilation of insight, makes a certain degree of progress in disconfirming his pathogenic beliefs, he becomes less afraid of the repressed transference. He acquires more control of the transference, unconsciously decides that he can safely bring it forth, and so brings it forth and displays it prominently for various motives, including the unconscious wish to test his pathogenic beliefs more directly than he had tested them earlier. As the patient makes more progress in disconfirming his pathogenic beliefs, he develops more control over the previously repressed transference. He becomes able not to express the transference when it is inappropriate and to express it when it is appropriate. He thereby, to all appearances, abolishes it.

The following schematic example illustrates the above:

A patient, at the beginning of his treatment, suffered from an unconscious rivalry with the analyst based on a father transference. However, he was afraid of his rivalry with the analyst at first and so kept it repressed. Later, as a consequence of analytic work, he succeeded in partially disconfirming his pathogenic belief in the danger of competing with the analyst. As he became unconsciously less afraid to compete with the analyst and hence more in control of his competition with him, he did compete unconsciously with him. He displayed his competitiveness with the analyst in order, among other motives, to assure himself that he would not endanger himself by competing with him. With further analytic work, he became even less afraid of his rivalry with the analyst and even more in control of it. He became conscious of his rivalry. Moreover, as he became conscious of it and more in control of it, he expressed it appropriately. He competed with the analyst when it was appropriate to do so, and he did not compete with him when it was not. He thereby, to all appearances (and for all practical purposes) abolished the transference.

The assumption that a patient does not truly abolish his transferences but instead gains control over them is born out by the remarkable follow-up studies of analytic patients originally carried out by Pfeffer (1959, 1961, 1963) and replicated by Norman et al. (1976). Each patient studied by these investigators had successfully finished his analysis at least five years before he was studied. Each patient reported to a follow-up analyst for (usually) five weekly 1-hour sessions. The follow-up analyst encouraged the former patient to talk freely about his analysis but did not comment on the patient's productions. Instead, he listened to them in a neutral way. In each case the former patient developed powerful transferences to the follow-up analyst similar to the ones he had developed to his treating analyst. Moreover, he brought them out and resolved them rapidly and approximately in the same order as in his original analysis. The fact that the patient rapidly developed these powerful transferences to the follow-up analyst shows that he had not truly abolished them. The fact that he rapidly brought them forth and rapidly resolved them shows that he had acquired a great deal of unconscious control over them. The powerful control which he exerted over his transferences to the follow-up analyst attests to the value that his analysis had for him in helping him to overcome his pathogenic beliefs and by doing so to gain control of his transferences.

EXPERIENCE VERSUS INSIGHT

The theory proposed in Part I reconciles two assumptions about the nature of the therapeutic process that are sometimes thought to be discrepant. According to one assumption, the therapeutic process is in essence a process by which the patient benefits primarily by new experiences with the analyst. According to the other, it is a process by which the patient benefits primarily by insights he acquires by assimilating the analyst's interpretations. According to the theory proposed here, it is both. It is in essence a process by which the patient becomes aware of his pathogenic beliefs. Moreover, it is a process by which the patient works to change his beliefs in two ways: (1) by testing them unconsciously in relation to the analyst, and (2) by assimilating insight into them conveyed by the analyst's interpretations.

The two processes complement one another. A patient may achieve insight from both. In the first (with which I am mainly concerned here) the patient, by unconsciously testing his pathogenic beliefs, also tests the analyst. By such testing the patient seeks experiences with the analyst that he may use in his struggle to disconfirm his pathogenic beliefs. He seeks experiences that are new in that they are different from the traumatic experiences with his parents (or other significant individuals) from which he had inferred his pathogenic beliefs.

In the *Outline* (1940a), Freud made explicit that the patient may and indeed should have experiences with the analyst different from those he had with his parents. Freud led up to this idea by discussing the patient's transference to the analyst. He wrote: "If the patient puts the analyst in the place of his father (or mother) he is also giving him the power which his superego exercises over his ego, since his parents were, as we know, the origin of his superego. The new superego now has an opportunity for a sort of *after-education* of the neurotic; it can correct mistakes for which his parents were responsible in educating him" (p. 175). Freud then warned the analyst not to misuse this power by attempting to make the patient over in his own image, adding that were he to do so, he would be repeating a parental error: "He [the analyst] will only be repeating a mistake of the parents who crushed their child's independence by their influence, and he will only be replacing the patient's earlier dependence by a new one. And in all his attempts at improving and educating the patient, the analyst should respect his individuality" (p. 175).

The patient's new experiences with the analyst are, in my view, essential to the success of his treatment. As in Freud's example, if the analyst were to attempt, like the patient's parents, to make the patient over in his image, he would crush the patient's independence. I would add that if the analyst were to be as dominating to the patient as his parents had been, the patient might not remember his parents' domination of him. It is because the analyst maintains his neutrality and so behaves differently from the parents that the patient may safely remember his parents' domination. If the analyst were to behave as the patient's parents had behaved, the patient would be no more inclined to lift his repressions in the treatment than he had been with his parents in his childhood.

Rangell (1981), using the language of Alexander and French (1946), stated that the patient in his analysis does receive corrective emotional experiences, but more from what the analyst does not do than from what he does do. In my opinion the patient, by his unconscious testing, seeks and receives corrective emotional experiences. However, he does not receive them (as Alexander and French assumed), because the analyst, by taking various roles, offers them to the patient. Rather, the analyst may provide the patient with corrective emotional experiences (i.e., he may pass the patient's tests) by being a good analyst and by attempting to understand the patient, to empathize with him, and to interpret his understanding of the patient to him.

A patient may make considerable progress in changing pathogenic beliefs and gaining insight into them (as did Mrs. C) by testing them in relation to the analyst. He may attain a great deal of insight (as did Mrs. C) without interpretive help. However, a patient is sometimes unable, by testing alone—that is, without help from interpretation—to disconfirm certain pathogenic beliefs. Or he may—without help from interpretation—attain insights, but these remain partial, not completely conscious, and lacking in cogency, power, and scope.

THE THERAPEUTIC ALLIANCE

The theory proposed in Part I changes and adds meaning to the concept of the therapeutic alliance. Ordinarily, the quality of a patient's alliance with the analyst is conceptualized, more or less, in terms of the patient's conscious attitudes to the analyst. Ordinarily, therefore, a patient who consciously hates the analyst, who wishes to terminate, or who is manifestly bored and indifferent to his treatment is thought to have a poor therapeutic alliance with the analyst. However, from the perspective of the theory proposed here, such is not the case. A patient who threatens to stop treatment, who consciously hates the analyst and acts hateful toward him, or who is manifestly bored and indifferent to the analyst may be unconsciously working closely with the analyst and, by his manifest feelings and behavior, be testing him. Indeed, a patient's wish to stop treatment, his hatred of the analyst, or his boredom may indicate that he has made considerable progress in his treatment and is working with the analyst more directly than before.

Such was the case with Miss P, the lawyer presented in Chapter 1. Her threats to stop treatment marked considerable progress in her analysis. She could permit herself to make these threats only after she had, as a consequence of analytic work, developed a certain degree of trust in the analyst. By making these threats, Miss P was working more directly and ultimately more successfully than earlier to test her beliefs that she did not deserve help from the analyst and would, by demanding help from him, drain him.

This concept applies equally well to Professor T, the bored patient presented in Chapter 6. Professor T's display of intense boredom did not reflect a poor alliance with the analyst. In displaying his boredom, the patient was working effectively and well. He was unconsciously testing the analyst by treating him as, in his opinion, his mother had treated him. He had felt squelched and constricted by what he experienced as his mother's bland indifference. He was, by his own bland, indifferent attitude to the analyst, testing him, hoping to assure himself that he would not squelch the analyst as his mother had squelched him. When Professor T inferred that he had not squelched the analyst, he made progress. He produced dreams of adventure, and he took more initiative in his work, showing that unconsciously he was not bland and indifferent. While consciously displaying indifference, he was unconsciously working well with the analyst to overcome his sense of constriction.

PSYCHIC DEPTH

As Hartmann (1951) has pointed out, Freud's ego psychology provides a new conception of psychic depth based on the concept of unconscious regulation by the criteria of danger and safety. The old concept of psychic depth (e.g., as evolved by Reich, 1949) assumes that the depth of an impulse depends upon its being in a particular psychic layer. However, according to Freud's structural model and to the theory proposed here, the psychic depth of an impulse is a function of the ego's evluation of the threat posed by the impulse. An impulse that the ego assumes it may experience safely is closer to the surface than an impulse that the ego assumes would endanger it if experienced. Thus, the analyst works from the surface when he helps the patient (or his ego) to bring forth those impulses the patient assumes he may safely experience and when he does not attempt to induce the patient (or his ego) to face those impulses the patient assumes would, if expressed, put him in a situation of danger.

IMPLICATIONS FOR TECHNIQUE

I shall end this chapter by briefly presenting certain implications of the theory proposed here for the psychoanalytic theory of technique. My presentation will indicate the outline of a theory of technique based on the concepts of ego psychology discussed earlier, which, along with the ideas about technique presented below, are based on the higher mental functioning hypothesis developed in Part I. Therefore, they differ somewhat from certain technical ideas presented by Freud in the *Papers on Technique* (1911–1915), many of which are based on the automatic functioning hypothesis.

The *Papers on Technique* assume, more or less, that unconscious mental life is regulated automatically in accordance with the pleasure principle and the repetition compulsion. They assume that the various repetitions that mark the behavior of the analytic patient are brought about automatically (beyond the ego's control) by the pleasure principle and the repetition compulsion. The *Papers on Technique* assume, too, that the patient's primary unconscious motivation in analysis is the attainment of certain infantile gratifications. Finally, the *Papers on Technique* assume that the analyst's principal task is to induce the patient to relinquish his infantile gratifications, and thereby to induce him to go where unconsciously he does *not want* to go.

The assumptions underlying the technical ideas presented below are in contrast to the assumptions of the *Papers on Technique*. We assume that the ego (1) exerts considerable control over unconscious mental life, (2) regulates unconscious mental life by the criteria of danger and safety, (3) brings about the various repetitions that mark the behavior of the analytic patient, and (4) brings these about, among other purposes, to test pathogenic beliefs. The assumptions presented here assume that the analyst's primary task is to help the patient in his struggle to disconfirm his pathogenic beliefs and thus to help the patient to go where unconsciously he *wants* to go.

THE ANALYST SHOULD HELP THE PATIENT TO CARRY OUT HIS PLANS

How, then, should the analyst approach his task of helping the patient? Since his task is to help the patient to go where he unconsciously wants to go, the analyst should, at each point of the treatment, infer the patient's unconscious plans for solving his problems and help the patient to carry them out. For example, he should help a patient who is working unconsciously to overcome his irrational worries about his wife, to understand and overcome his worries about her. He should help a patient who is struggling to retrieve certain painful memories to understand why he has repressed them and so retrieve them. He should help a patient who is struggling to overcome his fear of competition to understand this fear and overcome it.

This approach adds meaning to Anna Freud's idea (1936) that since the analyst has no access to the patient except through his ego, the analyst must work with him through his ego. This approach, which has been developed by Settlage (1974), makes explicit how the analyst makes an alliance with the patient's ego: He infers the ego's goals, including its unconscious goals, and helps the ego to carry them out. The analyst, in using the approach advocated here, works from the surface, if surface is defined as that which the patient may safely experience. This is because in general the patient (or his ego), at any particular period of his treatment, plans to bring forth only those mental contents that he may safely experience.

HOW THE ANALYST MAY DETERMINE WHETHER HE IS ON THE RIGHT TRACK

The analyst (as shown by the research presented in Chapters 19, 20, and 22) may check on whether he is in fact working in accordance with the patient's unconscious plans by observing the patient's reactions to his comments and interpretations. The analyst may assume that he is on the right track if the patient reacts to his interpretations and interventions by moving toward his unconscious goals. The patient may become less anxious and more insightful. He may become bolder (which, paradoxically, in some instances may mean more boldly testing the analyst by displaying weakness or incompetence, or by displaying indifference to the analyst, anger toward him, or lack of trust in him). By the same token, the analyst may in most instances assume that he is off course if the patient reacts to his interpretations by becoming stalemated, less confident in the analyst, more anxious and defensive, more inhibited, and less insightful.

The patient's unconscious affective and behavioral reactions to the analyst's interpretations are often a better guide than his conscious agreement or disagreement with them. If a patient repeatedly reacts to a certain kind of interpretation with which he consciously agrees by becoming more anxious and defensive, the analyst should consider the possibility that the patient is accepting the interpretation out of compliance. On the other hand, if a patient repeatedly reacts to a certain kind of interpretation which he consciously repudiates by becoming more insightful and by moving toward his goals, the analyst should assume that he is on the right track.

HOW THE ANALYST'S INTERPRETATIONS MAY HELP THE PATIENT

The analyst, by his interpretations, should help the patient to develop a broad conceptual map that tells him where he has come from, where he wants to go, and how he is working to get there. The analyst should help the patient to understand his motives not as isolated entities, but in relation to his ego goals, his pathogenic beliefs and the feelings of fear, anxiety, guilt, shame, and remorse which stem from them, and his assessments of the analyst.

Consider, for example, a patient who, as a consequence of his castration anxiety, developed a homosexual attachment to the analyst in order to placate the analyst. Such a patient may be helped by interpretations which make him aware of his unconscious homosexual attachment to the analyst. However, he may be helped considerably more by interpretations that make him aware that he maintains his homosexual attachment to the analyst out of anxiety, that he intends by it to placate the analyst, and that he would rather overcome his anxiety and relinquish his homosexual attachment to the analyst (and compete with him) than maintain this attachment to him. Such a patient may find that the more complete interpretation guides him more reliably in his unconscious efforts to disconfirm the pathogenic belief in castration and to pursue those goals he had relinquished in obedience to this belief. The more complete interpretation, if accurate, tells the patient not only where he is but where he wants to go. Moreover, it points to the barriers he must overcome to get there, and it indicates how he may go about overcoming these barriers, in this case by overcoming his irrational fear of castration by the analyst.

Or consider, for a second example, a patient who unconsciously maintains an infantile attachment to his mother for fear that if he pursues his goal of becoming more independent of her he will hurt her. Such a patient may find the interpretation, "You are sexually attached to your mother" lacking in context. It does not include the pertinent psychological fact that the patient unconsciously does not like being sexually attached to his mother, has a strong unconscious wish to overcome his attachment to her, and is maintaining his attachment to her primarily so as not to hurt her. The patient may experience the interpretation above as implying that he is a childish person who selfishly wishes to extract infantile gratification from his mother, whereas in his unconscious experience he is, because of his worry about his mother, making a painful sacrifice of his independence for her sake. Thus, though the patient may benefit from learning that he is sexually attached to his mother, he may benefit more if he learns, in addition, that he does not approve of being sexually attached to her and that he is maintaining his attachment to her in obedience to the irrational belief that if he becomes independent of her he will hurt her.

The analyst, by his interpretations, should help the patient to understand how by his symptoms, inhibitions, and character traits he is maintaining infantile ties to his parents either by complying with them or by identifying with them. For example, in treating a patient with castration anxiety such as the one discussed above, an analyst should help the patient to become aware that in order to avoid castration by his father he both repressed his sexuality and developed a passive feminine attitude. The analyst of Miss P, the lawyer discussed in Chapter 1, helped her by making her aware that it was out of compliance to her parents that she experienced herself as someone who did not deserve to be taken care of. The analyst of Miss D (a patient with separation guilt discussed in Chapter 3) helped her by making her aware that she had relinquished her wish to become independent of her mother in order to protect her mother. The analyst of Mr. S (the patient described in Chapter 4 who was sent to his uncle and aunt's when he was 2½) helped him by making him aware that he had experienced being sent away as a punishment for being rowdy and that he had given up his rowdiness in order to avoid a repetition of such punishment.

THE ANALYST SHOULD MAINTAIN A STEADY FOCUS

I shall, before ending this chapter, present one more implication for technique of the theory proposed in Part I. The theory assumes that a patient may work for a long period of time to disconfirm a few interrelated pathogenic beliefs and thus to reach just a few important interrelated goals. Since the patient may work in a variety of ways and may draw on a variety of present and past experiences, he may appear, at first glance, to be concerned with a number of unrelated problems. However, on closer examination, he will be seen to be working single-mindedly on the same few important problems (to disconfirm the same few pathogenic beliefs). The implication for technique is that the analyst should be as single-minded as the patient. Once the analyst has developed a line of interpretation that the patient finds helpful, the analyst should stick with it until the patient clearly changes direction. The analyst need not fear that the patient will find him repetitive or boring. As long as the patient is working unconsciously on a particular problem, he will be glad for the analyst's help with it and will find the analyst's comments about it fresh and interesting. Moreover, the patient may well be unresponsive if the analyst introduces a new theme unrelated to the patient's ongoing persistent concerns.

22

THE RESEARCH: A BROAD VIEW

JOSEPH WEISS
HAROLD SAMPSON

In this chapter we will examine from various vantage points the research presented in Part II. Our purpose will be to put it in a broad context. We will begin with a brief description of the patient and of our findings and conclusions.

THE PATIENT AND THE CONCLUSIONS

Our research was carried out on a single analytic case. We studied from transcripts and process notes the first 100 sessions of the analysis of Mrs. C, a married woman in her late 20s. Mrs. C came to treatment at the insistence of her husband. She came primarily for sexual problems; she was unable to have orgasms during sexual intercourse. She also felt driven and unable to enjoy life. She had an obsessive–compulsive character structure.

According to our formulation, Mrs. C was guilt-ridden. She suffered not only from Oedipal guilt but also from survivor guilt and separation guilt. She was burdened by the unconscious pathogenic belief that she was better off than the other members of her family and that by being better off she had deprived them and made them envious of her. She also believed that if she were to assert her independence of her family she would hurt them, especially her father. She unconsciously assumed omnipotent responsibility for them.

Mrs. C attempted to placate her conscience (and to protect her family) in various ways. She tried to protect her parents (and express her loyalty to them) by identifying with their worst traits. She became grim, puritanical, and self-sacrificing like her mother. She became irascible and bullying with subordinates as her father had been with her. She attempted to protect her siblings by becoming envious of them. For example, she developed a strong conscious envy of her younger brother for his possession of a penis.

Mrs. C's unconscious plan, according to our formulation, was to work to change the pathogenic beliefs underlying her feelings of guilt by testing them in relation to the analyst. She could test them in various ways. She could, for example, display her various abilities and her independence to the analyst in order to assure herself that by being capable, strong, and independent she would neither hurt the analyst nor incur his disapproval. Or she could complain about the analyst and imply that he was hurting her in order to assure herself that she would not, by such complaining, make him worry about her, as in childhood she had worried about her parents.

During the first 100 sessions of her analysis, Mrs. C's analyst remained relatively inactive. His comments were addressed primarily to Mrs. C's resistances. He would, for example, direct Mrs. C's attention to her hesitating to free-associate, to her lapsing in her free associations, or to her apparently attempting to avoid certain topics. Otherwise he made few interpretations.

Nonetheless, during her first 100 sessions Mrs. C made considerable progress. Both our research group and two experienced analysts who did not know our impressions studied the first 100 sessions and found that during these Mrs. C became increasingly more relaxed and less driven. She became more comfortable both with her husband and with the analyst. She also began to enjoy herself more and to have orgasms during intercourse.

Our formal research studies help fill out the picture of Mrs. C's behavior during the first 100 sessions. From these studies we concluded the following:

• Mrs. C, without interpretive help, became conscious of important previously repressed memories, ideas, feelings, and other mental contents. She became conscious of these previously repressed mental contents, not primarily because they pushed forth to the surface propelled by their own thrusts, but because she unconsciously decided that she could safely experience them, and so brought them forth (Chapter 12).

• Mrs. C, without interpretive help, became increasingly aware of previously repressed irrational omnipotent feelings of responsibility for others and irrational fears of hurting them (Chapter 14).

• Mrs. C, with little interpretive help, made significant changes in her behavior. She became increasingly able directly to oppose, criticize, and fight with others, including the analyst. She also became increasingly able directly to cooperate with, like, and express friendliness and affection toward others, including the analyst (Chapter 13).

• Mrs. C made a number of unconscious transference demands on the analyst, not primarily to satisfy unconscious transference impulses, but rather to test the analyst in an effort to change her pathogenic beliefs (Chapters 17 and 18).

• Mrs. C worked, during these 100 sessions, in accordance with an unconscious plan for solving her problems. This plan was to change her pathogenic beliefs and thereby overcome her guilt about being independent of and better off than others, and to overcome, too, her omnipotent sense of responsibility for others. Independent judges familiar with Mrs. C's intake interview and the process notes of the first 10 sessions of her treatment agreed reliably on her plan (Chapter 16).

• Mrs. C demonstrated (in the process notes study) an immediate favorable reaction to interventions that, according to our raters, should help her to carry out her plan. She became bolder and more insightful. She did not, however, demonstrate such a reaction to interpretations that, according to our raters, should not help her (or which should hinder her) in her efforts to carry out her plan. (This finding was only partially supported by the replication study [Chapter 19].)

• During the terminal period of her treatment, Mrs. C worked in accordance with a plan much like the one that guided her efforts during the first 100 sessions. The plan was to change the pathogenic beliefs underlying her guilt about separation from the analyst. Mrs. C demonstrated immediate favorable reactions to interventions that, according to our raters, should help her to terminate by becoming more ready to terminate (Chapter 20).

Taken together, the various studies of Mrs. C's behavior during the first 100 sessions support the following conclusions: She entered analysis burdened by the pathogenic beliefs (and the feelings of guilt and responsibility which stemmed from them) that if she were independent, successful, and happy, she would hurt her parents and siblings. She worked unconsciously by testing the analyst to change her pathogenic beliefs. As she succeeded by such testing in changing them, she permitted herself, largely without help from interpretation, to gain insight into them. She became more conscious, without their being interpreted, of her irrational pathogenic beliefs about her power to hurt others and about her sense of responsibility for them. She became able, largely unhelped by interpretation, both to bring forth important mental contents that she had repressed in obedience to these beliefs, and to behave in ways which she had inhibited in obedience to them. She became more able both to fight with the analyst and others and to feel close to them. These findings support the theory proposed in this book.

SOME IMPLICATIONS OF OUR FINDINGS

The findings reported above support the psychoanalytic concept of repression against an alternative hypothesis proposed by certain critics of psychoanalysis (e.g., Grünbaum, 1979). Grünbaum has written that the psychoanalytic theory of repression has not been demonstrated scientifically and has urged analysts to tackle the problem of demonstrating it. According to Grünbaum, analysts have not refuted the thesis that there is no such thing as repression and that those observations that the analyst and the patient regard as evidence for repression are based on the patient's compliance with the analyst. According to this thesis, the analyst deduces his ideas about the patient's repressions (including his ideas about the mental contents that the patient has repressed) from his theories about repression, rather than from his observations of the patient. The analyst conveys these ideas to the patient through his interpretations and other comments. The patient (perhaps unconsciously) takes the analyst's comments as suggestions, complies with them, and produces the requisite mental contents. The analyst then takes the patient's productions as evidence for his theory of repression.

We have taken a step in the direction recommended by Grünbaum. We have tested what may be called the compliance hypothesis against the repression concept and have found good evidence against the compliance hypothesis. The evidence is that Mrs. C, as reported above, became conscious of certain mental contents that the analyst had not interpreted or suggested in any way but, according to reliable independent ratings, were repressed by her at the beginning of her treatment. Moreover, the contents of which she became conscious were of the kind that our research group predicted would become conscious if her treatment was successful.

Our research lends strong support to the particular version of the higher mental functioning hypothesis presented in Chapter 1. It shows that Mrs. C, during the 100 sessions we studied, did a number of things unconsciously which she could have done only through the use of higher mental functions. For example, she controlled both the coming forth of previously repressed mental contents and the expression of previously inhibited behavior. She also devised an unconscious plan for changing her pathogenic beliefs and worked to carry it out by testing the beliefs in relation to the analyst.

Our findings, even if replicated repeatedly, would not rule out all unconscious automatic functioning. However, they would indicate that if such unconscious functioning does exist, its part in mental life is limited.

Our findings have significant implications for the theory of motivation. They point to the importance of the analytic patient's (and indeed of everyone's) wish to change his pathogenic beliefs and by doing so to overcome his problems. They also support the idea that the patient unconsciously may make plans for changing his pathogenic beliefs and that he may work unconsciously with the analyst to carry out these plans. They support the hypothesis that the psychoanalytic process is in essence a process by which the patient works in accordance with unconscious plans directed toward overcoming pathogenic beliefs. Since Mrs. C's plans during the last 100 sessions of her analysis were essentially the same as in the first 100 sessions of her analysis, our findings suggest that a patient may work for an entire analysis to change just a few pathogenic beliefs.

Our findings indicate the kinds of analytic interventions that are likely to help the patient, as well as those that are not. They also offer the analyst a guide as to when his interpretations are helpful and when they are not. Our findings suggest that the analyst may best help the patient by inferring his unconscious plans and helping him to carry them out. They suggest, too, that the analyst may assume that his interpretations are helpful if the patient reacts to them by moving toward his goals.

OUR RESEARCH METHOD: TESTING HYPOTHESES

In our investigations of psychoanalytic theory, we have tested particular psychoanalytic hypotheses, as opposed to testing a psychoanalytic theory that presumes to represent a consensus of what psychoanalysts believe. We have not tested a consensus theory for several reasons: First, there is no such thing; analysts today do not agree even about certain of the fundamental tenets of psychoanalytic theory. Second, the psychoanalytic theory (or, rather, the various versions of that theory) that comes closest to a consensus theory is organized in such a way that it cannot rigorously be tested. As pointed out in Chapter 2, the psychoanalytic theory that comes closest to a consensus theory is an omnibus theory, that is, a loosely organized mixture of hypotheses that are to varying degrees compatible with one another. Most analysts, for example, make use in their work of some concepts based on the automatic functioning hypothesis and some concepts based on the higher mental functioning hypothesis. Such an omnibus theory may be tested crudely against a nonpsychoanalytic theory, as, for example, a theory that denies the existence of unconscious mental life. However, an omnibus theory does not lend itself to being tested rigorously, because an omnibus theory, with its diverse and loosely organized set of concepts, is capable with certain *ad hoc* adjustments of explaining almost any finding.

We have not tested an omnibus psychoanalytic theory but rather two psychoanalytic theories, each of which is more logically consistent and highly organized than an omnibus theory. The one theory is a logically consistent clinical theory based on the automatic functioning hypothesis as this hypothesis is defined in the early theory. It assumes that all or almost all unconscious mental life may be derived from the interplay of psychic forces, which interact without regard for thought or current reality and are beyond the patient's control. It is more or less the same as the theory presented by Freud in the *Papers on Technique*. The other theory we tested (the one we favor) is a logically consistent clinical theory based on the higher mental functioning hypothesis. It is the theory developed by Weiss and presented in Part I. Though it does not rule out all automatic functioning, it assumes that a person exerts considerable control over his unconscious mental life, and that he regulates it in accordance with thoughts, beliefs, and assessments of current reality. The fact that the two theories we have tested are each more or less internally consistent and tightly organized has contributed to our being able rigorously to test the one against the other and to obtain evidence agianst the automatic functioning hypothesis. The fact that the theory based on the higher mental functioning hypothesis is relatively consistent and tightly organized has allowed us to test it in its own right (not against another theory but against observation) and to obtain support for it.

The disconfirmation of a broad, major scientific hypothesis is not possible, according to Thomas Kuhn (1962), until an alternative hypothesis has been developed. Until that point, findings that run counter to a prevailing and accepted theory (or hypothesis) are either attributed to poor measurement or accounted for by certain *ad hoc* explanations or certain *ad hoc* adjustments in the theory, as opposed to fundamental changes in it. If, however, contrary findings are repeatedly found to fit well with another theory, they may be judged to support the new theory and to disconfirm the old one.

We did what, according to Kuhn, an investigator must do if he is to begin to disconfirm a broad and established theory. That is, we tested a clinical theory based on the automatic functioning hypothesis against an equally evolved clinical theory based on the higher mental functioning hypothesis. We showed that the clinical theory based on the higher mental functioning hypothesis consistently fits observations better than the one based on the automatic functioning hypothesis.

The hypotheses we tested are derived from Freud's work and intended to explain those observations the analyst makes in his treatment of patients. They are hypotheses that underlie the concepts used by psychoanalysts today. This is because all psychoanalytic concepts are based, implicitly or explicitly, either on the automatic functioning hypothesis, on the higher mental functioning hypothesis, or on some combination of these. The fact that our findings challenge the automatic functioning hypothesis and support the higher mental functioning hypothesis should be of interest to all analysts.

EVIDENCE THAT A PATIENT MAY CHANGE OVER A LONG PERIOD OF TIME

A finding that does not fit the main theme of this book, but is of considerable practical as well as theoretical interest, is that Mrs. C made steady progress in a particular direction over a long period of time. She came, over the first 450 sessions of her treatment, to feel progressively more in control of her behavior.

We reported in Chapter 13 that Mrs. C came to feel progressively more in control of her behavior during the first 100 sessions of her analysis. This finding was based on the Drivenness Scale (Appendix 4), developed by Leonard Horowitz and applied to the first 100 sessions (Horowitz et al., 1978). This scale provides a direct measure of the patient's experience of conscious control over her behavior. It contains two kinds of complaint statements. According to the one kind, Mrs. C felt compelled to do something she did not consciously want to do. According to the other, she felt unable to do something she consciously wanted to do. This scale measures the frequency of such complaints over intervals of time. In the first 100 sessions, the number of Drivenness items per 20-hour block declined from 91 in sessions 1–20 to 52 in sessions 81–100. We[1] later applied the Drivenness Scale to two arbitrarily selected blocks of 20 hours. The findings, shown in Table 22-1, indicate a continuing

---

1. This study was carried out by Frances Sampson.

Table 22-1. Decline in Drivenness over Time as Demonstrated in 20-Hour Blocks

Blocks of sessions	Number of Drivenness items	Frequency per hour
1–20	91	4.5
21–40	83	4.1
41–60	58	2.9
61–80	67	3.3
81–100	52	2.6
$\chi^2 = 15.48, p < .01$		
191–210	38	1.9
434–453	29	1.5

decline in the patient's experience of drivenness well beyond the first 100 sessions. These findings demonstrate that the analytic patient may make continuing progress in overcoming problems for long periods of time.

FURTHER RESEARCH

Since the completion of this book, we have been replicating in various ways the research presented here. We have been studying the therapeutic process over Mrs. C's entire analysis. We have also been studying the therapeutic process in brief psychotherapy. Our recent research may be termed second-generation research in that it is derived from the work presented here but employs somewhat improved methods. We have, in our present work, obtained stronger findings than in the work presented here.

In this section we will comment on the brief psychotherapy studies, being carried out under the direction of George Silberschatz and John Curtis.[2] They are studying a large number of audio-recorded psychotherapies (of 16 sessions each) conducted by a number of therapists using a variety of psychodynamic approaches. In investigating these therapies, Curtis and Silberschatz have obtained transcripts of the patient's 16 ses-

2. Our brief psychotherapy studies were initiated by Saul Rosenberg in collaboration with George Silberschatz (NIMH Grant MH-34052). The reader interested in learning more about our current brief therapy studies may write to John Curtis and George Silberschatz, Department of Psychiatry, Mount Zion Hospital and Medical Center, P.O. Box 7921, San Francisco, CA 94120.

sions with the therapist, and of an intake interview and three follow-up interviews (at the end of therapy and at 6 and 12 months after termination).

Curtis, Silberschatz, and Saul Rosenberg have adapted Caston's plan diagnosis procedure (see Chapter 16) to the study of brief dynamic psychotherapies. They develop plan formulations for each of the brief therapies they study; these formulations are then used to determine, for example, the accuracy of therapist interventions (see below). As a first step in developing a plan formulation, a team of experienced clinicians (the clinical team) studies the verbatim transcripts of the intake interview and first two therapy hours and from these arrives at an agreed-upon written plan formulation for each case. Each formulation contains a description of the patient's presenting problems and history, as well as the following components: the patient's *goals* for therapy, the inner obstacles (*pathogenic beliefs*) preventing the attainment of these goals, the means by which the patient will work in therapy to disconfirm his pathogenic beliefs (*tests*), and the *insights* that will help the patient to attain his goals.

Next the clinical team, working from the written formulation, develops a list of concise statements of the patient's goals, his pathogenic beliefs, the tests he will use to work at disconfirming these beliefs, and the insights that will help him attain his goals. The clinical team then expands each list of components by adding less relevant items. To ensure the plausibility of the additional items the team uses the transcripts of the intake interview and the first two sessions to develop alternate case formulations and chooses the additional items from these. The clinical team also creates additional items by including some that are highly pertinent to other cases but not to the particular case.

After this, the clinical team rates all of the plan components in the expanded lists for their relevance to the particular case. Then a set of independent judges other than those on the clinical team (the reliability judges), after reading the same verbatim transcripts as did the clinical team, independently rates the expanded lists of items for their relevance to the case. The reliability of the plan formulation is determined by comparing the ratings of the reliability judges with one another and as a group with the ratings of the clinical team. Silberschatz, Curtis, and Rosenberg have found high levels of agreement for each of the plan components both among the reliability judges and between the reliability judges as a group and the clinical team. Thus, Silberschatz, Curtis, and Rosenberg have demonstrated that Caston's plan diagnosis method may be applied, with minor changes, to brief psychotherapies. Moreover, their method defines the components of the plan formulation more precisely, and assures that the alternative items rated by the judges are all plausible.

As noted, the plan formulation developed for each case is used to study the therapeutic process in that case. A study by Fretter (1984),[3] the theoretical significance of which has been highlighted by Silberschatz, Fretter, and Curtis (1986), illustrates one method by which this is done. Three brief psychotherapies were studied to investigate the effect on the patient's immediate progress of the therapist's interpretations. The hypothesis was that interpretations that the patient would experience as in accord with his unconscious plan for therapy would result in immediate progress, while other interpretations would not result in immediate progress or might, if the patient experienced them as contrary to his plan, even hinder him in making immediate progress.

Fretter began her investigation of this hypothesis by using a first set of independent judges to rate all the interpretations (selected as described below) of each therapy hour for their plan compatibility, that is, for the degree to which the interpretations were in accord with the patient's plan. The plan compatibility judges were "blind" to the patient's responses. Fretter used a second set of independent judges, blind to the analyst's interpretations, to study the patient's immediate response to each interpretation. She measured the patient's response by the change it produced in the degree to which the patient experienced the affects and ideas with which he was concerned. (She determined this change by comparing the level of experiencing that the patient manifested before and after each interpretation as measured by the Experiencing Scale [Klein et al., 1970]. This scale is considered a good measure for the study of the patient's progress in psychotherapy. A low score on the Experiencing Scale indicates that the patient is highly defensive and not progressing, a high score that he is not defensive and is progressing [see Chapter 12].)

Fretter now had the data to correlate the degree to which an interpretation was plan-compatible with the degree to which the patient, in response to the interpretation, was making progress as measured by the Experiencing Scale. She calculated the correlation of these two variables for each therapy hour, using the mean score for that hour for each variable. Significant correlations ranging from .6 to .8 between the plan compatibility of the therapist's interpretations and the Experiencing Scale scores in the responses were obtained for the three cases. These

---

3. This study was supervised by Silberschatz and Curtis.

results strongly support the hypothesis that the degree to which the therapist's interpretations are in accord with the patient's plan predicts the patient's subsequent capacity to discuss and experience feelings and ideas.

In the work cited above, Fretter demonstrated that certain of the methods used to study the therapeutic process in the first 100 sessions of Mrs. C's analysis can be applied, with certain changes, to the study of the process in brief psychotherapies. In this work Fretter improved upon the original methods of Caston *et al.* (Chapter 19) and Bush and Gassner (Chapter 20) in studying the impact of therapist interventions. Fretter carefully defined and selected the types of interventions studied, rather than trying to investigate the impact of *all* types of interventions. She eliminated all interventions that were not interpretive. By controlling for this source of variance, she identified significant interventions, that is, interventions to which the patient may be expected to react, and that judges may be expected to rate reliably. Moreover, Fretter not only compared individual interpretations with the subsequent patient responses but also (in contrast to Caston *et al.* and Bush and Gassner) correlated for each therapy hour the *mean* score of the patient's responses. By looking at hourly means, Fretter measured the patient's reactions not just to the last interpretation heard but to *all* of the therapist's recent interpretations. Thus, she measured what the patient in all likelihood responds to: the therapist's overall approach.

The work of Silberschatz *et al.* lends further support to the idea that the patient in either psychoanalysis or brief psychotherapy develops an unconscious plan for working with the therapist to overcome certain problems and to achieve certain goals. It supports the thesis that the patient during treatment is struggling to carry out plans for changing his pathogenic beliefs.

APPENDICES

APPENDIX 1. "D" SCALE; INSTRUCTIONS FOR RATING TYPE D BEHAVIORS

This study is based on the psychoanalysis of Mrs. C, a 28-year-old married woman. The passages you will see are excerpts from transcripts of her analytic sessions; they occur in random order. Each passage is a description or an instance of an episode in which Mrs. C blamed, criticized, disagreed with, opposed, or disapproved of someone (the analyst or some other person). Your task is to rate each behavior along a 4-point scale telling how directly the behavior was expressed. The scale values range from 1 to 4 as follows:

- "1" means that the behavior was only implied, not explicitly expressed, or was expressed with extreme uncertainty, tentativeness, or discomfort.
- "2" means that the behavior was expressed but then immediately undone (e.g., the patient changed her mind, excused the other person, criticized herself, etc.).
- "3" means that the behavior was expressed to some third person (e.g., the analyst), not to the offending party.
- "4" means that the behavior was expressed directly to the offending party.

Details about the scoring and examples of each score value follow. Please read the rules and examples first. Then rate each passage.

1. IMPLIED BLAME AND CRITICISM

Passages of this type contain hints of blaming, criticizing, etc., but the message is not explicit. The patient does not directly acknowledge the blaming and instead may seem to blame herself or be confused, vague, uncertain, and/or frustrated. A key word is *troubled*. She says that she is troubled by what someone (e.g., the therapist) does. Another variation is when the patient states her criticism as a vague generality rather than directing it towards any one person.

Examples of 1

She was also troubled with not getting any reactions from me, no interaction. She was afraid she needed approval.

It is very hard for her to suddenly be stopped when I call the time. When she gets to talking, her feelings well up and it is hard for her to get them under control. So, she feels somewhat upset.

Then she recalled her reaction to my question yesterday about what word she had used. She felt very uncomfortable and uncertain. When she knows somebody very well and they question her, she gets angry with them; otherwise, she tends to get defensive and is very tentative.

2. BLAME OR CRITICISM AND THEN UNDOING

In passages of this kind the patient blames or criticizes someone but then immediately undoes it by excusing the offender or criticizing herself for blaming. Typical comments that reflect the undoing are "Maybe it's all in my mind," "Maybe I'm wrong," "But then again, everybody does that," "But then again, I do that too," "Maybe I'm just using that as an excuse." Undoing is also assumed to occur when the patient blames someone but the passage indicates that she then became unsure, uncertain, or found herself wavering. The undoing may also occur in advance (e.g., "She's friendly, but she talks too much").

Examples of 2

Her father didn't understand how much that idea of feeling ugly meant to her. But then, that wasn't unusual, because he thought about himself first, and she thought about herself first, and so on.

When she goes home to visit her, her mother seems to her to be a rather critical person. But, the odd thing is that she cannot remember incidents of her mother being especially hard and critical. It was more as if she was silently disapproving much of the time except in cases where it was rather clear-cut that she had to disapprove. So the patient wondered if some of her attitude might be in herself more than in her mother.

Yesterday she just felt very frustrated. It's as though she's not getting anywhere. She felt almost "antagonistic," as though it is "your fault," but it isn't. She feels she is being totally unrealistic in her expectations of having all her problems solved in two weeks. That obviously cannot be so.

Next, the thoughts turned to the director at the agency, and the essence of this was that the director wanted the program run in a different fashion. She thinks she disagrees with him on this, but then, maybe she's wrong.

3. BLAME OR CRITICIZE A THIRD PERSON

In passages of this type, the patient complains about, criticizes or blames, or feels oppositional to some third person (her parents, a friend, a co-worker, etc.). The passage may report that she would like to confront the person or retaliate, but she has not yet done so.

Thus, it is important to differentiate between *feeling* oppositional or critical and *acting* in this manner. As explained below, acting defiant or hostile would be scored higher. Feeling oppositional or critical, as told to a third party, is scored 3. Sometimes the passage will say that she "was mean to" or "was angry at," and it will be unclear whether she was feeling or acting mean. When in doubt, assign the lower score of 3.

Examples of 3

She would like to retaliate. She would like to confront her parents with herself as a miserable example of what they have done. She was the way she was, and their smug self-congratulations made her quite angry when she thought about it.

When she was in the second grade, her eyesight was quite bad, and it wasn't known. She thinks in retrospect that the teacher should have known because she couldn't see the blackboard.

Then her other thoughts are about Barbara and how Barbara raises her own children. Barbara gets easily exasperated with the kids. Patient wonders how Barbara can really enjoy them. Mostly patient has the idea that Barbara treats her children as though they were a job, a duty, and it's duty that gets in the way.

She does not want to go because her parents will be there and friends of theirs. The trouble with going there is that she will fall into the role of the daughter of the house, and she anticipated being annoyed by her parents.

4. DIRECT CONFRONTATION OF SOMEONE

In this category, the patient reports that she directly confronted, criticized, defied, disagreed with, or acted harmfully toward someone; or she does so to the therapist.

Examples of 4

Then she mused about how the things that I do affect her differently at different times. She thought that on Friday as she was getting ready to leave, I stood way back in the room. It is such a small room anyway, as though I were trying to get away from her.

She began talking by saying that she had realized she had a certain feeling of anger toward me yesterday. Here she brings me all these ideas that she had, and I didn't give her any direction. It makes her feel like a child when she realizes this, and that distresses her also. She seems to feel that either she has to feel complete responsibility for everything that she does and that happens to her, or else she has to be a complete follower. She said she hadn't wanted to tell me about having felt angry with me; she was afraid of what my reaction might be.

Then she remembered a time when she wouldn't eat some turnips, and it just turned into a real battle with her mother. Patient went three meals without eating these turnips.

(I pointed out to her that referring to him as a male lead is even a way of removing herself from it.) She thinks it is more that he was a boy, and she would be interested in a boy, not a man.

APPENDIX 2. "C" SCALE; INSTRUCTIONS FOR RATING TYPE C BEHAVIORS

This study is based on the psychoanalysis of Mrs. C, a 28-year-old married social worker. The passages you will see are excerpts from transcripts of her analytic sessions; they occur in random order. Each passage is a description or an instance of an episode in which Mrs. C felt close or affectionate toward another person (the analyst or someone else). This includes feeling sympathetic, admiring, or wishing to be loved; as well as complimenting, agreeing with, cooperating with; or acting friendly or loving. Your task is to rate each behavior along a 4-point scale to tell how directly the behavior was expressed. The scale values range from 1 to 4 as follows:

- "1" means that either the feeling was only *implied* or it was expressed with extreme uncertainty, tentativeness, or discomfort.
- "2" means that the feeling or behavior was *expressed* but was then immediately *undone*, e.g., the patient changed her mind, retracted it, or shifted to some other feeling or behavior.
- "3" means that the feeling was expressed to a *third person* (e.g., the analyst) but not to the individual in question.
- "4" means that the behavior was expressed *directly* to the individual in question.

Details about the scoring and examples of each scale value follow. Please read the rules and examples first. Then rate each passage.

1. FEELING OF CLOSENESS IS IMPLIED BUT DISCREDITED OR EXPRESSED WITH DISCOMFORT

Passages of this type indicate some hint that the patient was probably feeling close, but she expressed confusion, uncertainty, or discomfort about the feeling or could not acknowledge it or carry it through.

This category is used to indicate that she is afraid of some feeling of closeness, feels it is weak, passive, or defective. The patient may passively need someone and feel dysphoric over that feeling: She is afraid of needing to feel close and regards it as a defect.

This category is also used when she indicates that to need another person, or to turn to or consult someone, makes her feel weak, defective, debased, or out of control.

If the patient stated that she wants to submit or needs to submit, that would *not* be a 1; but if she said that she gets uncomfortable observing this need in herself, it would be scored 1.

Examples of 1

She was also troubled with not getting any reactions from me. No interaction. She was afraid that maybe she needed approval.

It seems like only when Henry threatens to leave does he really seem to take on importance for her and then she feels some respect for him and that is very disturbing because she then has to admit that she needs him.

She said she is afraid of making me into some kind of a father figure which would answer all her needs.

Today she arranged to see her supervisor, which she doesn't very often do. She realized she never took problems to her supervisor. Patient feels that it is a weakness or that she is complaining.

2. FEELING CLOSE AND THEN IMMEDIATELY UNDOING

In passages scored 2, the patient states that she feels close to someone or expresses closeness behaviorally, but then she immediately undoes it by taking back the feeling or by shifting to an oppositional feeling or behavior. The following kinds of phrases often signal an undoing: "On the other hand," "But then again," "However."

Undoing is also assumed to occur when the patient feels close to someone and then becomes unsure, uncertain, or finds herself wavering.

Occasionally, the undoing occurs in advance (e.g., "If I can provoke my husband, then I can get close to him.")

Examples of 2

She referred to a woman that she had to dinner and how nice and free this woman was and yet how she felt compelled to think of something critical.

At the end of this past summer she had orgasms twice during intercourse. Since then she has simply been afraid to ever do it again because she will always be disappointed, and she has pushed Henry away much of the time since.

What she said at the end of the hour was trying to please me, she thought, but then she wondered why that should be necessary.

Her mother has been very affectionate and often is when she's there now. But she thinks it is too late for her mother to hug her now.

3. FEELING CLOSE TO SOMEONE EXPRESSED TO A THIRD PERSON

In passages of this type, the patient tells the therapist that she feels close to some third person (e.g., her husband, parents, a friend, a co-worker). She may state that she cares about, trusts, feels empathy for, or needs someone. She may compliment or admire and wish to emulate someone, or she may wish to comply and cooperate with someone.

In many cases that would be scored 3, the patient tells the analyst that she *felt* friendly or affectionate toward someone. On the other hand, if the patient *acted* in a friendly or affectionate way towards that person, the score would be higher, as explained below. Thus, it is important to differentiate between *feeling* friendly and *acting* friendly. Feeling friendly, as to a third party, is scored 3. Sometimes the item will say that she "was friendly," and then it will be unclear as to whether she was feeling friendly or acting friendly. When in doubt, assign the lower score, 3. In the same way, differentiate between the *feeling* "she wanted intercourse" and the *behavior* "she had intercourse." The *feeling* is scored 3, the *behavior* will be scored 4.

Examples of 3

On the other hand, Betty's parents were great. She just loved Betty's father, who was very genuine and sincere.

She's thinking about whom she has ever trusted. She had one close friend in high school that she had real feeling for.

She had a funny reaction to Henry this weekend, needing him in contrast to before.

Then she said she wanted Henry to want to have intercourse with her.

4. FEELING CLOSE DIRECTLY EXPRESSED

In passages of this type, the patient, through her verbal or nonverbal behavior, directly expresses her feeling of closeness to somebody (e.g., she directly expresses her concern for someone; she compliments directly, laughs with, or acts affectionately toward another person). Passages in this category reflect a shared mutuality with the other person. If she consults someone's advice, that would be scored 4. Likewise, when she reports agreeing with, dancing with, getting along with, or having intercourse with someone, the item should be scored 4.

Examples of 4

She said I looked very tired. She was thinking if I am tired, what would make me so, and then she felt concern about me.

Then she said she just realized that actually she had intercourse Sunday morning.

She recalled again asking her father how should she behave when she wanted to date as a teenager, how should a girl be with a boy?

(I said I thought that the issue which she had forgotten at the end of the hour yesterday was relevant here.) She immediately said it was true, that as a matter of fact, when she had first thought of whatever it was, she thought it was really there in her mind until she tried to work out what it was.

APPENDIX 3. FREEDOM VERSUS BELEAGUERMENT SCALE; INSTRUCTIONS TO RATERS

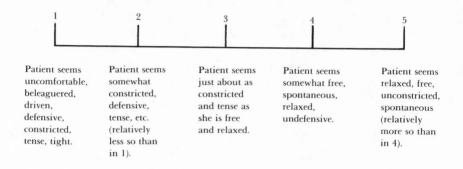

1	2	3	4	5
Patient seems uncomfortable, beleaguered, driven, defensive, constricted, tense, tight.	Patient seems somewhat constricted, defensive, tense, etc. (relatively less so than in 1).	Patient seems just about as constricted and tense as she is free and relaxed.	Patient seems somewhat free, spontaneous, relaxed, undefensive.	Patient seems relaxed, free, unconstricted, spontaneous (relatively more so than in 4).

The enclosed pages contain verbatim segments from the first 100 hours of a psychoanalysis. The patient is an attractive 28-year-old married social worker whose major presenting problem is her inability to enjoy and unwillingness to have sexual relations with her husband. In addition to her sexual problem, the patient also complains of feeling chronically tense, self-critical, overly serious, and unable to relax and be lighthearted. As a result, she feels that she has trouble interacting comfortably with other people.

You will be asked to rate each segment along a dimension of how free or relaxed the patient is as opposed to how anxious or driven she seems. This dimension represents an inferred state of the patient, so you will need to incorporate a variety of cues in making your ratings. The following are cues for inferring *freedom and relaxation*:

a. When the patient is able to associate freely, easily, and flexibly.
b. When the patient is able to be playful with ideas and explore connections between thoughts in an uninhibited, spontaneous manner.
c. When she is able to experience and explore her feelings freely and undefensively.

The following are cues for inferring anxiety, beleaguerment, and drivenness:

a. When the patient is defensive, constricted, or narrow in her associations.
b. When she feels beleaguered or compelled by things beyond her control.
c. When the patient feels anxious, tense, rigid, tight, or grim.
d. When she seems halting, timid, or bothered by her train of thoughts, and when her associations come with difficulty.
e. When she seems stuck, without vitality or hope.

Please read the rating scale carefully and then study the examples below (try to rate each example yourself before looking at the correct rating). The scale is a 5-

point continuous rating scale. If you are rating a segment that falls between a rating of 2 and 3, for example, then you may rate it 2.5. If you feel the segment is closer to a rating of 2 then you may rate it 2.2. or 2.3; similarly, if you feel the segment is closer to a 3 then you may rate if 2.7 or 2.8. In other words, you are free to use the entire range of the rating scale.

(All of the examples are taken from process notes, so that they read like a narrative rather than like a direct transcript. When you actually do the task, you'll be reading from transcripts.)

Example 1

The mother was tall and attractive. The thing that occurred to the patient was that the mother and the son seemed to be truly affectionate with one another. Silence again. Again she thought about her playgroup and how she treats the members of the playgroup and how much she feels that she herself is doing what she had said her mother did. It is true that at times she does enjoy the children but most of the time she doesn't enjoy them. She must seem very grim. The mother of one of the boys requested that she do something and she had completely forgotten about it. Again silence. It's strange, usually by Friday she feels she has so much to say but not today. She feels she's resisting something. Another silence. (Rating: 3.0)

Example 2

It's just that she's so rigid; even if she knows what she's supposed to do, she's rigid. It just shouldn't be that important. Then she laughed and said that actually in point of fact, she had walked through some place and her skirt had knocked over a box of paints and she had made more of a mess than the kids had. This is just exactly like her father. They could break something and he would be very angry and upset with them; on the other hand, he could clown around and then take some dishes out to the kitchen and drop something and break it and that was perfectly all right. But if the kids did it, it was a horrible offense. What bothers her is that all this should be so important and she knows she was upsetting the children and she knows she was in the wrong.

She contrasted this with the feeling she has had recently. Sometimes when she feels she's doing the right thing, that even if it doesn't work out and she's firm, she doesn't feel upset. However, this whole week she's been picking on the kids, she's been finding fault all week with them and it seems that is all she has been doing; maybe not, but that's what it feels like. (Rating: 4.0)

Example 3

She doesn't imagine anything. She just feels tense, tight, nervous and upset. Then she said if someone is not interested in her she makes special efforts to be friendly. If she feels they are interested then she doesn't do that. Then more about how she just always felt disapproved of at home and she supposed she earned it because she was unpleasant. Then she returned to the notion of her not having anything to say, not doing what she was supposed to do, etc. (Rating: 1.0)

Example 4

On the other hand, she does get relief sometimes when she just goes ahead and says it. She realizes that it won't be magical, it is not going to be any cure like that. It's as though she has learned what is not going to happen but she is not at all sure what will happen. Silence. And she also said she feels passive and has the idea if she breaks something down she has to build it up again. She has certain responsibilities. Silence. And she said she finds this being silent upsetting. She thinks I must be bored with her. She just wants to withdraw. She'd like to be interested as well as to be interesting. Silence.

She went to a party last night with Henry. It was the kind of party where you had to walk around and talk to many different people. She didn't want to burden people so she made it easy for them to get away from her. This fellow was somehow hard to talk with. It would have been better if she could have thought of something to say. He finally did so to break the silence but it was just difficult and it ought to be her responsibility. (Rating: 2.5)

Example 5

She saw herself with a stick and yet she remembers her brother having a stick once. The main point of this was that she had the idea of wanting to kill her brother and hitting him is in the same category. It just horrifies her to see how powerful such things are in her. Then she was silent. Then she said, there's a thought that occurred to her now that she has had before and she has elected to not say it before, but now she is going to say it. This has to do with her feelings about touching herself in her vagina. She wonders if it is because of the accident, but she finds it extremely hard to touch herself or for Henry to touch her. She thinks it is just ugly and it makes her extremely uncomfortable. (Rating: 5.0)

In the segments that you will be rating, there is apt to be a good deal of range on this rating scale; that is, there will probably be at least a few ratings of 1, 2, 3, and so on through 5. In some of the material, there will also be fluctuations within the segments. Your task is to *assign one overall rating to each segment*, so try to form a *general impression of the segment as a whole.*

Before beginning the rating procedure, please turn to the *last* eight segments and read them quickly (without making any ratings) so that you will get some idea of the range of segments. After reading these segments turn to the *first* segment, read it carefully, and then record your rating on the scoring sheet provided. *Please be sure to enter the code from the upper right-hand corner of each segment in the space provided on the scoring sheet.* You should try to work for about an hour at a time whenever possible with a copy of the rating scale in front of you. It is essential that you begin each new rating session by carefully reading the scale and looking over the last few segments you rated.

The segments were selected without regard for length, so don't let mere length affect your ratings.

APPENDIX 4. DRIVENNESS SCALE; INSTRUCTIONS TO RATERS

These are the instructions used by Leonard Horowitz and his group of judges, with additional refinements made by Frances Sampson based on a second group of judges' experience in trying to duplicate Horowitz's application of his instructions. The modifications are intended to simplify the task of others who may want to apply this scale.

Your task is to find all passages that indicate that Mrs. C was having poor control over her behavior. At times, for example, she complains that she has some disability—that she can't focus on a topic, or that she can't enjoy her work, make decisions, or end a conversation when she wants to. Phrases like "I can't," "It is hard to," and "It feels too selfish to" are important kinds of markers of such disabilities. Other less direct expressions will occur to you, too. For example, in one passage the patient asked the analyst "if it was better to force herself to say things if she doesn't feel ready to say them." This passage can be taken to mean: She finds it hard to say things.

Other examples of poor control occur when the patient reports a compulsive or obligatory behavior. She may report that she *has to* tell what is on her mind, or that she *has to* find fault with another person. This kind of passage may take alternate forms (e.g., "She found herself being harsh and abrupt, and she wishes she didn't have to be").

The goal is to find all instances in which the patient says she *can't* do something or *has to* do something. Look for "can't (do)," "am afraid to (do)," "have difficulty (doing)," "have to (do)," or "need to (do)." Also look for "wishes" she could do. Be sure that it involves a behavior (a *do*), which can include thoughts and ideas, since the point is that she has difficulty translating some impulse into *behavior* (e.g., "I am afraid to be unclear, to let my thoughts just ramble.") Treat the following as equivalent:

- "I am afraid to be unclear."
- "I am afraid for my thoughts to be unclear."
- "I have difficulty being unclear."
- "I can't be unclear."

FORMS NOT TO INCLUDE

In applying these we tried to get the sense of what was intended by each, and how Horowitz's judges had actually applied them by studying his items.

I. Statement of strong wishes
   a. "I need to know where I stand with a person."
   b. "I need your approval."
   c. "I am afraid I need your approval."

(The relevant issue seems to be that none of these include a behavior by the patient; they would be counted if stated as "need to ask," "need to seek," "need to get"; "need to have" would not count.)

II. Dislikes
  a. "I can't stand that feeling."
    ("Have to feel" or "can't let self feel" would count.)
  b. "I worried about crying during the hour."
  c. "I am afraid that I shall be late."
  (If this is a matter of style, politeness in speech, or external circumstances, or just an expression of concern without the force of an internal compulsion either to be late or not to be, exclude it; same with the rest here.)
  d. "I don't like to be late."
  e. "I was troubled being the center of attention."
  f. "Sometimes I gossip but I hate myself for that."
  g. "Naming people makes it all too close."

III. Don't know fact or don't know how to
  a. "I can't remember whether I told you this before, but . . . ."
  (As opposed to "can't let self remember" a certain thing, which she must state pretty directly or make the inference unavoidable that she feels it as a compulsion.)
  b. "I was troubled being the center of attention; I didn't know what to say."

IV. Refusal to believe or denial of something
  (Decision hard when referent is own behavior; include it if it has a sense of a positive or negative compulsion and isn't excluded on other grounds, e.g., VI, XI, or XII.)
  a. "I could not believe that he really wanted me."
  b. "When we broke up, I couldn't accept it."

V. Conflict
  a. "I am always in conflict: Should I do this or that?"

VI. Conditionals
  (These are sometimes hard to decide; base your decisions on which element seems predominant: the compulsion or some element of simply spelling out conditions of behavior—"When someone says this I *have to* say that, or when someone says this I say that.")
  a. "If X, then I will feel foolish or then I won't be able to do X."
  b. "If X, I can, but if Y, I cannot."
  c. "If I had more confidence, then maybe I would be able to criticize them."
  d. "Here's what will happen: First A, then B, then I will feel foolish."

VII. Question
  a. She asked if she should force herself to talk if she's not ready.

VIII. Self-description as trait: regularity rather than compulsion
  a. "I tend to forget things.
  b. "I feel stupid."

    c. "I am always worrying about things."

    d. "I feel guilty if I enjoy myself."

IX. Comment on an unexplained relationship

    a. "I can't figure out why that should be."

    b. "I chose social work because I couldn't think of anything else."

X. Statement of behavior

    a. "I found myself stifling their question."

       (Not a "can't" or "have to.")

    b. "For so long, I was hostile to my mother."

    c. "I have nothing to say."

XI. Overcame a disability

    a. "I forced myself to talk in the meeting."

       (Not *had to* force.)

XII. Formerly I couldn't but now I can

    a. "In the past I had to work, but now I do not."

XIII. A disability is itself the subject or object of a sentence

    (Exclude if it really seems subordinate to some other point she's making.)

    a. "I use my inability to express feeling as a way of . . . ."

XIV. Uncertainty about some disability

    a. "I don't know where I could . . . ."

XV. Ought to and should

"I should control my feelings."

XVI. Specific detail, not a general disability: Couldn't do a specific thing at a specific time and place

    (The point here is whether the barrier was an internal compulsion or something external, circumstantial, or such, e.g., don't exclude if phrasing really says "I couldn't *let* myself find her, or understand him.")

    a. "I looked for my mother and couldn't find her."

    b. "The Negro boy said something she couldn't understand."

In general, exclude anything that seems too inferential, even though the inference seems sound, or where the phrasing leaves doubt as to whether she's referring to an *internal* prohibition–compulsion. We are not interested here in clinical inferences (e.g., don't infer that if she says she likes to do something it's because she's really afraid not to, etc.).

Count as one item any item which is repeated many times in a single session, or a couldn't/had to expressed as a single thought with the same referent behavior. Count as separate items any items with separate referent behaviors (e.g., couldn't think, do, speak, handle, etc.) that appear as separate disabilities, even though contained in the same content sequence. For example:

- "I couldn't do it" repeated many times in various words = 1 item.
- "I couldn't do it, I couldn't think about it" = 2 items.

- "I had to do it because I couldn't do it" = 1 item.
- "I couldn't sing and I couldn't dance either" = probably 2 items. (In each case if she's talking about an inhibition, not a lack of talent, opportunity, or whatever.)
- "I had to do *this* because I couldn't do *that* = 2 items if both are compulsions or prohibitions.

APPENDIX 5. INSTRUCTIONS FOR SELECTING ITEMS CONCERNING IRRATIONAL IDEAS

1. An "item" is a discrete unit. Even though the theme of an entire hour may be "insight into omnipotence," the entire hour is not an item. Each discrete instance in which she discusses the problem is an item.

2. Do not use inference in selecting items. The unconscious expression of an impulse is not insight. It is not an item if she mentions some derivative form of controlling others that you know is theoretically related to omnipotence. *She* must state it. If she does not, then she does not have insight into the behavior. For example, do not select items in which she mentions *only* her difficulty getting close to people. Although *you* know that this is related to her fear of controlling them, *she* does not know it at that point.

3. An item involves her explicit discussion of an incident in which she was involved and her concern about its interpersonal effects. Therefore,

a. It is not an item if the analyst brings up the subject, and she merely agrees with him (e.g., "You must have been angry." "Yes, I was angry.").
b. It is not an item if she talks about someone else's control.
c. It is not an item if she says she was controlling herself.

4. The expression of anger or aggression *per se* is not insight. Do not select items in which her only comment is "I feel angry." The item should show some additional thought on her part, such as "I don't know why I feel angry; it bothers me to feel angry." The important element in these items is her increasing *insight* into her difficulties with omnipotence.

5. You must consider the context.

a. Just because she uses the word "fighting" or "controlling" does not mean she is talking about hostility or aggression. (For example, when she mentions "fighting something coming into her mind," that is not fighting, that is withholding or resistance.)
b. Do not include items that discuss criticism, but where the focus is on her difficulty *being criticized* rather than her difficulty criticizing. Similarly, do not include items that discuss fighting, but where the focus is on her difficulty submitting rather than on her difficulty fighting.

6. Not all unpleasant emotions are related to her fears of hurting or controlling others. This scale deals with her problems around fighting, blaming, and criticizing. Feelings of jealousy, possessiveness, or competiveness are not fighting; they are related to fears of being left out or deprived. Therefore, do not include these items.

APPENDIX 6. LEVEL OF AWARENESS INTO IRRATIONAL FEELINGS OF RESPONSIBILITY AND GUILT

This scale is concerned with the patient's increasing insight into issues of omnipotence and control of others during the first 100 hours of her analysis.

STAGE 1

Patient feels that she is weak, helpless, impotent, or unable to exert control in interpersonal situations, so that she cannot do things she wants to, or feels compelled to do things that she does not want to. She does not experience guilt because she doesn't feel responsible or in control of her thoughts or actions.

Examples

    a. Although she did not want to visit her aunt, she just couldn't say no.
    b. She wanted to behave differently, but she found herself doing the same old thing.
    c. She just had to be argumentative.

STAGE 2

Patient still feels unable to exert control, but she recognizes a vague sense of guilt and/or responsibility for others that she cannot account for or knows is unreasonable. The guilt is connected to (1) something she didn't do, but thought she should have or (2) something she did or thought but doesn't know why she should feel so guilty. Her insight at this stage is that she feels guilty for "something" but she is unaware of the omnipotent thoughts that are causing the guilt.

Examples

    a. 1. She feels disturbed that she wasn't nicer to her friend.
       2. She feels responsible when people criticize someone close to her.
       3. She feels bothered when she thinks of herself as selfish.
    b. 1. She's bothered by the thought that her girlfriend is not very pretty.
       2. She thinks she feels guilty because she went to the movies alone.

STAGE 3

Patient now feels that she can control others and is bothered by that feeling. She may express concern that she can harm others by this control. She may talk of feeling guilty, worried, frightened, or uncomfortable about controlling or harming others by her thoughts, actions, or lack of actions. She now has insight into the cause of her feelings of excessive responsibility (i.e., her idea that she can control and thus harm people).

Examples

   a. She can hurt people, if she isn't careful.
   b. She remembers once thinking she wanted to kill her best friend, and that is just awful.
   c. She thinks it is terrible that she can make people obey her.

STAGE 4

Patient feels she can control others without being bothered by that feeling. She feels powerful without guilt. She may even enjoy feeling powerful, strong, or controlling.

Examples

   a. She can make people obey her.
   b. She really enjoys making people obey her.

STAGE 5

Patient is engaged in an attempt to assess realistically the extent of her ability to control others. As part of this assessment she may distinguish between her thoughts and her actions, or she may attempt to anticipate the realistic consequences of her actions, even if this assessment is difficult for her to make.

Examples

   a. She's trying to figure out just how much control she really has over others.
   b. She realizes it's not what she did that bothers her, but rather what she was thinking.

APPENDIX 7. PLAN DIAGNOSIS RELIABILITY MEASURES; DETERMINATION OF PLAN FOR ACCOMPANYING CLINICAL MATERIAL

I. GOALS

In this section you are presented with a list of specific *concrete* behaviors which the patient may possibly want to attain. In each case, you will designate to what degree the itemized behavior is likely to be either an immediate or eventual goal. You will rate each item in *both* categories. You may use intermediate values if you wish.

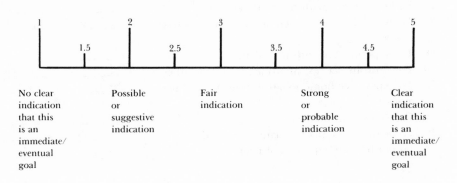

1	2	3	4	5
	1.5	2.5	3.5	4.5
No clear indication that this is an immediate/eventual goal	Possible or suggestive indication	Fair indication	Strong or probable indication	Clear indication that this is an immediate/eventual goal

	Immediate goal	Eventual goal
1. To think clearly.	_____	_____
2. To express doubts about the validity of psychoanalysis.	_____	_____
3. To not be preoccupied with somatic symptoms.	_____	_____
4. To be dependent.	_____	_____
5. To let herself feel confused.	_____	_____
6. To become conscious of her penis envy.	_____	_____
7. To enjoy being the center of attention.	_____	_____
8. To masturbate without guilt.	_____	_____
9. To actively get the analyst to respond.	_____	_____
10. To not care what her parents think about her.	_____	_____
11. To become pregnant.	_____	_____
12. To be arrogant.	_____	_____
13. To accept the analyst's observations as true.	_____	_____
14. To tell her parents they have been inadequate.	_____	_____
15. To respond to the analyst's activity.	_____	_____
16. To be in control in her marriage.	_____	_____
17. To leave other people without worrying about them.	_____	_____

18. To admire people. _____ _____
19. To be modest. _____ _____
20. To compete with her mother. _____ _____
21. To give her husband control in the marriage. _____ _____
22. To be firm with her clients. _____ _____
23. To acknowledge her sense of being physically defective. _____ _____
24. To face her envy of the analyst. _____ _____
25. To enjoy sex with her husband. _____ _____
26. To be stubborn with the analyst. _____ _____
27. To enjoy the idea of men being sexually attracted to her. _____ _____
28. To be permissive with her clients. _____ _____
29. To confront her sexual attraction to her father. _____ _____
30. To experience homosexual feelings toward her mother. _____ _____
31. To criticize the analyst. _____ _____
32. To be the good girl her parents wanted. _____ _____
33. To not be contemptuous of people. _____ _____

II. OBSTRUCTIONS

In the following list of possible obstructions indicate the degree to which each is likely to be operative in the patient, according to the following scale:

1	2	3	4	5
1.5	2.5	3.5	4.5	
Unlikely	Possibly likely	Fairly likely	Strongly or probably	Definitively operative

Rating

1. Defensive need to defer to men in order not to devastate them. _____
2. Defensive identification with her mother. _____
3. Guilt about being stimulating if she exhibits herself. _____
4. Guilt about hurting people if she excludes them. _____
5. Defensive need to defy the analyst. _____

6. Defensive need to conceal feelings of superiority. _____
7. Defensive need to share pleasure with others. _____
8. Defensive need to make men omnipotent. _____
9. Shame about being physically defective. _____
10. Fear of unconscious homosexual impulses. _____
11. Fear of being in control. _____
12. Fear of criticism because of narcissistic injury. _____
13. Guilt about omnipotent fantasies of power over the analyst. _____
14. Fear about sexual excitement. _____
15. Defensive need to submit to the analyst. _____
16. Defensive need to dominate men. _____
17. Shame of revealing weakness. _____
18. Fear of being out of control. _____
19. Defensive need to establish a relationship with analyst. _____
20. Fear of being competitive with other women. _____

III. SUMMARY STATEMENT OF MRS. C'S IMMEDIATE GOAL

For this task, refer to Chapter 16 under the section "The Second Study: The Case of Mrs. C".

IV. TESTS AND INTERVENTIONS

In this exercise, actual references to the text indicate possible testing by the patient. Based on the summary immediate goal which you chose in the preceding section, decide whether the patient's testing activity is relevant to this immediate goal (i.e., is powerful and plan-relevant or not). The most powerful and plan-relevant instance is one which is either a clear-cut hero's or coward's choice in terms of the immediate goal (means). Rate the "test" on this 5-point scale:

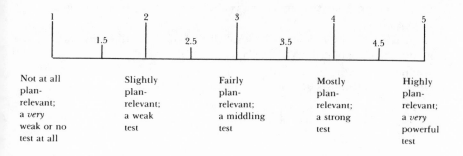

1	2	3	4	5
1.5	2.5	3.5	4.5	

Not at all plan-relevant; a *very* weak or no test at all	Slightly plan-relevant; a weak test	Fairly plan-relevant; a middling test	Mostly plan-relevant; a strong test	Highly plan-relevant; a *very* powerful test

Test

Secondly, you will rate actual interventions or analyst's responses to the test, and some hypothetical ones, in terms of whether they are facilitative toward the specific goal (means) which you have designated, on the following scale:

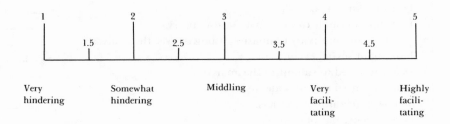

| Very hindering | Somewhat hindering | Middling | Very facilitating | Highly facilitating |

Intervention

1. (P. 1, top) Patient's hesitancy and difficulty focusing.　　Test _____
2. (P. 1, middle) Analyst comments lack of focus enables her not to talk.　　Intervention _____
3. (P. 1, further down) Analyst comments her difficulty accepting freedom of situation.　　Intervention _____
4. (P. 1, bottom and 1A, top) Patient describes parents' ignoring her, then refers to her own competitiveness.　　Test _____
5. (P. 1A, top) Analyst does not comment on #4.　　Intervention _____
6. (P. 1A, middle) Patient asks if she can raise question about time of meeting.　　Test _____
7. (P. 2, about lines 13–14) In response to patient's stated fear of needing approval, what if the analyst had responded, "Perhaps instead you are afraid of *not* needing the approval?"　　Intervention _____
8. (P. 2, bottom) Patient describes pushing thoughts out of her mind and being guilty about silence.　　Test _____
9. (P. 2, bottom) Analyst suggests she is afraid rather than guilty.　　Intervention _____
10. (P. 2, bottom) In relation to #8 above, what if the analyst had responded, "You mean, you feel like you don't have the freedom to *not* talk?"　　Intervention _____
11. (P. 2A, about lines 7–16) Patient's discussion about being ugly.　　Test _____
12. (P. 3, top) Patient's query about the ladies room.　　Test _____

13. (P. 3, top) Patient is late and talks about fighting against letting things come to her mind.   Test _____

14. (P. 3, middle) After being silent, patient asks if she should force herself to say things even if she does not feel ready.   Test _____

15. (P. 3, middle) Analyst responds by asking patient if she remembers the rule.   Intervention _____

16. (P. 3, middle) What if analyst had said, "You are implying you need me to tell you what to do."   Intervention _____

17. (P. 3, middle) What if analyst had said, "Yes. You should try to say what comes to mind even if it is difficult to do so."   Intervention _____

18. (P. 3, middle) In response to patient's pleasure that the other girl had panicked, what if analyst had said, "So, feeling stronger than the other person felt good to you?"   Intervention _____

19. (P. 3B, middle) Patient talks about being an unconscious flirt and worries about leading a man beyond the point where he will stop.   Test _____

20. (P. 3, near bottom) In response to patient's concern about becoming upset with "lack of response" with her husband, and by implication in the sessions, what if analyst had observed, "Yet, you don't *seem* very upset about my lack of response today."   Intervention _____

21. (P. 4A, top) Patient refers to having been late last session and asks what she should do.   Test _____

22. (P. 4A, top) Patient's question about the people in the front office leaving and how would the analyst know she was there.   Test _____

23. (P. 4A, middle) Patient talks about being afraid of crying in the hour and successfully controlling that.   Test _____

24. (P. 4A, middle) Analyst comments in relation to #23 that the patient felt as if she were in the presence of her father.   Intervention _____

25. (P. 4A, middle) What if the analyst had suggested she was uncomfortable controlling herself.   Intervention _____

26. (P. 4B, top) Patient talks about parents' smug self-congratulations and her wish to retaliate by confronting them with herself as a miserable example of what they have done.   Test _____

27. (P. 4B, top) Analyst comments on #26 that she might be uncertain whether to tell her parents she is in analysis.   Intervention _____

28. (P. 4B, bottom and 4C, top) Patient's discussion about past ills and somatic issues. Test _____

29. (Sessions 3 & 4) Analyst does not interpret or inquire into patient's lateness. Intervention _____

30. (Sessions 3 & 4) Patient refers to feelings of physical illness during the hours. Test _____

31. (P. 4C, top) Patient says before analysis she had many things she wanted to talk about, now she notices her tendency to forget them. Test _____

32. (P. 5, top) Patient is troubled because people at the agency criticize her colleague. Test _____

33. (P. 5, top) Patient describes wanting reassurance about the phone call with her parents and going to her husband. Test _____

34. (P. 5, top) Analyst points out she did not mention her concern in analysis but went to her husband instead. Intervention _____

35. (P. 5B, bottom) Patient is silent, then mentions her need to find fault with people before she can be close to them. Test _____

36. (P. 5B, bottom) Analyst wonders whether she has criticisms of him she has not mentioned. Intervention _____

37. (P. 5C, middle) Patient falls silent after talking about grabbing instructor's nubby tie. Test _____

38. (P. 5C, middle) Analyst does not comment on silence. Intervention _____

APPENDIX 8. PATIENT SCALE OF KEY UNCONSCIOUS WISHES (APPLIED BY THE AF JUDGES)

0	1	2	3	4	5	6
Segment is *not an example* of the patient's expressing a wish or attempting to elicit a response from the analyst.	Segment is a *rather poor example* of the patient's expressing a wish or attempting to elicit a response from the analyst.	Segment is a *weak example* of the patient's expressing a wish or attempting to elicit a response from the analyst.	Segment is a *moderate example* of the patient's expressing a wish or attempting to elicit a response from the analyst.	Segment is a *good but somewhat weak example* of the patient's expressing a wish or attempting to elicit a response from the analyst.	Segment is a *good example* of the patient's expressing a wish or attempting to elicit a response from the analyst.	Segment is an *excellent, clear-cut example* of the patient's expressing a wish or attempting to elicit a response from the analyst.

APPENDIX 9. ANALYST SCALE OF GRATIFYING VERSUS FRUSTRATING KEY UNCONSCIOUS WISHES (APPLIED BY THE AF JUDGES)

0	1	2	3	4	5	6
Analyst's response is *clearly non-neutral*; the analyst in effect gratifies the patient's wish. He may console the patient when she seeks consolation, reassure her, punish her, etc.	Analyst's response is *non-neutral*; he gratifies the patient's wish albeit in a somewhat subtle fashion. His consolation, reproach, punishment, etc., is more subtle than in 0.	Analyst's response is *mildly non-neutral*; his gratification of the patient's wish is extremely subtle, but his response remains more non-neutral than neutral.	Analyst's response is either ambiguous or falls midway between neutral and non-neutral. The response may contain both neutral and non-neutral aspects, *but these are not explicit enough to warrant a higher or a lower rating.*	Analyst's response is *mildly neutral*; there are no non-neutral aspects to his response, but the neutral aspects are not sufficiently explicit or clear to warrant a higher rating.	Analyst's response is *neutral*; it contains the elements described in 6 but it is less clear.	Analyst's response is an *excellent, clear-cut example of a neutral intervention*; the patient's wish is in effect frustrated. The analyst may ask for clarification, he may remain silent, interpret the patient's wish or demand, etc., but he does not gratify the patient's wish.

APPENDIX 10. PATIENT SCALE OF KEY TESTS (APPLIED BY THE HMF JUDGES)

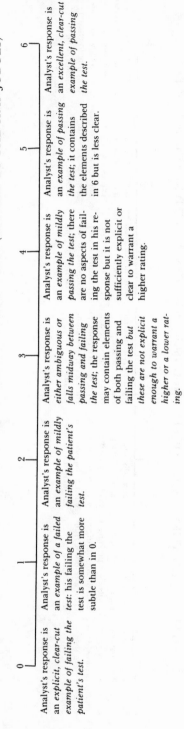

0

Segment is *not an example* of the patient testing the analyst.

1

Segment is a *rather poor example* of the patient testing the analyst.

2

Segment is a *weak example* of the patient testing the analyst.

3

Segment is a *moderate example* of the patient testing the analyst.

4

Segment is a *good but somewhat weak example* of the patient testing the analyst.

5

Segment is a *good example* of the patient testing the analyst.

6

Segment is an *excellent, clear-cut example* of the patient testing the analyst.

APPENDIX 11. ANALYST SCALE OF PASSING VERSUS FAILING TESTS (APPLIED BY THE HMF JUDGES)

0

Analyst's response is an *explicit, clear-cut example of failing the patient's test.*

1

Analyst's response is an *example of a failed test:* his failing the test is somewhat more subtle than in 0.

2

Analyst's response is an *example of mildly failing the patient's test.*

3

Analyst's response is *either ambiguous or falls midway between passing and failing the test;* the response may contain elements of both passing and failing the test *but these are not explicit enough to warrant a higher or a lower rating.*

4

Analyst's response is an *example of mildly passing the test;* there are no aspects of failing the test in his response but it is not sufficiently explicit or clear to warrant a higher rating.

5

Analyst's response is an *example of passing the test;* it contains the elements described in 6 but is less clear.

6

Analyst's response is an *excellent, clear-cut example of passing the test.*

APPENDIX 12. INTERCORRELATIONS AMONG THE PATIENT MEASURES ($N = 102$)

	Experiencing	Boldness	Relaxation	Love	Satisfaction	Fear	Anxiety
Experiencing	1.00	.22*	.05	.23*	.22*	−.07	.17
Boldness	.22*	1.00	.26*	.12	.05	.29*	.04
Relaxation	.05	.26*	1.00	.21*	.18	.02	−.31*
Love	.23*	.12	.21*	1.00	.54*	.15	−.07
Satisfaction	.22*	.05	.18	.54*	1.00	.08	−.03
Fear	.13	.29*	.02	.15	.08	1.00	−.11
Anxiety	.17	.04	−.31*	.07	−.03	−.11	1.00

*$p < .05$, two-tailed test.

APPENDIX 13. PLAN COMPATIBILITY OF INTERVENTIONS SCALE (CASTON; PILOT STUDY[1] AND REPLICATION STUDY)

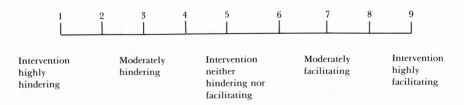

| 1 | 2 | 3 | 4 | 5 | 6 | 7 | 8 | 9 |

Intervention highly hindering | Moderately hindering | Intervention neither hindering nor facilitating | Moderately facilitating | Intervention highly facilitating

EFFECTS OF THERAPEUTIC INTERVENTIONS: INSTRUCTIONS TO RATERS

We are studying the immediate effects of analyst's interventions on a patient in psychoanalysis. Essentially, your task will be to rate the analyst's interventions according to a 9-point scale which indicates whether these are likely to have facilitated or hindered the patient's progress toward given therapeutic goals. You will, of course, not know what the patient's actual *response* to each intervention was.

The criteria for rating an intervention as either facilitating or hindering are *specific* for the case used in this study. The criteria were developed from the actual

1. A 5-point version of this scale was used for the pilot study.

context of the first 100 hours of this case. The therapeutic goal which was actually realized and the specific process by which it was achieved have been conceptualized and set forth below. It is necessary to famliarize yourself very well with this summary, because your judgment of an intervention as faciliating or hindering is entirely based on whether the intervention serves the *specific* process, as outlined, which leads to the goal.

THE PATIENT AND PRESENTING PROBLEM

The patient is a 28-year-old married woman complaining of sexual frigidity, trouble with sense of self-respect, and difficulty with pleasurable feelings. She is the second of four children, with an older sister and a younger sister and brother. The family of origin as a unit has always been intact. Both the patient's father and husband are businessmen. Patient is a social worker.

THE BASIS FOR THE PROBLEM

At the beginning of the analysis, the patient was unable to respond sexually, get close to others, be spontaneous and productive in her work, or tolerate and express strong affects, because she could not let down or relax her controls. She was so vulnerable to feeling criticized, humiliated, put down by others, or guilty and submissive toward them, that she had to be defensively on guard, tight, and overcontrolled. She overcontrolled herself because she could not defend herself against others.

Correspondingly, these anxieties were initially reflected in the analytic relationship, such that she had difficulty liking, and collaborating comfortably with, the analyst (i.e., "getting close to him"). These anxieties were based primarily on her relation to her mother. On the one hand she could not defend herself against the mother, or else felt guilt toward her. Consequently, at the outset she unconsciously feared that she would be "owned" by the analyst, just as by the mother; that she would become homosexually attached to him, just as to her mother; that she would have to believe what the analyst said whether she believed it was true or not, as with mother's judgments of her; and that she would have to feel identified with him (out of guilt) in ways that she felt like her mother—messy, disgusting, a victim.

THE GOALS AS ACHIEVED

The patient, in fact, reduced enough of the above anxieties in the first 100 hours to achieve a new, if limited capacity to respond sexually; free-associate and reveal symptoms and preoccupations; think and work more spontaneously and productively; tolerate and express strong affects—especially anger—more readily; and exercise control more appropriately over her clients.

HOW THE GOALS WERE ACHIEVED

The patient reduced the above anxieties by establishing an ego-syntonic capacity to defend herself against others (i.e., to "oppose" them), in particular the analyst, in various ways. That is to say, oppositional behavior first had to become integrated harmoniously with other existing ego regulations. In becoming able to "oppose," she became thus able to protect herself from criticism, humiliation, guilt, and submission to others (i.e., was less vulnerable). This achievement then made her able to *allow* herself to yield, get close, relax controls, enjoy sex, free-associate, reveal symptoms, etc., because whenever she might feel too blame-worthy, or too submissive, or too guilty, she knew that she could always switch to the "attack." She could do this (i.e., oppose) by blaming others, criticizing or disagreeing with them, resisting guilt and submission through stubbornness, withholding, refusing to give in, etc.

That the patient achieved "increasing integration" of the above behaviors and attitudes meant that she became more aware of these oppositional tendencies and gained greater control over them. They became abilities, such that she could then express them at will and in harmony with her overall intentions.

THE ANALYST'S INTERVENTIONS IN RELATION TO THE PATIENT'S PROGRESS IN HER INTEGRATION OF OPPOSITIONAL TENDENCIES

Whether the analyst's interventions are categorized as faciliating or hindering therefore depends on whether what he says or does, or doesn't say or do, helps the patient in her analysis and integration of the so-called "oppositional" behaviors.

Hindering interventions by the analyst are those comments (as well as some omissions and silences) in which the *patient perceives the analyst* as being critical (toward her); humiliating; guilt-provoking; encouraging of submission, dependence; patronizing, condescending; *or* threatened, defensive (in response to her); frustrated, angry; weakened, injured (increasing her guiltiness); superior, mocking; uninterested, aloof.

In such instances the patient is more likely to feel vulnerable, and thus have more anxiety and reluctance to become aware of, test, and integrate the various oppositional behaviors and attitudes.

Facilitating interventions by the analyst are those in which he seems to her to not oppose her tendency to be oppositional, and/or those which aid her tendencies to be independent and separate from the analyst and others, as for instance, when:

1. The analyst makes comments or asks questions which pull for further elaboration of material in which the patient is presenting herself as oppositional in its various forms. The analyst also should not, in doing so, appear to be threatened or threatening.

2. The analyst ignores and does not pull for elaboration of material in which the patient is presenting herself as put down, childish, etc.
3. The analyst makes observations or interpretations that, how, or why the patient is defending against inclinations to be oppositional (e.g., to blame, accuse, be separate and independent).

In general, the patient's progress is facilitated if she feels encouraged in her trials of oppositional tendencies because the analyst hasn't opposed them. In this, she is enabled to become more aware of and test these tendencies, and integrate them so they become abilities.

RATING THE INTERVENTIONS

In making your ratings of the analyst's interventions, you will have to empathize with how the patient is likely to perceive him and his remarks at that point in time. The emphasis is on how the patient will consciously or unconsciously appraise what the analyst says or does in each instance with respect to the goal of oppositionalness. For example, even though it may seem to you as clinical judge that the analyst was "objectively" neutral and/or accurate in his comments, the patient may have heard it as hindering for many possible reasons (e.g., because of its ambiguity, timing, or tone, it might appear to be mocking, authoritative, impatient, etc.).

To establish the context for this judgment, each item provides you with the patient's productions which precede the analyst's intervention. Following the context is the section containing the analyst's responding interventions, which you will rate on the scale provided. You will notice that in many cases the analyst's verbalizations are interspersed with brief interactions with the patient. In making scaled judgments of how facilitative the response is, you are to review the meaning of the entire "package" of what the analyst has said, just as you assume that the patient will review and appraise all of what the analyst has just said at that point in time.

APPENDIX 14. PSYCHOANALYTIC INTERPRETIVENESS SCALE (PILOT STUDY AND REPLICATION STUDY)

This scale categorizes the therapist's utterances by the extent to which they are psychoanalytically (and nontrivially) interpretive. The range extends from comments of low or extratherapeutic content to deep interpretations. The rationale behind the scale assumes that the directing beacon of the therapist—even when he makes no proposition, but merely says something like "Notice *this*"—generates associations and attempts at new organization on the part of the patient. Such assertions may have enlightenment value without necessarily delineating the final gestalt. This scale, therefore, may be viewed as spectrum of the naming of what is relatively not available to the patient, of what is warded off.

The interventions are judged in the light of the immediately preceding production by the patient. How far beyond the patient's material the cognitive content of the intervention reaches is, of course, one consideration in the assessment. At the same time, since the therapy hour is a time of fresh and ever-shifting warding-off activities in the patient's mind, even a therapist's statement which is a mere direct paraphrase of what the patient said may have enlightenment impact; rather than being experienced as "nothing new," it may be received, utilized, and assimilated in the development of further integrations and insights.

Level	Category of intervention	Example
1	Extratherapeutic or content-containing assertion (i.e., a comment not part of, or contributing minimally to, the exploration in the therapy)	1. "I have a schedule change." 2. "Sorry, I have to answer the phone." 3. "Oh, yes, yes."
1	Request for material already verbalized	1. "Huh? What?" 2. "Would you repeat that please? I didn't catch all of it."
2	Request for material not recently verbalized, but which is not likely to have been withheld or warded off	1. "At what age did that happen?" 2. "Which girl did you mean?" 3. "And what was the name of the book?"
3	Request for associations to specific material (i.e., rather than free associations)	1. "What comes to mind when you think about that incident?" 2. "And what about boys wearing bell-bottoms?"
3	Echoing paraphrase or assertion (therapist repeats closely a part or all of what patient has just said)	1. Paraphrase example A: PATIENT: "It's not that I'm not thinking of anything, it's that sometimes it doesn't seem so important to me, or to you maybe, and that it won't lead to anything, and so I don't talk about it."

THERAPIST: "So you won't talk about it because you think it won't lead to anything. . . ."

2. Paraphrase example B:

PATIENT: "And if I ever do have a son, I think I probably wouldn't let him have the gun to play with, I'd probably just bully him and make him docile like his sisters."

THERAPIST: "You'd take away, not let him have his gun to play with."

3	Assertion of significance (of some area or material, without specifying in what way)	1. "That's a striking way to put that." 2. "You've mentioned that three times today."
4	Request for material likely to have been withheld or warded off	1. "Maybe when you said 'sexual organs,' you were really thinking of the street word?" 2. "Did this business about the garbage remind you of what you said about mother yesterday?" 3. "Perhaps you felt excited when he said that to you?"
4	Naming or focusing assertion or paraphrase (or same disguised as a request) especially for material withheld, warded off, or not noticed (Inference very near to the available verbal or nonverbal source. Pointing out affects and defenses are appropriate here. For focused paraphrase, the therapist makes heightened clarification in his reverbalization.)	1. "You're guilty about this." 2. "You seem hesitant." 3. "Why are you chuckling when you said you were disappointed?" 4. "You're leaving out that the same is true of your father." 5. Paraphrase example A:

PATIENT: "It's not that I'm thinking of anything, it's that sometimes it doesn't seem so important to me, or to you maybe, and that it won't lead to anything, and so I don't talk about it."

THERAPIST: "So, essentially, you're editing." (or) "Making omissions so as to always seem pertinent."

6. Paraphrase example B:

PATIENT: "And if ever I do have a son, I think I probably wouldn't let him have the gun to play with; I'd probably just bully him and make him docile like his sisters."

THERAPIST: "Not wanting your boy to have the equipment his sisters can't have."

5   Enlarging paraphrase or assertion (or same disguised as a request) (Here, while the inference is still moderately near to the manifest source, it carries the implications in the derivatives a step beyond, adding something novel or revelatory in content or organization.)

1. Paraphrase example A:
   PATIENT: "It's not that I'm thinking of anything, it's that. . . ." (etc., as in previous paraphrase A patient quote).
   THERAPIST: Leaving me to admire your best products."

2. Paraphrase example B:
   PATIENT: "And if I ever do have a son. . . ." (etc., as in paraphrase B patient quote).
   THERAPIST: "Making men equal with you by making them like your concept of women, who don't have any powerful equipment."

6   Deeply interpretative paraphrase or assertion (or same disguised as a request) (Here the symbolic transformation or new organization spelled out in the inference is at a greater distance from the manifest source.)

1. Paraphrase example A:
   PATIENT: 'It's not that I'm not thinking of anything, it's that. . . ." (etc., as in paraphrase A patient quote).
   THERAPIST: "So mother can beam admiringly into your potty and say, good job!"

2. Paraphrase example B:
   PATIENT: "And if I ever do have a son. . . ." (etc., as in paraphrase B patient quote).
   THERAPIST: "To castrate him to make him like what you believe girls are."

APPENDIX 15. ADDITIONAL GUIDELINES FOR RATING ANALYST'S RESPONSES FOR PLAN COMPATIBILITY (REPLICATION STUDY)[1]

In making your ratings of the analyst's interventions, you will have to empathize with how the patient is likely to perceive him and his remarks at that point in time. The emphasis is on how the patient will consciously or unconsciously appraise what the analyst says or does in each instance with respect to the goal of oppositionalness. For example, even though it may seem to you as clinical judge that the analyst was "objectively" neutral and/or accurate in his comments, the patient may have heard it as hindering for many possible reasons (e.g., because of its ambiguity, timing, or tone, it might appear to be mocking, authoritative, impatient, etc.).

1. Plan compatibility instructions to replication study judges use *same* description of plan that is contained in Appendix 13, but different guidelines for making the ratings (sorting into piles).

To establish the context for this judgment, the data in each item provides you with the patient's productions which precede the analyst's intervention. Following the context is the section containing the analyst's responding interventions, which you will rate on the scale provided.

These items are excerpts from the transcripts of tape-recorded sessions and are presented in random order.

Familiarize yourself with the style of the analyst and the patient before making any ratings. Look at a handful of the responses you will be rating which fall at the beginning, middle and at the end of the material in order to get a sense of pace, language use, and style of interactions.

Next, take these responses and group them into three piles, according to whether you believe they are minimally, moderately, or maximally facilitative to the patient. This will provide you with your own anchor points for going through the rest of the material in order to rate it.

It would be useful to rate about half the material and then check on yourself for consistency. A good method is simply to take a spot check of every fifth item you rated and see whether your second rating falls within a point (in either direction) of your first rating before continuing with the second half of the items.

With material as complex as this, it's generally not a good idea to complete the ratings at one time. Returning to the material and becoming more immersed in it will help you make the ratings more accurately.

CLINICAL EXAMPLES FOR PLAN COMPATIBILITY RATINGS

Patient's production preceding the analyst's intervention (fictitious):

Well it happened like that too, what I was talking about before, at the agency, I thought, she might've been doing case work a long time, all right, but so why didn't she speak up about the matter at the conference? She could have, but—maybe I'm making too much of it too, I, I, like the pot calling the kettle black, I guess, I shouldn't . . . I don't even know why I'm talking about this today, maybe I've strayed. (*Pause.*) I just remembered the day that you didn't say anything about the office move, which I had thought you were planning to announce that day.

Comment on Patient's Production

She has presented here a mixture of advancing and retreating postures. Initially she speaks critically of the co-worker, then begins to take it back, becoming concerned she will be too harsh, then self-blames, then claims she's weak or scattered ("straying from the topic"). After her pause, however, she returns to an advance. What will the analyst pick up from all this?

If he labels her as weak, needy, fearful or dependent, especially if he implies it is inherent in her or is tied to important gratifications, plan compatibility (PC) will be lowered.

Example 1a. You have a wish for me to tell you things, like whether you've strayed from the topic, or to make announcements. That's the real focus of your thoughts today. (PC = 1)

Example 1b. I wonder if it's that you preferred to have me talk, like about the office move, rather than other matters? (PC = 2, because he makes the same point as in 1a, but more tentatively.)

Example 1c. What else comes to mind about straying off the topic? (PC = 3. While the analyst doesn't say that he believes she has strayed with the implication that she's fearful or out of control, he seems to be very interested in it, to the exclusion of other important "advance posture" material. If he had referred to "*your* straying off the topic," it would seem clearer that he does believe that she has to and wants to stray and PC would = 2. "Straying" is also synonymous with withholding and resisting.)

If, however, he *observes* that her apparent needy state is a defense, particularly against an advance posture, it implies she needn't present herself as needy, and PC is raised.

Example 2a. You're talking about people who don't speak up, and yet you seem more comfortable about letting me talk. (PC = 5. Analyst directs attention to the defensive area, but ambiguously, because of the possible emphasis on her dependent wishes.)

Example 2b. You said, "The pot calling the kettle black." You seem guilty about some feeling about the other social worker. (PC = 6)

Example 2c. Your idea that you've strayed is a smoke screen for your feelings about a co-worker who doesn't speak up. (PC = 7. If it were clearer that he means critical feelings, we would certainly raise it to PC = 8.)

Example 2d. You're uncomfortable about letting me know, you're afraid to let me know I was remiss, just like the social worker was remiss to not speak up at the meeting. (PC = 9)

If the analyst invites exploration or airing of the distortions implied by a retreatful posture, PC may be raised. Putting such communications in the form of a question often functions this way. Thus if he *asks whether* she's needy, afraid, weak, etc., rather than asserting that she *is* such, the rating moves upward from possible lower ratings. However, each of these has to be judged on its own merits, as when the form of a particular question indicates that it is a thin disguise for an assertion.

Example 3a. Why must you think you've strayed? (PC = 7)

Example 3b. You think you may have strayed from the topic? (PC = 5)

Example 3c. How do you think you've strayed? (PC = 5)

Example 3d. Straying? Because of the jump around to these other topics? (PC = 4)

Example 3e. So then, you don't even know why you're talking about it today? (PC = 2)

If he responds to an apparently needy posture with a caretaking response, PC will be lowered.

Example 4. Just so it's straight in your mind, let me review what you've been talking about. (PC = 2)

If the analyst ignores the retreatful posture, e.g., by responding to nonretreatful aspects, or by not responding, PC may be raised.

Example 5. Today you seem interested in people who don't speak up. (PC = 6)

If he observes that she seems or wants to be oppositional, attacking, or exhibitionistic, *without* implying ridicule, shock, irritation, antagonism, insistence on his authority, or apparent injury, PC will be raised. Also, PC is raised considerably when he interprets defenses *against* oppositionalness, etc., implying she is not forbidden to be that way.

Example 6a. You apparently clearly thought the co-worker was slipshod, so I wonder why you backed away from the idea? (PC = 8)

Example 6b. You know, you really seem hesitant, really afraid to "let her have it," or me either. (PC = 9)

Example 6c. You seem guilty about painting critical pictures of all these people today, and maybe the idea of straying is to cloud over what makes you feel guilty. (PC = 9, provided that you believe it's clear to the patient that the analyst assumes the guilt is unwarranted or neurotic.)

If the analyst observes that the patient is oppositional, etc. but *implies* ridicule, shock, irritation, antagonism, insistence of his authority, or apparent injury, PC will be lowered. Also, if he indicates her oppositionalness, etc. is merely defensive or represents fearfulness or manipulation, with the implication that she should renounce it or not take it seriously, PC is lowered.

Example 7. Bringing up the announcement about the office move is probably your attempt to set up a struggle, or argument here. And then we wouldn't get to what is really troubling you. (PC = 2; not a "1" because analyst is apparently not greatly threatened by her need to set up a struggle, and that's important to the patient.)

Example 7b. You've left something out of all this, and you're aware of it to some degree, because you mention "straying." It's holding back associations, which will slow us down further. (PC = 1)

If the analyst is *irrelevant* relative to what she is talking about, even if the content of his intervention *is* facilitative, its PC rating should be lowered about one point. If the analyst is, in addition, "pushy" about it (such as riding his own "hobby horse"), PC should be lowered even more.

If the analyst is vague, windy, unclear, or ambiguous about an otherwise facilitative or hindering intervention, the PC rating will move toward the middle ranges.

APPENDIX 16. SCALE FOR EVALUATING TEST POWER

In this exercise, actual references to the test indicate possible testing by the patient. Based on the summary immediate goal that you chose in the preceding section, decide whether the patient's testing activity is relevant to this immediate goal (i.e., is powerful and plan-relevant or not). The most powerful and plan-relevant instance is one which is either a clear-cut hero's or coward's choice in terms of the immediate goal (means). Rate the "test" on this 5-point scale:

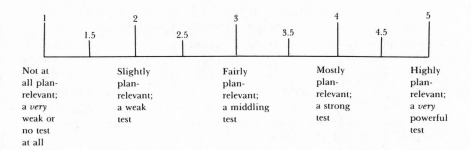

1	2	3	4	5
	1.5	2.5	3.5	4.5
Not at all plan-relevant; a *very* weak or no test at all	Slightly plan-relevant; a weak test	Fairly plan-relevant; a middling test	Mostly plan-relevant; a strong test	Highly plan-relevant; a *very* powerful test

APPENDIX 17. BOLDNESS SCALE (PILOT[1] AND REPLICATION STUDIES)

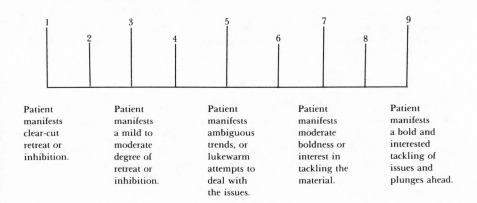

1	3	5	7	9
	2	4	6	8
Patient manifests clear-cut retreat or inhibition.	Patient manifests a mild to moderate degree of retreat or inhibition.	Patient manifests ambiguous trends, or lukewarm attempts to deal with the issues.	Patient manifests moderate boldness or interest in tackling the material.	Patient manifests a bold and interested tackling of issues and plunges ahead.

The Boldness Scale is used to rate the degree to which the patient pursues a deepening exploration of significant personal issues with boldness, ease, and interest.

1. In the pilot study, a 5-point version of this scale was used.

The judge combines two factors in making this rating: *Does the patient focus on important rather than trivial issues? Does the patient deal with these issues with ease?* The final rating indicates the degree to which we believe the patient is making a bold advance toward, rather than an inhibited or timid retreat from, self-discovery, understanding, and mastery of his or her conflicts.

SIGNIFICANCE VERSUS TRIVIALITY

Significant material focuses on conflict-related expressions regarding important impulse–defense derivatives and their associated affects, as these relate to important objects, the self, or the analyst. On the other hand, a trivial focus tends to allow defensive retreats; for instance, the patient may center on minor details in narratives or about procedures which are not conflict-related, and which are not likely to continue on toward other problem-related ideas and feelings. When a patient presents conflict-related material in disguised, displaced, and derivative ways, we would rate the focus as relatively *more* significant than non–conflict-related material (although, of course, it is not as optimally significant when it is conscious, direct, and self-related).

The following fictitious examples show an ascending order of significant focus for a given patient:

Example 1

I told my supervisor I didn't want to use the whole list, I didn't think it was necessary, because there are a lot of things on it that are too similar to the ones the group had just been using, and besides, the quality is so-so. I have a colleague who's used them too, and has not found them too useful. I know of a different list they've used at the XLM agency, that I've suggested to the administration here, but I don't think they'll do much with it really.

Example 2

My sister complains about her husband a lot that he's just a kind of show-off. It embarrasses her that he's always doing a theatrical comedian bit at these parties, you know, always telling these loud dirty jokes, and wears sexy shirts and tight pants and all. I can sort of see her point a little, you know, he even, she says, lets it all hang out and flaunts it in their bedroom, when there doesn't seem to be any point in doing it, because we know what he's got.

Example 3

My father was always putting his two cents in, I would barely get to say what I was thinking and he'd be sticking his opinion in, telling me what was what or that I was wrong and he was so damned articulate about it sometimes. At the same time, I mean. A pushy show-off know-it-all. Makes me think of what Max says about guys having, well, his word is "balls," and I don't know why I think of it except it's that I think, maybe, that men are always showing off their power and masculinity. I don't know if it's that I don't like it, or want to show-off myself. (*Pause.*) You know, I like it when you make comments, but sometimes it makes me—feel—feel cut off in my thoughts.

EASE VERSUS DIFFICULTY

The *ease* with which the patient approaches his or her subject matter, versus *difficulty*, can be ascertained from the following clues:

Ease
- Boldly tackles the material with interest.
- Develops, explores, expands material (e.g., raises and follows associations, memories, new ideas).
- Is clear, direct, unhesitating, purposive.
- May be playful or at ease with the material.
- Boldly confronts experiential (e.g., emotional) aspects when these dominate the material.

Difficulty
- Hesitation, speech disruptions present.
- Retreatful, timid, inhibited tone.
- Belabored delivery, repetitions, rambling.
- Ambiguity, obliqueness of reference, vagueness.

Example 3 above is an example of a high level of patient ease and development of subject matter. Examples 4 and 5 below will demonstrate increasing levels of difficulty using the basic issues from Example 3.

Example 4

My father did, you know, like to talk and uh, had his own—was pretty clear about his positions on things and all, and stated things pretty clearly too. He'd comment on my opinions, you know, if I was going on about something, if he had a good idea, he'd want to put it forth. (*Pause.*) Wanted you to know it. And, I don't know why, but Max said, I'm thinking of what Max said—about men who have, it sounds awful—balls. I suppose there's something I don't—I guess, that I don't like about it, all this stuff, or something about it. (*Pause.*) Anyway, I'm thinking about your making interpretations and I don't know why.

Example 5

Um—there's something that my father used to do about talking about things, uh, that was, that he would, would make it clear to you, you know, what he was thinking, uh, had an opinion about. Even if, you know, you had your own ideas about it, which is OK, I guess, that he might take a different, uh, tack, position on it. (*Pause.*) I'm thinking about Max, who talks about men who can do that, and say pretty much what they want, anytime. Uh, I don't even know if that relates to what I was talking about. (*Pause.*) There was a supervisor at the agency today who talked a lot.

PRESENCE OF AFFECT

Affect is an important guide to judging the degree of boldness in the material, *when* we can ascertain that *the affect expression is in the service of bold expansion and self-confrontation.* Indeed, it is a complex problem to decide this, but the point here is that the presence of more, versus less, affect *per se* should not invariably raise the boldness rating. The clearest instance of such a situation would be when the patient pursues trivial topics and is rambling and full of speech disruptions as well—hence, clearly retreatful, and not bold—*and then* expresses her sad, depressed, even weepy impression that she doesn't seem to be getting anywhere. The fact that she here is forthright and expressive about her feelings is insufficient to credit her with a high boldness rating, since this affect expression itself does not reflect or demonstrate the bold expansion of significant topics.

To summarize, the *presence of affect expression* will increase boldness ratings when it either (1) relevantly expands the material that is being explored (if that material is significant). For instance, in Example 3, more intense expressions of anger, or envy, or exhibitionistic wishes might have relevantly amplified different parts of what the patient was focusing on in the subject matter; (2) appears itself to be an emerging, previously warded-off content, which would then be a proper target of self-confrontation and exploration (e.g., the discovery of previously warded-off sadness or envy).

Using the 9-point scale given, we will now rate and discuss the foregoing examples.

Example 1. Boldness = 3

In this example, the patient appears to be delivering a number of relatively bland, trivial details with ease. At most, the conflict-related issues may relate to her being assertive with her supervisor, or critical of the administration, or to a vague transference hint that she doesn't like the analyst's agenda, but she does not actually focus on or explore these possible foci; and they are neither pronounced nor does the associated material "run deep." This example would have earned a rating of "2" or "1" if, using the same material, rambling, vagueness, and speech disruptions were additional characteristics.

Example 2. Boldness = 7

The conflict areas here appear to be exhibitionism and anger or envy about exhibitionism, or possibly an identification with it; but these foci are displaced to other actors (sister and brother-in-law). The patient gives a meek hint that she probably identifies with the sister, and if she had not done so the boldness rating would slip to "6" or "5." Hence, the issues run relatively deep in the derivatives, and are developed to some extent, but very little developed in terms of *her own* motives and conflicts. It does appear to be delivered with ease.

Example 3. Boldness = 8

The conflict areas at least include those in example 2, and add themes of castration and penetration. The range of associations are relevant and wide (genetic, transference, current), and the material more clearly relates to *her* motives and conflicts. The derivatives run deep and are very suggestive of warded-off material.

Some affect amplification relevant to these significant issues is present ("so damned articulate," "pushy show-off," etc.); and without these, the rating might have slipped to "7." The example would have earned a "9" if any of the following held true: (1) even more direct and relevant affects; (2) even more deliberated exploration of her own motives as implied by what she is saying—for instance, as by a more clear-cut development of the transference connection at the end.

Example 4. Boldness = 5

The material suggestively runs deep, but her handling is vague, hesitant, disrupted, making it harder to see connections. Self-exploration and self-confrontation are lukewarm.

Example 5. Boldness = 3

It is harder to infer how deep the material runs; the development is unimpressive and a little vague, with a mild degree of hesitation.

APPENDIX 18. INSIGHT SCALE (PILOT[1] AND REPLICATION STUDIES)

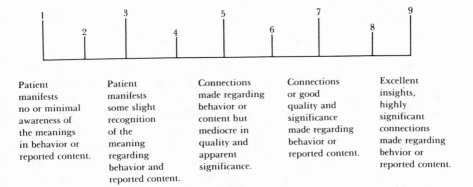

| 1 | 2 | 3 | 4 | 5 | 6 | 7 | 8 | 9 |

Patient manifests no or minimal awareness of the meanings in behavior or reported content.

Patient manifests some slight recognition of the meaning regarding behavior and reported content.

Connections made regarding behavior or content but mediocre in quality and apparent significance.

Connections or good quality and significance made regarding behavior or reported content.

Excellent insights, highly significant connections made regarding behvior or reported content.

The Insight Scale is used to rate the degree with which the patient develops insight into himself and his problems. At the high end of the scale the patient

1. In the pilot study, a 5-point version of this scale was used.

achieves excellent insight and awareness of the "how, what, and why" in significant areas of his personality. At the low end, the patient is minimally aware of significant connections. In making this rating, the judge will consider and combine several factors.

SIGNIFICANCE OF SUBJECT MATTER

Important areas for illumination include the patient's motives and defenses against motives, with respect to himself, important others, and the analyst, particularly when they have not been previously understood or have been warded off. Insight into what these motives and defenses are, how they function and how they originate are relevant. Insight into *im*personal tasks (e.g., concocting recipes, study projects) is not relevant to this rating. Insight into how others function psychologically is relevant, but only insofar as the patient appears to be aware of parallels with himself, or if the insight about the other person had been previously warded off.

INTEGRATION OF MATERIAL EXPLORED

The patient tends to make or improve his map of himself by linking ideas, behaviors, feelings, memories, or experiences in a meaningful way. At a simpler level, the linkage is merely associative (i.e., two things are newly considered as a juxtaposition). At a more insightful level, the connection tends to be causal or functional (e.g., "This is because of that," "This prevents or facilitates that.").

DEGREE OF AWARENESS OF POTENTIAL INSIGHTS

Evidence that the patient is carrying out the work of self-observation in making associative or causal connections increases the insight rating, as opposed to material which appears to be *merely* reported or experienced without any sense of the patient seeing the connections. Cues to this aspect may appear as direct comments (e.g., "I've never thought [or felt] this before," "I think it's an important idea," "I'm surprised I said [felt] this."). Some of these involve the emergence of warded-off ideas, memories, affects, or attitudes, which carry or imply significant relations and connections with other material, and which would likely be rated high. More common indicators of self-observation which may accompany less-understood or less-powerful material include: "Makes me think of . . . ," "I'm wondering why I thought this," "Now I'm feeling like . . . ." On the other hand, we would lower the ratings of instances where the patient has, or almost has, an insight, but loses the thread or becomes scattered or confused.

EXTENT OF INSIGHT

We would tend to raise the ratings of an instance when the insights involved show depth, power, complexity, amplitude, or specificity of focus, when these appear to be in the service of understanding.

GENERAL COMMENTS

It is useful in rating a segment of process to paraphrase in summary from the one or few points of insight the patient makes, then judge them according to significance, integration, awareness, and extent. Also, we pay attention to the insights acquired, and not whether it is easy or hard for the patient to arrive at them. The following fictitious examples will give an idea how the ratings are made.

Example 1

I told my supervisor I didn't want to use the whole list, I didn't think it was necessary, because there are a lot of things on it that are too similar to the ones the group had just been using, and besides, the quality is so-so. I have a colleague who's used them too, and has not found them too useful. I know of a different list they've used at the XLM agency, that I've suggested to the administration here, but I don't think they'll do much with it really.

(Insight = 1. The patient at most may be talking about having critical feelings towards others, but even so, the material is not relatively significant. No linkages of any weight are made. If the patient had continued and also said, "I'm reminded of telling my sister—that I already had my own recipe for chocolate mousse, and I didn't need hers at all for the dinner party," then we might increase the rating to a "2." While this latter addition does not illuminate very much more significantly, the patient demonstrates some self-observation, e.g., "I'm reminded of . . . ," and *may* alert herself to the theme of rejecting the ideas of others.)

Example 2

My sister complains about her husband a lot that he's just a kind of show-off. It embarrasses her that he's always doing a theatrical comedian bit at these parties, you know, always telling these loud dirty jokes, and wears sexy shirts and tight pants and all. I can sort of see her point a little, you know, he even, she says, lets it all hang out and flaunts it in their bedroom, when there doesn't seem to be any point in doing it, because we know what he's got.

(Insight = 3. The patient offers a monologue on her sister's irritation with latter's husband's phallic exhibitionism, or potentially more significant area, but what parallels exist with the patient are not crystal clear. However, there are two suggestive points of entry: ". . . can sort of see her point a little . . ." and ". . . because *we* know what he's got.")

Example 3

Um—there's something that my father used to do about talking about things, uh, that was, that he would, would make it clear to you, you know, what he was thinking, uh, had an opinion about. Even if, you know, you had your own ideas about it, which is OK, I guess, that he might take a different, uh, tack, position on it. (*Pause.*) I'm thinking about Max, who talks about men who can do that, and say pretty much what they want, anytime. Uh, I don't even know if that relates to what I was talking about. (*Pause.*) There was a supervisor at the agency today who talked a lot.

(Insight = 4. Patient appears to be talking about her father's verbal forcefulness, probably vis-à-vis herself, an area of likely relative significance. She consciously connects father and men who are like father in this way, though somewhat vaguely and meagerly. She shows minimal awareness when she almost negates this connection. While the last idea of the quote is likely thematically connected, she does not seem aware of it. The fact that the patient stumbles and stutters is of no consequence for this rating.)

Example 4

My father did, you know, like to talk and uh, had his own—was pretty clear about his positions on things and all, and stated things pretty clearly too. He'd comment on my opinions, you know, if I was going on about something, if he had a good idea, he'd want to put it forth. (*Pause.*) Wanted you to know it. And I don't know why, but Max said, I'm thinking of what Max said—about men who have, it sounds awful—balls. I suppose there's something I don't—I guess, that I don't like about it, all this stuff, or something about it. (*Pause.*) Anyway, I'm thinking about your making interpretations and I don't know why.

(Insight = 6. This is the same material as in the preceding example, and it has deepened, e.g., "men who have balls," become more specific, i.e., about father's forcing his ideas on her, and widened to include a transference reference.)

Example 5

My father was always putting his two cents in, I would barely get to say what I was thinking and he'd be sticking his opinion in, telling me what was what or that I was wrong and he was so damned articulate about it sometimes. At the same time, I mean. A pushy show-off know-it-all. Makes me think of what Max says about guys having, well, his word is "balls," and I don't know why I think of it except it's what I think, maybe, that men are always showing off their power and masculinity. I don't know if it's that I don't like it, or want to show-off myself. (*Pause.*) You know, I like it when you make comments, but sometimes it makes me—feel—feel cut off in my thoughts.

(Insight = 8. Again using the same material, this example shows even greater specificity regarding the father, men's exhibitionism and power, and her potential envy, with the depth of her attitudes and motives bared by her affectively colored choice of words. If she had added, for one possibility, that all this focus on her father and men was also serving as an easy way to express the same feelings about the analyst without designating him as the target, the rating would surely be worth a "9.")

APPENDIX 19. INSTRUCTIONS FOR APPLYING THE BOLDNESS AND INSIGHT SCALES (REPLICATION STUDY)

The following items are excerpts from the tapescripts of the patient's productions from the first 100 hours of an analysis. The patient is a 28-year-old married woman complaining of difficulty with pleasurable feelings. She is the second of four children, with a sister 2 years older, a sister 5 years younger, and a brother 6 years younger. The family of origin as a unit has always been intact. Both the patient's father and husband are businessmen. Patient is a social worker.

The patient's productions will be rated according to two 9-point scales: how much the patient boldly tackles issues versus retreats from them, and to what extent insightful connections are made.

You will rate the patient's production in each item. In general, you will consider whether there are significant (i.e., nontrivial) developments in terms of the two scales.

Since the process in analysis is partly free-associative and partly responsive to interventions, the patient's productions may continue along one line of exploration, but need not necessarily do so. The appearance of a shift in material may represent a retreat, *or* it may represent important, newly emerging contents. Likewise, silences may either be reflective (i.e., potentially productive) or they may be retreatful. You can best decide on the basis of the accompanying verbal material and behavior.

The presence of painful, distressing, guilty or other material marked by negative affect is not evidence of "retreat" in itself; rather, when the patient confronts such material, it is evidence of bold advance. However, when the patient expresses genuine dissatisfaction, disappointment, guilt, depression, etc. *about* her handling and exploration of the material, this is *usually* evidence for retreat.

The scales are self-explanatory. Read them over before you begin.

APPENDIX 20. RATING THE SHIFT IN BOLDNESS OR INSIGHT AFTER AN INTERVENTION (REPLICATION STUDY)

After you have made judgments of single segments using the Insight Scale, you will be shown how the items pair up in terms of preceding, or "context" segments, and succeeding, or "effect" segments with respect to the analyst's interventions. Using the first of each pair as an anchoring context, make a global judgment in terms of how much the patient has shifted ahead or back in her level of insight in the segment which follows the intervention.

SHIFT SCALE

+3 = Notable increase
+2 = Moderate increase
+1 = Small increase
 0 = No change
−1 = Small decrease
−2 = Moderate decrease
−3 = Notable decrease

APPENDIX 21. PLAN COMPATIBILITY SCALE (BUSH)

The purpose of making this rating is to estimate the likelihood that the patient will experience a particular intervention as supporting or opposing her immediate efforts at mastery. How the patient hears an intervention will be determined not only by the type of test she may currently be posing for the therapist, but also by how that intervention fits into other things the therapist has said, or not said, earlier in the session. Therefore, in order to make this rating, it will be necessary for you to form some impressions about what the patient is currently working on, how she is trying to use the therapeutic relationship, and how she has interpreted the therapist's prior interventions in that session.

The highest scale score should be reserved for interventions which strongly and unambiguously support the patient's current efforts at mastery. Conversely, the lowest scale score should be reserved for interventions which strongly and unambiguously oppose the patient's current efforts at mastery. Intermediate scores should be given to interventions which are, to varying degrees, neutral, irrelevant, or contradictory in terms of their implications for the patient's current efforts at mastery. Feel free to make between-point ratings (e.g., −2.5, −1.5, +1.5, +2.5, etc.) and to use only as many scale points as actually apply to this set of interventions.

−3 The therapist's intervention *strongly and unambiguously opposes* the patient's current efforts at mastery. It is *very anti-plan.*

−2 The therapist's intervention *moderately opposes* the patient's current efforts at mastery. It is *moderately anti-plan.*

−1 The therapist's intervention *mildly, or somewhat ambiguously, opposes* the patient's current efforts at mastery. It is *mildly anti-plan.*

  0 The therapist's intervention is highly ambiguous in terms of how it relates to the patient's current efforts at mastery. It may contain *contradictory implications* for what the patient is working on, or it may be *irrelevant.*

+1 The therapist's intervention *is mildly or somewhat ambiguously supportive* of the patient's current efforts at mastery. It is *mildly pro-plan.*

+2 The therapist's intervention is *moderately supportive* of the patient's current efforts at mastery. It is *moderately pro-plan.*

+3 The therapist's intervention is *strongly and unambiguously supportive* of the patient's current efforts at mastery. It is *very pro-plan.*

APPENDIX 22. ATTITUDE TOWARD TERMINATION SCALE

This scale is to be used for the purpose of assessing short-term fluctuations in the patient's *subjective feelings of readiness* (and *resistance*) with respect to the idea of termination. You will be applying it to references the patient makes to termination during the last 100 hours of a recorded analysis.

We assume that *any* of the following items would, depending on the context, probably be an indication of some feeling of readiness with respect to the idea of termination:

1. The patient seems comfortable or matter of fact in referring to termination.
2. She seems accepting of the idea of termination and feels *appropriately sad* (as opposed to *anxiously depressed*) about it.
3. She feels confident of her ability to handle conflicts on her own.
4. She feels optimistic about the future.
5. She feels she can find healthy replacements for the functions that the analyst and the analysis have been serving.

In contrast to the foregoing indications of feelings of readiness for termination, we assume that any of the following items, depending on the context, would probably be an indication of some feelings of resistance or lack of readiness with respect to the idea of termination:

1. The patient seems uncomfortable, conflicted, apprehensive, or despairing in referring to termination.
2. She seems unaccepting of the idea of termination and is either defiantly angry or *anxiously depressed* (as opposed to *appropriately sad*) about it.
3. She feels extremely helpless, dependent, and unsure of her ability to handle conflicts on her own.

4. She feels worried and pessimistic about the future.

5. She feels she cannot replace the analyst or be happy without him.

In applying this scale to segments of the transcript, feel free to use between-point ratings (e.g., +1.5, +.5, −.5, −1.5).

SCALE POINTS

−2 The patient is giving strong indications that she does not feel ready to terminate and *no* indications that she is simultaneously having any opposite kinds of feelings (i.e., feelings of readiness to terminate). She is expressing unequivocal resistance to the idea of termination, which may be conveyed in a variety of ways. For example, she may be expressing a desire to just avoid the whole issue altogether by postponing termination or by seeing the analyst on a reduced basis following termination; she may be expressing a strong refusal to give up the analyst and/or her infantile demands and wishes with respect to him; or she may be conveying a sense of utter despair and fearfulness about her ability to function independently of the analyst or to be happy without him.

−1 Although the patient is clearly conveying a strong feeling that she neither feels ready nor wishes to terminate her analysis, she is also indicating that she may simultaneously be having some weaker feelings of an opposite kind (i.e., tentative feelings of readiness for termination). She is expressing resistance to the idea of termination, but it is not unequivocal. Her dominant feelings are in the direction of wanting to hold on to the analyst, wanting to avoid facing the need to give him up, and being fearful, worried, and pessimistic about her ability to function and enjoy her life on her own. However, there are suggestions that she may also be aware of wanting, or even of starting, to prepare herself for termination or of having positive thoughts about the idea of termination.

 0 This score should be used to reflect either (a) a statement the patient makes that is too ambiguous in its implications to rate; or (b) a statement which has contradictory implications of equal valence. In the latter case the patient would be expressing to an equal degree both resistant, apprehensive feelings and accepting, confident feelings about termination.

+1 Although the *dominant* feelings the patient is conveying are that she feels ready for termination, she is also, to a lesser degree, experiencing feelings of resistance to and apprehension about the idea of ending her analysis. The patient is primarily expressing tentative feelings of readiness to terminate that momentarily seem to outweigh her resistance to giving up the analyst and her apprehension about being able to function well independently of him. She may be feeling cautiously optimistic about her future, but also may be experiencing some hesitation, worry and self-doubt. She may be showing her acceptance of and sadness about a final separation from the analyst, but not without some expressions of regret and reluctance.

+2 The patient is giving *strong* indications that she feels ready to terminate. There are *no*, or only minimal, indications that she is simultaneously experiencing opposite kinds of feelings. This may be conveyed in a variety of ways depending on the context: She may be feeling matter-of-fact and comfortable in talking about termination; she may be showing her acceptance of a final separation from the analyst and expressing appropriate sadness about it; she may be feeling confident of her ability to solve conflicts on her own and to make good life decisions for herself; she may be feeling optimistic about the future; she may be expressing a healthy sense of resolution about her treatment and preparedness for termination; she may be expressing a desire and readiness to reinvest her emotional energies elsewhere.

APPENDIX 23. EXCERPTS THAT ILLUSTRATE HOW MRS. C EXPRESSED HER RESISTANCE TO TERMINATION

(All excerpts are taken from the analyst's process notes of the last 114 sessions.)

SEGMENT 1, FROM HOUR 1015

ANALYST: It seems to me that what you feel is consistent. You don't feel like a mother. You feel you're no good as a social worker. You can't relate to Henry. You're not interested in sex. It's as if what you're saying is that you're not ready to stop, that the whole idea is ludicrous, that you haven't changed.

PATIENT: (*Silence.*) She is wondering what I think about it. What does she want to hear me say? She wonders if everything will fall into place if she just comes to terms with finishing here. Or is there something more? (*Silence.*) Today, she was feeling that her cold and flu were much worse. Even though she had thought it wouldn't be so bad until today. She used to just give herself up to these things. But after she saw Mrs. Harrington [her daughter's[1] teacher] today, she just felt awful. And when I just spoke, she felt as though she would cough and felt so much worse immediately. She wants to get too sick to think. She just wants to go to bed and withdraw.

ANALYST: It sounds to me as though this mood is like what you felt for so many years as a girl. You felt sick and depressed and unloved and worthless. And you're feeling this as a reaction to anticipating losing me. Even my mentioning finishing makes you immediately feel sicker.

PATIENT: (*Pause.*) That's the way she remembers feeling. Now she feels she has

1. Mrs. C had a daughter after several years of analysis.

never stopped feeling that way and that she will go on feeling this way forever. What if I tell her, she'll just try to live up to that. Or else she'll resist it. But, in any case, she will be trapped and caught. She doesn't want to feel this way. If she does feel this way, she must not be ready.

SEGMENT 2, FROM HOUR 1016

PATIENT: She just suddenly became very aware of me. It's as if she's thinking that she is really going around the point, that she's aware of something else. It's this, she wants me to notice her as a lover, as well as a favorite child, but how can I notice her if she's not here? (*Silence.*)

This morning she felt that the time is coming closer. After the summer she'll never see me again. Ready or not. She is very aware of the time or the lack of it. It's a deadline she didn't want. It's easier to stand somehow, if she keeps reminding herself how much time is left. That's the way she's always done everything. To think it's only 8 weeks, then 4, then 2. Last night, Henry was in a funny mood. He was kind of nervous. He really didn't know why. She feels it's because it's the last month of his analysis.

ANALYST: You're making the point that you feel more angry than you would like to be and that you're saying no. I think what you'd really like to say no about is that you want to say no, you don't want to stop. Your whole reaction is as though I'm rejecting you. As though you are really what you felt from your father. As though I am really turning away from you, kicking you out. Rejecting you. This is the same assumption you had about what your mother and father were doing.

SEGMENT 3, FROM HOUR 1017

PATIENT: Henry has said a lot about the fact that he doesn't really care what she wants to do. He doesn't want her to just sit around and hole up at home. She does less of that now than she used to. She still feels resistant to his pushing her. She remembers her mother doing the same thing to her. Then she feels, if she resists everything, she is not ready to finish. If she is not ready, how can she finish? She feels she's saying something.

ANALYST: Yes. You are giving me a message.

PATIENT: If others are pushing her like her mother used to and Henry does, if she doesn't respond, then she loses something. But here she feels she cannot respond and still she can be safe. She wants me to let her do this and not push her. She's remembering a feeling that she really could just come here and not push or be pushed. Now, she feels that I too am pushing her. She wonders why she feels that because she was the one to bring up the whole idea of this being her last year here. She introduced the subject and all I did was discuss it with her. When we discussed it, she felt ready. But now, she feels that my pushing is worse than anybody else's. If she can't come here and get away from that feeling, where can she go? (*Silence.*)

SEGMENT 4, FROM HOUR 1017

PATIENT: Now she's thinking about working for another year and the fact that she doesn't like Arnold Spencer [the possible assistant she would have at the agency]. She feels it's her last year, so she doesn't care. Everything's a big mess. So she will just stop then and have another child and life will go on and on. She will be depressed. She can't get out of whatever it is she's caught up in. She wonders if she wants to ask me if she can come back next year and not finish. (*Pause.*) Then she thought of the arguments she makes to herself about how happy she would be to finish. Life would be so much easier practically. Now things like that don't matter. If she asked to come back next year, what would happen? She really has to set a time limit or she will never finish. What does she have to do to get ready?

ANALYST: Maybe you're getting ready right now. You really sound as if you were mourning our separating before we're separated. It's as if I had died and you're feeling bereft.

PATIENT: That certainly is the feeling. (*Pause.*) She is afraid that she will do this until the last day. That frightens her. She has no feeling of being able to handle things. She's just hopeless. Everything is insurmountable. (*Pause. By now she's crying softly.*) She's thinking of the way she has been feeling while coming here. She feels that she will never have that feeling again. It doesn't seem possible to replace it.

ANALYST: Which is just what one feels when one loses someone one loves, that they can never be replaced.

As she got up to leave, tears were streaming down her face.

SEGMENT 5, FROM HOUR 1022

Again, she struggles with wanting to make something of her vacation. She'll be taking Emily to school each day. But that doesn't really count. That's just a cover-up because it involves no effort. What will she do next year? Or will everything fall apart? She wallows in her emptiness and loss. And now she's thinking of her reaction when I put into words that we're getting a divorce. What she had been thinking was that she was interested in reading about divorce because of she and Henry. It never occurred to her that her interest might be because she's separating from me. Nonetheless, it's as if it was my idea and she felt angry. It was better than killing me. But, it's as though it's a threat to me, that she might kill me. (*Silence.*)

SEGMENT 6, FROM HOUR 1038

(*Pause.*) She understands what I say, but she still had this strong desire. It's very hard to think about. (*Silence.*) What I said is simple, but she can't take in that she hasn't gotten what she wanted. For her, everything has always been big or little. When she has decided she has wanted something, she has been consumed by it. She feels that with each disappointment, the feeling has gotten stronger. Now she has such a strong feeling of wanting me to say that she can stay with me forever, that she can't stand it. If this is disappointment, then where is she? She feels everything has accumulated. If even this last wish is disappointed, she can't just suddenly come to terms with herself. (*Silence.*)

SEGMENT 7, FROM HOUR 1055

PATIENT: Yes. There's something she wants that's still missing. She's practically finished here. She wonders if she can go on and do it on her own. The trouble is that in the past, she must have always counted on my doing it for her. It's her desires and it won't just happen to her. So she felt overwhelmed and depressed. Will she make it?

ANALYST: In other words, will you find this inner core that's missing?

PATIENT: She chuckled. She said it's like a penis that's really not there.

SEGMENT 8, HOUR 1055

That reminds her of a dream. When she woke up she was thinking that in the dream, what she was really trying to do was to find some way to find a penis, quite literally. Then, when that didn't work, there was the second part of the dream when she was looking for a substitute. Now it makes sense to her because her whole feeling was one of "I want, I want, I want." So the question is, will she give up what she wants. She knows now that all these attempts won't work. That as long as she continues them she would always be unhappy and unsatisfied. She felt scared because she feels now she has to go through giving me up before she can do these other things.

As much as she longs for these solutions, she now feels more deeply than ever that none of them will be an answer. She knows that she can't ever have a penis. She also knows that if she had money, it really wouldn't give her what she envies in the others. It's not the real thing. A baby is not the answer. Does she have to go through life feeling so jealous? She knows that she has to be true to herself.

APPENDIX 24. ILLUSTRATIVE TERMINATION INTERVENTIONS

FROM HOUR 1001

Yes. As though you have it one moment, and the next moment it's gone. (*Pause.*) But the main point is how strongly, even now, you remember in this way what a traumatic experience it was for you when Daniel [her younger brother] was born. And your father turned away from you. Now when we're talking about finishing, you feel I'm turning away from you and you feel jealous of others connected with me. And you feel that you'll be damned if you will admit that you want anything from me, which is what you felt about your father.

FROM HOUR 1010

Well, another way to think about your feeling is that what you're missing is not a penis, but what you felt you lost when you turned away from me in the dream. You felt that after that nothing would be the same. We would stay together for a while and see each other, but what you wanted you would never get. What's lost is not the styrofoam, but the chance to have a special relationship with me, to be my lover, and to be mine alone. You would never have that any more than you could get rid of your mother and have your father replace her with you. What hurts is to feel that what you've always wanted can never be.

FROM HOUR 1019

Well. I think you are saying what you think would replace me—our baby. I think your preoccupation with dying was because you were really preoccupied by wanting a birth. And that's what accounts for your change in feeling today when you got the gerbils.

FROM HOUR 1025

Yes. And I think you are wishing to be pregnant now to get rid of the emptiness that you feel in leaving me. Feeling rejected by me. And when you were a girl I think it must have seemed like a solution to the same feelings. It is as if you were saying to yourself, if you could have a baby like your mother, then your daddy would have loved you. And so I think your stomach expressed that feeling then last night.

FROM HOUR 1034

ANALYST: Well, so it sounds as though instead of telling me how angry you are feeling that I'm kicking you out, you're telling me instead how sick you are.

[Intervening patient material omitted.]

ANALYST: What you really seem to be struggling with is feeling jealous. You were talking about Betty and Joanne yesterday and feeling excluded from them. You obviously felt excluded from your mother and father's special relationship. You feel excluded from my relationships with others. Especially last week when you found me laughing with the other woman. Right now the only exception seems to be your feeling about your husband. And you explain that by saying that Dr. X [her husband's analyst] is gone. Your rival is no longer around. So the central feeling that you're struggling with is being jealous.

PATIENT: She feels that what she's doing, though, is dispersing it all toward all these irrelevant things. It's as if she can't stand being excluded from anything.

ANALYST: And especially now when we're talking about stopping. You feel excluded from my life. The fact that I'm even talking with you about finishing you take as proof that I'm kicking you out and excluding you. Otherwise, I would go on with you forever.

FROM HOUR 1038

Yes. It's as though you came to me hoping that you would have another chance to be born, this time a boy. And now you're afraid that you will be born prematurely, before you're a boy. So you'll leave feeling dumb, stupid, inadequate, no good. All the things that mean you're female and that you don't have a water fountain. (*Pause.*) It also seems that this is connected with the strong feeling you had of wanting to give me the money on Friday. The point is you didn't want to give me something, you wanted me to give you a gift for your birthday. You wanted me to give you what you have always wanted, which is to be reborn a boy, or some alternative such as to stay on with me forever, or to have your daddy's love, or to be pregnant and go away with a gift inside you. So I think you're really terribly disappointed over the fact that you have not gotten a water fountain. Your father didn't love you. You didn't get a boy baby. And you really can't stay pregnant forever. You feel nothing has worked.

FROM HOUR 1038

I think these are technicalities. The point is really simple. These are all things that you have really wanted desperately and you feel you haven't gotten. I think your point is to convince me how lonely, lost, bereft, alienated and depressed you are, hoping that this will make me say, OK you can stay on forever. I think this is your strong secret hope. When you were a little girl, you said you set it up so that your mother would kick you out. Now you feel I'm kicking you out just as you hoped then that she really wouldn't. You hope, now, that I will say it's OK, you can stay, as though you really are a little girl and that you really do need to be taken care of.

FROM HOUR 1055

Well, recently you've been talking about substitutes for a penis too. You've emphasized that what Joanne and Dorothy and Arnold Spencer all have is money. That it gives them this basic confidence. Then there's Joanne and Mary and others who are pregnant. And you feel if you could just stay permanently pregnant that would do it, and you did come here hoping that you would get what's missing from me.

FROM HOUR 1061

In the background is your feeling about Arnold Spencer. You were wondering about how you can deal with the confidence which you attribute to his being a man. And your complaint is not just that I haven't given you a baby, but that I haven't given you a penis. So you're really feeling that you haven't gotten anything you wanted. You wanted to be changed into a boy, and I didn't do that. And I haven't made you pregnant. So your complaining really means that I haven't done these things. It's essentially the same complaint that you have about your mother. That she turned you out unfinished, a female, that she could have babies and you couldn't. And you're angry with me because I haven't undone that.

FROM HOUR 1067

Let me recapitulate what you've been saying. You started saying you were afraid I would think that you were defiant, as though I had said, "Stop being late," and this happens at a time when you are feeling very insecure and hopeless about stopping. And then you tell me that Alice [her assistant at the agency] tried to make you feel guilty for what you hadn't done. I think the reason you were so sensitive to that and upset about it was because that's your message to me. You feel that I haven't given you what you want. That I haven't made you feel better, and now I'm turning you out. I think you want to make me feel guilty about it so I will change my mind and get even with me. (*Silence.*) And you said that Alice was motivated by not feeling special, and that's what's motivating you.

FROM HOUR 1074

Right. We have talked about how it is necessary to acknowledge what you want before you can really give it up. I think it was true that yesterday you felt very strongly how it would really be to not have breasts and to have a penis.

FROM HOUR 1086

It seems to come down to your feeling that nothing is worthwhile without me. (*Pause.*) You endow me with all of the power to frighten everyone, and you're astonished that John [the analyst's research assistant] would talk back to me. But that's because you endow me with this great power. And that's why you don't want to leave. So all will be lost if you have to give it up.

FROM HOUR 1096

[This was a speech of some length—here, again, inadequately summarized.] I'm struck by the fact that you find yourself again looking at women for the clues as to what makes them seem to accept being women. It reminds me of all the times that you have looked at women's personalities for their clues and the tricks that they use that you could copy. Again, as though you're wondering how can they accept being women or hide it? And you're searching for that right now at a time when we're about to finish. The paradox is though that you feel you have to have my strength, that you have to have this penis in order to accept being a woman.

FROM HOUR 1110

Well. I have an idea. Last week you seemed to be wanting to replace me with Arnold. I think in the dream it's as though you're saying if you can't have me, then you can become me and make love to yourself. That if you really can't have me, you can dream it.

APPENDIX 25. PLAN FORMULATION FOR THE LAST 100 HOURS

From the very outset of the last 100 hours, Mrs. C is actively engaged in trying to work through what for her are the central termination issues: She is very worried about her power to hurt the analyst by making him unimportant in her life, no longer needing or wanting his help, making clear that her primary emotional attachments and loyalties are to her husband and daughter, and being eager to terminate. We expect that she will be continually testing the analsyt throughout this period to disconfirm her unconscious belief in her power to narcissistically devastate him by independently and assertively leading her own life, loving her husband and daughter, having confidence in her own opinions, taking credit for her own accomplishments, feeling proud of her femininity, freely enjoying her sexuality, and emotionally disengaging from him.

Her deep-seated fear of her power to injure the analyst in these ways are central unresolved features of the father transference. She believes that her father was an extremely narcissistic, insecure, and possessive individual who had an intense need to unfairly demean anyone who was different from him and to be admired and envied by others. He was contemptuous and degrading towards his wife, and continually solicited reassurance from his children that his actions and beliefs were right in every respect. He not only demanded that his children agree with his ideas, but that they also share his preferences, to the point of liking the same flavor of ice cream. Mrs. C felt that her father desperately needed his children to demonstate their loyalty to him by deferring to his authority, by modelling themselves after him, and by having him be the central and most important figure in their lives. She felt that he envied even their attachment to the family cat and therefore did not want it around.

Mrs. C unconsciously believes that the analyst is very much like her father in terms of being narcissistically needy and vulnerable to being hurt by her. She has taken his penis envy interpretations to mean that he needs her to admire him, feel inferior to him, and to want to be just like him. Similarly, she has taken his interpretations about how desperately she wanted her father's love, and now wants his love, as an indication that he needs to feel that he is very important to her, in fact, irreplaceable. She fears he will not be able to tolerate her preferring her husband to him, her not needing him anymore, and her looking forward to ending her analysis. She unconsciously believes that the analyst wants her to feel helpless, empty, unprotected, and bereft at the thought of living without him. She fears her termination is actually going to be a very painful loss for *him*, rather than for her. Consequently, we assume that Mrs. C has a lot of guilt over feeling that she is rejecting and abandoning a weak, needy, vulnerable father figure, and that she will therefore be inclined to punish herself and to placate the analyst by making the termination process into a huge ordeal and acting like she longs to cling to him and dreads the prospect of leaving him.

We believe that a key part of Mrs. C's plan for the last 100 hours is to be able to feel ready to terminate and to have a confident and optimistic attitude about the future. We also assume that the kinds of feelings she expresses about the idea of termination will be largely a function of how she is testing the analyst and how guilty and worried about hurting him she is at any given point in time.

We predict that Mrs. C will feel freer to experience and express feelings of readiness for termination whenever the analyst makes interpretations which imply that he is not possessive of her, does not require her to give him or his ideas an exalted position of importance in her life, and does not need her to remain dependent on him, attached to him, or involved with him. In short, we expect her to feel more confident, relaxed, and matter-of-fact about the idea of termination whenever the analyst's behavior suggests that he is ready, willing, and able to let her go. Such interventions on the analyst's part would be considered pro-plan in that they would help the patient achieve her therapeutic goals. Conversely, we predict that the patient will demonstrate a greater resistance to the idea of termination when the analyst makes interventions which connote to her that he cannot tolerate being replaced in her affections, and that he still needs her to admire and envy him, to remain dependent upon him, to pay allegiance to his ideas, and to make the termination process into a painful experience of mourning and renunciation. In short, we expect her to feel more reluctant, apprehensive, and pessimistic about the idea of termination when the analyst's behavior implies that he is not yet ready to let her go. Such interventions on the analyst's part would be considered anti-plan in that they would impede the patient's efforts to terminate her analysis with a sense of readiness, confidence, optimism, and accomplishment.

It should be noted that the analyst is working with a very different theory about what the patient needs to accomplish during the termination phase of her analysis. He is not aware of her guilt toward him, of her perception of him as being highly vulnerable to narcissistic injury, or of her fear of her power to hurt him by making him or his interpretations unimportant. He instead believes, in accordance with traditional analytic theory, that the patient needs to more completely acknowledge her deepest infantile Oedipal longings within the father transference so that she can renounce them in a definitive way and fully mourn the loss of the analyst as an infantile love object. We expect him to inadvertently make both pro-plan and anti-plan interpretations, as well as interpretations which contain both pro- and anti-plan elements.

APPENDIX 26. DESCRIPTION OF A TESTING SEQUENCE IN HOURS 1015–1024

We will describe here two interrelated tests that Mrs. C simultaneously and successfully carried out with the analyst over a block of 10 sessions (the first 10 of the last 100 hours of her analysis). The first test involved an attempt to disconfirm her belief that the analyst desperately needed her to remain dependent upon him and involved with him. She carried out the test by claiming that she did not feel ready to terminate and by repeatedly asking if she could rescind the termination date or continue seeing the analyst after termination on a once-a-week basis. The second test involved a form of turning passive into active in an attempt to disconfirm her unconscious belief that she was cruelly rejecting and abandoning the therapist by terminating her analysis. She carried out this test by accusing the analyst of heartlessly rejecting and abandoning her. The ostensible rationale for this accusation was that if the analyst really cared about her, he would actively oppose her termination instead of agreeing to it.

The analyst passed both tests by acting perfectly comfortable with the patient's demands and accusations. In other words, he acted as though it was reasonable and appropriate for her termination to proceed as scheduled even though she was expressing painful feelings of rejection and requesting a postponement. He never responded to her questions about the possibility of changing the termination date or continuing to see him on a different basis after termination. Moreover, he told her that she was trying to manipulate him into letting her stay on by attempting to make him feel guilty and sorry for her.

Following this testing sequence the patient started to feel better, to express feelings of readiness for termination, and to become aware of thoughts about the analyst dying as a consequence of her leaving.

The analyst believed that he was frustrating the patient's central unconscious striving, her desire to consummate her childhood Oedipal wishes in the transference. We believe that he was passing a very crucial test. Given the actual clinical circumstances, had he agreed to postpone her termination, or to continue to see her following termination, the patient would likely have thought that it was very difficult and painful for the analyst to part with her. Her pathogenic belief in her power to hurt the analyst by terminating would have been reinforced, and she would have become more guilty and reluctant to terminate. We thought that the patient was also very relieved that her hurt feelings did not induce the analyst to shift his course. Part of her unconscious purpose in carrying out these tests had been to combat her unconscious guilt feelings about termination by identifying with the analyst's ability to not worry about making her feel worthless and rejected by adhering to their agreed-upon termination date.

REFERENCES

Abrams, S. Freudian models and clinical stance. *Bulletin of the Philadelphia Association for Psychoanalysis*, 1971, *21*(4), 279–282.

Alexander, F., & French, T. M. *Psychoanalytic therapy: Principles and application.* New York: Ronald Press, 1946.

Arlow, J. The structural hypothesis—theoretical considerations: The first annual Bertram D. Lewin memorial symposium on the ego and the id after fifty years. *Psychoanalytic Quarterly*, 1975, *44*(4), 509–525.

Arlow, J., & Brenner, C. *Psychoanalytic concepts and the structural theory.* New York: International Universities Press, 1964.

Asch, S. Varieties of negative therapeutic reaction and problems of technique. *Journal of the American Psychoanalytic Association*, 1976, *24*, 383–407.

Bachrach, H. M. Analyzability: A clinical-research perspective. *Psychoanalysis and Contemporary Thought*, 1980, *3*, 85–116.

Balson, P. *Dreams and fantasies as adaptive mechanisms in prisoners of war in Vietnam.* Unpublished paper written in consultation with M. Horowitz and E. Erikson, 1975. (On file at the San Francisco Psychoanalytic Institute)

Bellak, L. Studying the psychoanalytic process by the method of short range prediction and judgment. *British Journal of Medical Psychology*, 1958, *31*, 249–252.

Bellak, L., & Smith, M. B. An experimental exploration of the psychoanalytic process. *Psychoanalytic Quarterly*, 1956, *25*, 385–414.

Beres, D. Certain aspects of superego functioning. *Psychoanalytic Study of the Child*, 1958, *13*, 324–351.

Brenner, C. In J. Marmor (Reporter), Validation of psychoanalytic techniques (Panel report). *Journal of the American Psychoanalytic Association*, 1955, *3*, 496–505.

Brenner, C. *Psychoanalytic technique and psychic conflict.* New York: International Universities Press, 1976.

Buxbaum, E. Technique of terminating analysis. *International Journal of Psycho-Analysis*, 1950, *31*, 184–190.

Calef, V. The unconscious fantasy of infanticide manifested in resistance. *Journal of the American Psychoanalytic Association*, 1968, *16*, 697–710.

Caston, J. Manual on how to diagnose the plan. In J. Weiss, H. Sampson, J. Caston, & S. Gassner, *Further research on the psychoanalytic process.* The Psychotherapy Research Group, Department of Psychiatry, Mount Zion Hospital and Medical Center, Bulletin #4, June 1980, pp. 31–55.

Cohen, J., & Cohen, P. *Applied multiple regression/correlation analysis for the behavioral sciences.* Hillsdale, NJ: Erlbaum, 1975.

Colby, K. M. On the greater amplifying power of causal–correlative over interrogative inputs on free association in an experimental psychoanalytic situation. *Journal of Nervous and Mental Disease*, 1961, *133*, 233–239.

Coltrera, J., & Ross, N. Freud's psychoanalytic technique—from beginnings to 1923. In B. Wolman (Ed.) *Psychoanalytic techniques: A handbook for the practicing psychoanalyst.* New York: Basic Books, 1967, pp. 13–50.

Compton, A. (Reporter). Aspects of psychoanalytic interventions. *Kris Study Group of the New York Psychoanalytic Institute*, Monograph VI. New York: International Universities Press, 1975.

Cronbach, L. J., Gleser, G. C., Nand, A. H., & Rajaratnam, N. *The dependability of behavioral measures.* New York: Wiley, 1972.

Dahl, H., & Stengel, B. A classification of emotion words: A modification and partial test of de Rivera's decision theory of emotions. *Psychoanalysis and Contemporary Thought*, 1978, *1*, 269–312.

Dahl, H. The appetite hypothesis of emotions: A new psychoanalytic model of motivation. In C. E. Izard (Ed.) *Emotions in personality and psychopathology.* New York: Plenum, 1979, pp. 201–225.

Davis, D. R. Clinical problems and experimental researches. *British Journal of Medical Psychology*, 1958, 74–82.

de Rivera, J. *A decision theory of the emotions.* Unpublished doctoral dissertation, Stanford University, Stanford, CA, 1962.

Dewald, P. A. *Psychotherapy, a dynamic approach.* New York: Basic Books, 1971.

Dewald, P. A. The clinical assessment of structural change. *Journal of the American Psychoanalytic Association*, 1972, *20*, 302–324.

Dewald, P. A. Transference regression and real experience in the psychoanalytic process. *Psychoanalytic Quarterly*, 1976, *45*(2), 213–230.

Dewald, P. A. The psychoanalytic process in adult patients. *Psychoanalytic Study of the Child*, 1978, *33*, 323–332.

Ebel, R. L. Estimation of the reliability of ratings. *Psychometrika*, 1951, *16*, 407–424.

Erikson, E. H. *Childhood and society.* New York: Norton, 1950.

Erikson, E. H. The problem of ego identity. *Journal of the American Psychoanalytic Association*, 1956, *4*, 56–121.

Erikson, E. H. *Identity, youth and crisis.* New York: Norton, 1968.

Fenichel, O. *Problems of psychoanalytic technique* (D. Brunswich, Trans.). New York: The Psychoanalytic Quarterly, 1941.

Ferenczi, S. The problems of the termination of the analysis (1927). In M. S. Bergman & F. R. Hartman (Eds.), *The evolution of psychoanalytic technique.* New York: Basic Books, 1976, pp. 207–215.

Firestein, S. K. *Termination in psychoanalysis.* New York: International Universities Press, 1978.

Fisher, S., & Greenberg, R. P. *The scientific credibility of Freud's theories and therapy: VIII.* New York: Basic Books, 1977.

Fiske, D. W. Methodological issues in research on the therapist. In A. S. Gurman & A. M. Razin (Eds.), *Effective psychotherapy: A handbook of research* (2nd ed.). New York: Pergamon Press, 1977, pp. 23–43.

French, T. *The integration of behavior* (Vol. 2: *The integrative process in dreams*). Chicago: University of Chicago Press, 1954.

Fretter, P. B. The immediate effects of transference interpretations on patients' progress in brief, psychodynamic psychotherapy (Doctoral dissertation, University of San Francisco, 1984). *Dissertation Abstracts International*, 1984, *46*(6). (University Microfilms No. 85-12112)

Freud, A. *The ego and the mechanisms of defense* (1936). New York: International Universities Press, 1946.

Freud, S. Project for a scientific psychology (1895). *Standard Edition, 1*, 283–398. London: Hogarth Press, 1966.

Freud, S. The interpretation of dreams (1900). *Standard Edition, 4*, 1–338; *5*, 339–627. London: Hogarth Press, 1953.

Freud, S. Freud's psycho-analytic procedure (1904). *Standard Edition, 7*, 249–254. London: Hogarth Press, 1953.

Freud, S. On psychotherapy (1905a). *Standard Edition, 7*, 255–568. London: Hogarth Press, 1953.

Freud, S. Jokes and their relation to the unconscious (1905b). *Standard Edition, 8*, 9–181. London: Hogarth Press, 1960.

Freud, S. Analysis of a phobia in a five-year-old boy (1909). *Standard Edition, 10*, 3–149. London: Hogarth Press, 1955.

Freud, S. Formulations on the two principles of mental functioning (1911). *Standard Edition, 12*, 213–226. London: Hogarth Press, 1958.

Freud, S. Papers on technique (1911–1915). *Standard Edition, 12*, 83–171. London: Hogarth Press, 1958.

Freud, S. The dynamics of transference (1912). *Standard Edition, 12*, 97–108. London: Hogarth Press, 1958.

Freud, S. On beginning the treatment (1913). *Standard Edition, 12*, 121–144. London: Hogarth Press, 1958.

Freud, S. Remembering, repeating and working-through (1914). *Standard Edition, 12*, 147–156. London: Hogarth Press, 1958.

Freud, S. Observations on transference-love (1915). *Standard Edition, 12*, 157–171. London: Hogarth Press, 1958.

Freud, S. Introductory lectures on psycho-analysis (1917). *Standard Edition, 15*, 1–239; *16*, 241–465. London: Hogarth Press, 1963.

Freud, S. Beyond the pleasure principle (1920). *Standard Edition, 18*, 3–64. London: Hogarth Press, 1955.

Freud, S. The ego and the id (1923). *Standard Edition, 19*, 3–66. London: Hogarth Press, 1961.

Freud, S. Inhibitions, symptoms and anxiety (1926a). *Standard Edition, 20*, 77–175. London: Hogarth Press, 1959.

Freud, S. Psycho-analysis (1926b). *Standard Edition, 20*, 259–270. London: Hogarth Press, 1959.

Freud, S. Civilization and its discontents (1930). *Standard Edition, 21*, 57–243. London: Hogarth Press, 1961.

Freud, S. New introductory lectures on psychoanalysis (1933). *Standard Edition, 22*, 3–182. London: Hogarth Press, 1964.

Freud, S. Analysis terminable and interminable (1937). *Standard Edition, 23*, 209–253. London: Hogarth Press, 1964.

Freud, S. An outline of psychoanalysis (1940a). *Standard Edition, 23*, 141–207. London: Hogarth Press, 1964.

Freud, S. Splitting of the ego in the process of defence (1940b). *Standard Edition, 23*, 272–278. London: Hogarth Press, 1964.

Friedman, M. Toward a reconceptualization of guilt. *Contemporary Psychoanalysis,* October 1985, *21*(4), 501–547.

Garduk, E. L., & Haggard, E. A. Immediate effects on patients of psychoanalytic interpretations. *Psychological Issues,* 1972, *7*(4), Monograph 28.

Gassner, S., Sampson, H., Weiss, J., & Brumer, S. The emergence of warded-off contents. *Psychoanalysis and Contemporary Thought,* 1982, *5*(1), 55–75.

Gill, M. Metapsychology is not psychology. In M. M. Gill & P. S. Holzman (Eds.), *Psychology vs. metapsychology. Psychological Issues,* 1976, *9*(4), 71–105.

Gitelson, M. The curative factors in psychoanalysis. *International Journal of Psycho-Analysis,* 1962, *43*, 194–205.

Glover, E. *The technique of psycho-analysis.* New York: International Universities Press, 1955.

Glover, E. *The birth of the ego: A nuclear hypothesis.* New York: International Universities Press, 1968.

Gottschalk, L. A., & Gleser, G. C. *The measurement of psychological states through the content analysis of verbal behavior.* Berkeley: University of California Press, 1969.

Gottschalk, L. A. The application of a method of content analysis to psychotherapy research. *American Journal of Psychotherapy,* 1974a, *28*(4), 488–499.

Gottschalk, L. A. Quantification and psychological indicators of emotions: The content analysis of speech and other objective measures of psychological states. *International Journal of Psychiatry in Medicine,* 1974b, *5*(4), 587–610.

Greenberg, L. S. Psychotherapy process research. In C. E. Walker (Ed.), *The handbook of clinical psychology.* Homewood, IL: Dow Jones-Irwin, 1983, pp. 169–204.

Greenson, R. R. The working alliance and the transference neurosis. *Psychoanalytic Quarterly,* 1965, *34*, 155–181.

Greenson, R. R. *The technique and practice of psychoanalysis* (Vol. 1). New York: International Universities Press, 1967.

Grünbaum, A. Epistemological liabilities of the clinical appraisal of psychoanalytic theory. *Psychoanalysis and Contemporary Thought,* 1979, *2*, 451–526.

Guilford, J. P. *Psychometric methods* (2nd ed.). New York: McGraw-Hill, 1954.

Hartmann, H. *Ego psychology and the problem of adaptation* (1939). New York: International Universities Press, 1958.

Hartmann, H., Kris, E., & Loewenstein, R. M. Comments on the formation of psychic structure. *Psychoanalytic Study of the Child,* 1946, *2*, 11–38.

Hartmann, H. Technical implications of ego psychology. *Psychoanalytic Quarterly,* 1951, *20*, 31–43.

Hartmann, H. Notes on the reality principle (1956a). In *Essays on ego psychology.* New York: International Universities Press, 1964, pp. 241–267.

Hartmann, H. The development of the ego concept in Freud's work (1956b). In *Essays on ego psychology.* New York: International Universities Press, 1964, pp. 268–296.

Harway, N., Dittimar, A., Raush, H., Bordin, E., & Ringler, P. The measurement of depth of interpretation. *Journal of Consulting and Clinical Psychology,* 1955, *19*, 247–253.

Holt, R. Experimental methods in clinical psychology. In B. Wolman (Ed.), *Handbook of clinical psychology.* New York: McGraw-Hill, 1965, pp. 40–77.

Holt, R. The past and future of ego psychology: The first annual Bertram D. Lewin memorial symposium on the ego and the id after fifty years. *Psychoanalytic Quarterly*, 1975, *44*(4), 550–576.

Horowitz, L. M., Sampson, H., Siegelman, E. Y., Wolfson, A., & Weiss, J. On the identification of warded-off contents: An empirical and methodological contribution. *Journal of Abnormal and Social Psychology*, 1975, *84*, 545–558.

Horowitz, L. M., Sampson, H., Siegelman, E. Y., Weiss, J., & Goodfriend, S. Cohesive and dispersal behaviors: Two classes of concomitant change in psychotherapy. *Journal of Consulting and Clinical Psychology*, 1978, *46*, 556–564.

Kanzer, M., & Blum, H. Classical psychoanalysis since 1939. In B. Wolman (Ed.), *Psychoanalytic techniques: A handbook for practicing psychoanalysts*. New York: Basic Books, 1967, pp. 138–139.

Kernberg, O., Burstein, E., Coyne, L., Appelbaum, A., Horowitz, L., & Voth, H. Psychotherapy and psychoanalysis: Final report of the Menninger Foundation's psychotherapy research project. *Bulletin of the Menninger Clinic*, 1972, *36*, 1–275.

Kiesler, D. J. *The process of psychotherapy: Empirical foundations and systems of analysis*. Chicago: Aldine, 1973.

Klein, G. S. The emergence of ego psychology: A symposium. *Psychoanalytic Review*, 1969, *56*(4), 511–525.

Klein, G. S. *Psychoanalytic theory: An exploration of essentials*. New York: International Universities Press, 1976.

Klein, M. H., Mathieu, P. L., Gendlin, E. T., & Kiesler, D. J. *The experiencing scale: A research and training manual* (Vols. 1 & 2). Madison, WI: Psychiatric Institute, Bureau of Audio Visual Instruction, 1970.

Kline, I. *Fact and fantasy in Freudian theory* (2nd ed.). London: Methuen, 1981.

Knapp, P. H. Short term psychoanalytic and psychosomatic predictions. *Journal of the American Psychoanalytic Association*, 1963, *11*, 245–280.

Kris, E. Problems in clinical research (1947). In *The selected papers of Ernst Kris*. New Haven: Yale University Press, 1975, pp. 24–30.

Kris, E. On preconscious mental processes (1950). In *The selected papers of Ernst Kris*. New Haven: Yale University Press, 1975, pp. 217–236.

Kris, E. Ego psychology and interpretation in psychoanalytic therapy (1951). In *The selected papers of Ernst Kris*. New Haven: Yale University Press, 1975, pp. 237–251.

Kris, E. On some vicissitudes of insight in psychoanalysis. *International Journal of Psycho-Analysis*, 1956a, *37*, 445–455.

Kris, E. The recovery of childhood memories in psychoanalysis (1956b). In *The selected papers of Ernst Kris*. New Haven: Yale University Press, 1975, pp. 301–340.

Kuhn, T. S. *The structure of scientific revolutions*. Chicago: University of Chicago Press, 1962.

Levine, F., & Luborsky, L. The core conflictual relationship theme. In S. Tuttman, C. Kaye, & M. Zimmerman (Eds.), *Object and self: A developmental approach*. New York: International Universities Press, 1981, pp. 501–525.

Lipton, S. Later developments in Freud's technique (1920–1939). In B. Wolman (Ed.), *Psychoanalytic techniques: A handbook for practicing psychoanalysts*. New York: Basic Books, 1967, pp. 51–92.

Loewald, H. On the therapeutic action of psychoanalysis. *International Journal of Psycho-Analysis*, 1960, *41*, 17-33.

Loewald, H. Freud's conception of the negative therapeutic reaction, with comments on instinct theory. *Journal of the American Psychoanalytic Association*, 1972, *20*(2), 235-245.

Loewald, H. The waning of the Oedipus complex. *Journal of the American Psychoanalytic Association*, 1979, *27*, 751-775.

Loewenstein, R. M. Some remarks on defenses, autonomous ego and psychoanalytic technique. *International Journal of Psycho-Analysis*, 1954, *35*, 188-193.

Loewenstein, R. M. Some thoughts on interpretation in the theory and practice of psychoanalysis. *Psychoanalytic Study of the Child*, 1957, *12*, 127-150.

Luborsky, L. Measuring a pervasive psychic structure in psychotherapy: The core conflictual relationship theme. In N. Freedman & S. Grand (Eds.), *Communicative structures and psychic structures*. New York: Plenum, 1976.

Luborsky, L., Bachrach, H., Graff, H., Pulver, S., & Christoph, P. Preconditions and consequences of transference interpretations: A clinical–quantitative investigation. *Journal of Nervous and Mental Diseases*, 1979, *169*(7), 391-401.

MacCorquodale, K., & Meehl, P. E. On a distinction between hypothetical constructs and intervening variables. *Psychological Review*, 1948, *55*, 95-107.

Mahl, G. F. Disturbances and silences in the patient's speech in psychotherapy. *Journal of Abnormal and Social Psychology*, 1956, *53*, 1-15.

Mahl, G. F. Exploring emotional states by content analysis. In I. de S. Pool (Ed.), *Trends in content analysis*. Urbana: University of Illinois Press, 1959a.

Mahl, G. F. Measuring the patient's anxiety during interviews from "expressive" aspects of his speech. *Transactions of the New York Academy of Sciences*, 1959b, *21*(3), 249-257.

Mahl, G. F. Measures of two expressive aspects of a patient's speech in two psychotherapeutic interviews. In L. Gottschalk (Ed.), *Comparative psycholinguistic analysis of two psychotherapeutic interviews*. New York: International Universities Press, 1961, pp. 91-114.

Malan, D. *The frontier of brief psychotherapy*. New York: Plenum, 1976a.

Malan, D. *Toward the validation of dynamic psychotherapy*. New York: Plenum, 1976b.

Meehl, P. *Clinical and statistical prediction: A theoretical analysis and a review of the evidence*. Minneapolis: University of Minnesota Press, 1954.

Miller, G. A., Galanter, E., & Pribram, K. H. *Plans and the structure of behavior*. New York: Holt, Rinehart & Winston, 1960.

Modell, A. On having the right to a life: An aspect of the superego's development. *International Journal of Psycho-Analysis*, 1965, *46*, 323-331.

Modell, A. The origin of certain forms of pre-Oedipal guilt and the implications for a psychoanalytic theory of affects. *International Journal of Psycho-Analysis*, 1971, *52*, 337-346.

Modell, A. Self-preservation and the preservation of the self: An overview of some recent knowledge of the narcissistic personality. In *Narcissism, masochism, and the sense of guilt in relation to the therapeutic process*. The Psychotherapy Research Group, Department of Psychiatry, Mount Zion Hospital and Medical Center, Bulletin #6, June 1983, pp. 1-11.

Niederland, W. The survivor syndrome: Further observations and dimensions. *Journal of the American Psychoanalytic Association*, 1981, *29*, 413-423.

Norman, H. F., Blacker, K. H., Oremland, J. D., & Barrett, W. G. The fate of the transference neurosis after termination of a satisfactory analysis. *Journal of the American Psychoanalytic Association*, 1976, *24*(3), 471–498.

Nunberg, H. Therapeutic results of psycho-analysis. *International Journal of Psycho-Analysis*, 1937, *18*, 161–169.

Ornstein, A., & Ornstein, P. On the interpretive process in psychoanalysis. *International Journal of Psychoanalytic Psychotherapy*, 1975, *4*, 219–271.

Peterfreund, E. The need for a new general theoretical frame of reference for psychoanalysis: The first annual Bertram D. Lewin memorial symposium on the ego and the id after fifty years. *Psychoanalytic Quarterly*, 1975, *44*(4), 534–549.

Pfeffer, A. A procedure for evaluating the results of psychoanalysis: A preliminary report. *Journal of the American Psychoanalytic Association*, 1959, 7, 418–444.

Pfeffer, A. Follow-up study of a satisfactory analysis. *Journal of the American Psychoanalytic Association*, 1961, *9*, 698–718.

Pfeffer, A. The meaning of the analyst after analysis. *Journal of the American Psychoanalytic Association*, 1963, *11*, 229–244.

Rangell, L. The psychoanalytic process. *International Journal of Psycho-Analysis*, 1968, *49*, 19–26.

Rangell, L. The intrapsychic process and its analysis: A recent line of thought and its current implications. *International Journal of Psycho-Analysis*, 1969a, *50*, 65–77.

Rangell, L. Choice, conflict, and the decision-making function of the ego: A psychoanalytic contribution to decision theory. *International Journal of Psycho-Analysis*, 1969b, *50*, 599–602.

Rangell, L. The decision-making process: A contribution from psychoanalysis. *Psychoanalytic Study of the Child*, 1971, *26*, 425–452.

Rangell, L. Psychoanalysis and the process of change. *International Journal of Psycho-Analysis*, 1975, *56*, 87–98.

Rangell, L. From insight to change. *Journal of the American Psychoanalytic Association*, 1981, *29*, 119–141.

Rapaport, D. The autonomy of the ego (1951). In M. M. Gill (Ed.), *The collected papers of David Rapaport*. New York: Basic Books, 1967, pp. 357–367.

Rapaport, D. Some metapsychological considerations concerning activity and passivity (1953). In M. M. Gill (Ed.), *The collected papers of David Rapaport*. New York: Basic Books, 1967, pp. 530–568.

Rapaport, D. Present-day ego psychology (1956). In M. M. Gill (Ed.), *The collected papers of David Rapaport*. New York: Basic Books, 1967, pp. 594–623.

Rapaport, D. The theory of ego autonomy: A generalization (1957). In M. M. Gill (Ed.), *The collected papers of David Rapaport*. New York: Basic Books, 1967, pp. 722–744.

Rapaport, D. A historical survey of psychoanalytic ego psychology (1958). In M. M. Gill (Ed.), *The collected papers of David Rapaport*. New York: Basic Books, 1967, pp. 745–757.

Rapaport, D., & Gill, M. M. The points of view and assumptions of metapsychology. *International Journal of Psycho-Analysis*, 1959, *40*, 153–162.

Reich. A. On the termination of analysis (1950). In *Annie Reich: Psychoanalytic contributions*. New York: International Universities Press, 1973, pp. 121–135.

Reich, W. *Character analysis.* New York: Noonday Press, 1949.

Renik, O. Typical examination dreams, "superego dreams" and traumatic dreams. *Psychoanalytic Quarterly,* 1981, *50,* 159.

Rice, L. N., & Greenberg, L. S. (Eds.). *Patterns of change.* New York: Guilford Press, 1984.

Sampson, H., & Weiss, J. Testing hypotheses: The approach of the Mount Zion Psychotherapy Research Group. In L. Greenberg & W. Pinsof (Eds.), *The psychotherapeutic process: A research handbook.* New York: Guilford Press, 1986, pp. 591–613.

Sampson, H., Weiss, J., Mlodnosky, L., & Hause, E. Defense analysis and the emergence of warded-off mental contents: An empirical study. *Archives of General Psychiatry,* 1972, *26,* 524–532.

Sandler, J. The background of safety. *International Journal of Psycho-Analysis,* 1960, *41,* 352–356.

Sandler, J., & Joffe, W. Towards a basic psychoanalytic model. *International Journal of Psycho-Analysis,* 1969, *50,* 79–90.

Sargent, H. D., Horwitz, L., Wallerstein, R., & Appelbaum, A. Prediction in psychotherapy research: A method for the transformation of clinical judgements into testable hypotheses. *Psychological Issues,* 1968, *4*(1), Monograph 21.

Seitz, P. The consensus problem in psychoanalytic research. In L. A. Gottschalk & A. H. Auerbach (Eds.), *Methods of research in psychotherapy.* New York: Appleton-Century-Crofts, 1966, pp. 209–225.

Settlage, C. The technique of defense analysis in the psychoanalysis of an early adolescent. In M. Harley (Ed.), *The analyst and the adolescent at work.* New York: Quadrangle, 1974, pp. 3–39.

Settlage, C. Psychoanalytic developmental thinking in current and historical perspective. *Psychoanalysis and Contemporary Thought,* 1980, *3*(2), 139–170.

Sharpe, E. *Collected papers in psychoanalysis.* London: Hogarth Press, 1950.

Silberschatz, G., Fretter, P., & Curtis, J. How do interpretations influence the process of psychotherapy? *Journal of Consulting and Clinical Psychology,* in press, 1986.

Spiesman, J. C. Depth of interpretation and verbal resistance in psychotherapy. *Journal of Consulting and Clinical Psychology,* 1959, *23*(2), 93–99.

Strachey, J. The nature of the therapeutic action of psychoanalysis. *International Journal of Psycho-Analysis,* 1934, *15,* 127–159.

Strupp, H., Chassan, J. B., & Ewing, J. A. Toward the longitudinal study of the psychotherapeutic process. In L. A. Gottschalk & A. H. Auerbach (Eds.), *Methods of research in psychotherapy.* New York: Appleton-Century-Crofts, 1966, pp. 361–400.

Tinsley, H. E., & Weiss, D. J. Interrater reliability and agreement of subjective judgements. *Journal of Counseling Psychology,* 1975, *22,* 358–376.

Velleman, P. F., & Hoaglin, D. C. *Applications, basics, and computing of exploratory data analysis.* Boston: Duxbury Press, 1981.

Waelder, R. Inhibitions, symptoms and anxiety: Forty years later. *Psychoanalytic Quarterly,* 1967, *36,* 1–36.

Weinshel, E. The ego in health and normality. *Journal of the American Psychoanalytic Association,* 1970, *18,* 682–735.

Weinshel, E. M. The transference neurosis: A survey of the literature. *Journal of the American Psychoanalytic Association*, 1971, *19*, 67–88.

Weinshel, E. *Some observations on the psychoanalytic process.* Presentation given at a scientific meeting of the San Francisco Psychoanalytic Institute, September 19, 1983.

Weiss, J. Crying at the happy ending. *Psychoanalytic Review*, 1952, *39*(4), 338.

Weiss, J. The emergence of new themes: A contribution to the psychoanalytic theory of therapy. *International Journal of Psycho-Analysis*, 1971, *52*(4), 459–467.

Weiss, J., & Sampson, H. Testing alternative psychoanalytic explanations of the therapeutic process. In J. M. Masling (Ed.), *Empirical studies of psychoanalytical theories* (Vol. II). Hillsdale, NJ: Lawrence Erlbaum Associates, 1986, pp. 1–26.

Wolfson, A., & Sampson, H. A comparison of process-notes and tape-recordings: Implications for therapy research. *Archives of General Psychiatry*, May 1976, *33*, 558–563.

Zilboorg, G. The emotional problem and the therapeutic role of insight. *Psychoanalytic Quarterly*, 1952, *21*, 1–24.

INDEX